f

Pediatric Emergency Procedures

Pocket Atlas of Pediatric Emergency Procedures

Christopher King, M.D., F.A.C.E.P.
Assistant Professor of Emergency Medicine and Pediatrics
University of Pittsburgh School of Medicine
Attending Physician, Emergency Medicine
University of Pittsburgh Medical Center
Children's Hospital of Pittsburgh
Pittsburgh, Pennsylvania

Fred M. Henretig, M.D, F.A.A.P.
Professor of Pediatrics and Emergency Medicine
University of Pennsylvania School of Medicine;
Director, Section of Clinical Toxicology
Division of Emergency Medicine
The Children's Hospital of Philadelphia
Philadelphia, Pennsylvania

Illustrator
Christine D. Young, A.M.I

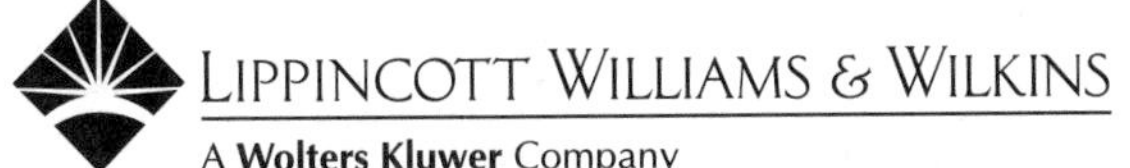

Philadelphia • Baltimore • New York • London
Buenos Aires • Hong Kong • Sydney • Tokyo

Acquisitions Editor: Elizabeth Greenspan
Cover Designer: Karen Quigley
Compositor: Maryland Composition Company, Inc.
Printer: Courier Westford

530 Walnut Street
Philadelphia, PA 19106 USA
LWW.com

Printed in the USA

Library of Congress Cataloging-in-Publication Data

King, Christopher, 1959–
Pocket atlas of pediatric emergency procedures/Christopher King, Fred M. Henretig; illustrator, Christine D. Young.
p. ; cm.
Derived from: Textbook of pediatric emergency procedures.
ISBN 0-683-30666-9
1. Pediatric emergencies—Atlases. 2. Pediatric intensive care—Atlases. I. Henretig, Fred M. II. Title.
[DNLM: 1. Emergency Medicine—methods—Child—Atlases. 2. Emergency Medicine—methods—Child—Handbooks. 3. Emergency Medicine—methods—Infant—Atlases. 4. Emergency Medicine—methods—Infant—Handbooks 5. Emergencies—Child—Atlases. 6. Emergencies—Child—Handbooks. 7. Emergencies—Infant—Atlases. 8. Emergencies—Infant—Handbooks. WS 39 K52p 2000]
RJ370 .K56 2000
618.92′0025—dc21 99-052482

Care has been taken to confirm the accuracy of the information presented and to describe generally accepted practices. However, the authors, editors, and publisher are not responsible for errors or omissions or for any consequences from application of the information in this book and make no warranty, expressed or implied, with respect to the currency, completeness, or accuracy of the contents of the publication. Application of this information in a particular situation remains the professional responsibility of the practitioner.

The authors, editors, and publisher have exerted every effort to ensure that drug selection and dosage set forth in this text are in accordance with current recommendations and practice at the time of publication. However, in view of ongoing research, changes in government regulations, and the constant flow of information relating to drug therapy and drug reactions, the reader is urged to check the package insert for each drug for any change in indications and dosage and for added warnings and precautions. This is particularly important when the recommended agent is a new or infrequently employed drug.

Some drugs and medical devices presented in this publication have Food and Drug Administration (FDA) clearance for limited use in restricted research settings. It is the responsibility of the health care provider to ascertain the FDA status of each drug or device planned for use in their clinical practice.

10 9 8 7 6 5 4 3 2 1

Contents

Preface •

This atlas is intended for physicians and other health professionals who care for children with acute illness or injury. It is designed to provide a stepwise presentation of procedures performed in the emergency department (ED) through the use of detailed illustrations, summaries and descriptions, and "Clinical Tips" for achieving optimal results. Because patient care in the ED covers a broad spectrum of clinical presentations—from minor to imminently life-threatening conditions—the procedures in this atlas likewise range from the simple (e.g., otoscopy) to the most complex and invasive (e.g., emergent endotracheal intubation). As such, the information in this atlas is applicable to pediatric care in a wide variety of clinical settings.

While we believe this atlas can serve as a valuable resource when used appropriately, we strongly emphasize that it is by no means a comprehensive text. It is a pocket atlas derived from the far more thorough and detailed *Textbook of Pediatric Emergency Procedures*. This atlas should not be the sole reference for the novice practitioner nor should it supplant bedside teaching under the supervision of a senior preceptor. For educational purposes, this book is intended only to augment the standard methods for training health care providers that are currently practiced. We hope that experienced clinicians will also find it useful as a brief "refresher" prior to performing a procedure or as a teaching tool for instructing students, residents, etc.

As a result of our decision to produce an atlas rather than a synopsis or summary, the reader will notice that not all chapters from *Textbook of Pediatric Emergency Procedures* are included here. As with any atlas, the primary purpose of this book is to offer a pictorial representation of the relevant material. Therefore, procedures possessing no real "visual" element, such as conscious sedation or rapid sequence induction, have been omitted. Similarly, sections which appear in all chapters of the larger text (that is, "Anatomy and Physiology," "Indications," and "Complications") have not been included. This book focuses specifically on the sequence of actions that a clinician must perform to successfully accomplish each procedure while minimizing complications. Those desiring further information on the procedures shown in this book are referred to the *Textbook of Pediatric Emergency Procedures* and other standard references.

We offer this atlas as an additional resource to those with whom we share the privilege and responsibility of providing health care to children.

Acknowledgments •

For Tammy, Jordan and Ashley—CK

For Marnie, Jon and Jeff; Elizabeth, Alice and Marcus; and in memory of Max—FH

As this atlas is derived from *Textbook of Pediatric Emergency Procedures*, we would like to thank all those who participated in the creation of that text. We express special appreciation to Mark Joffe, Brent King, John Loiselle, Rich Ruddy, and Jim Wiley, who served as associate editors. We also wish to acknowledge the masterful artwork of Christine Young. Finally, we thank the contributing authors listed below.

William Ahrens, M.D.
Peter J. Alderson, MA, M.B.A., M.B.
Michael F. Altieri, M.D.
Angela C. Anderson, M.D.
David T. Bachman, M.D.
M. Douglas Baker, M.D.
Judith C. Basher, M.D.
Courtney A. Bethel, M.D., M.P.H.
Mananda S. Bhende, M.D.
Douglas A. Boenning, M.D.
G. Randall Bond, M.D.
James M. Callahan, M.D.
Carolyn M. Carey, M.D.
Vidya T. Chande, M.D.
Jennifer Pratt Cheney, M.D.
Cindy W. Christian, M.D.
Mark C. Clarke, M.D.
Kathleen M. Connors, M.D.
Richard T. Cook, Jr., M.D.
Andrew T. Costarino, Jr., M.D.
Kathleen M. Cronan, M.D.
Holly W. Davis, M.D.
Joanne M. Decker, M.D.
Douglas S. Diekema, M.D., M.P.H.
Gregg A. DiGiulio, M.D.
E. Howard Dixon III, M.D.
Alfred T. Dorsey, M.D.
Ann-Christine Duhaime, M.D.
Robert Eberlein, M.D.
Joel A. Fein, M.D.
George L. Foltin, M.D.
Scott H. Freedman, M.D.
Susan M. Fuchs, M.D.
Ronnie S. Fuerst, M.D.
Angelo P. Giardino, M.D., M.S.E.D.
Timothy G. Givens, M.D.
Marc H. Gorelick, M.D.
John W. Graneto, D.O., M.Ed.
Michael Green, M.D.
Russell H. Greenfield, M.D.
Elliott M. Harris, M.D.
Mary A. Hegenbarth, M.D.
Mark L. Helpin, D.M.D.
Dee Hodge III, M.D.
Daniel J. Isaacman, M.D.
Jean Marie Kallis, M.D.
Zach Kassutto, M.D.
John J. Kelly, D.O.

Kathleen P. Kelly, M.D.
Hnin Khine, M.D.
Brent R. King, M.D.
Bruce L. Klein, M.D.
Jean E. Klig, M.D.
Susanne Kost, M.D.
Nanette C. Kunkel, M.D.
Natalie E. Lane, M.D.
Bernard J. Larson, D.D.S.
Jane Lavelle, M.D.
Alex V. Levin, M.D.
William J. Lewander, M.D.
Lisa S. Lewis, M.D.
Jordan D. Lipton, M.D.
John Loiselle, M.D.
Constance M. McAneney, M.D.
Robert M. McNamara, M.D.
Leo G. Niederman, M.D., M.P.H.
Ronald I. Paul, M.D.
Mary Clyde Pierce, M.D.
Shari L. Platt, M.D.
Michael P. Poirier, M.D.
J. Christopher Post, M.D.
Linda Quan, M.D.
Peter D. Quinn, D.M.D., M.D.
Scott Reeves, M.D.
Clark A. Rosen, M.D.
Steven G. Rothrock, M.D.
Richard M. Ruddy, M.D.
Seema Sachdeva, M.D.
Richard A. Saladino, M.D.
Richard J. Scarfone, M.D.
Robert W. Schafermeyer, M.D.
Gary Schwartz, M.D.
Michael Shannon, M.D., M.P.H.
Kathy N. Shaw, M.D.
Harold K. Simon, M.D.
Stephen A. Stayer, M.D.
Dale Steele, M.D.
Maria Stephan, M.D.
Gary R. Strange, M.D.
Thomas E. Terndrup, M.D.
Susan B. Torrey, M.D.
Patricia L. VanDevander, M.D.
Robert J. Vinci, M.D.
David K. Wagner, M.D.
Gary Seth Wasserman, D.O.
James F. Wiley II, M.D.
George Anthony Woodward, M.D.
Grace M. Young, M.D.
Stephen Zderic, M.D.

CHAPTER 1 •

Restraint Techniques

OVERVIEW

1. Assess potential for danger to patient or emergency department staff.
2. Use verbal intervention first.
3. Papoose for younger children, five-point restraint for others.
4. Form a standard restraint team with specific roles.
5. Chemical restraint when indicated and safe.
6. Monitor frequently: cardiopulmonary, neurovascular, and mental status.
7. Remove as soon as patient proves to be in control.
8. Document decisions, times, and monitoring.

CLINICAL TIPS

1. Have a plan of action before attempting restraint.
2. Remove stethoscopes, loose jewelry, or anything that might be used as a weapon before performing restraint procedure.
3. Once the decision to restrain has been made, do not "bargain."
4. Use the least amount of restraint necessary for patient and staff safety.
5. Protect yourself and other health care team members.
6. If a patient is able to pull his or her hand out of the leather restraints, roll a washcloth into a ball in his or her hand.
7. Never leave a restrained patient alone.

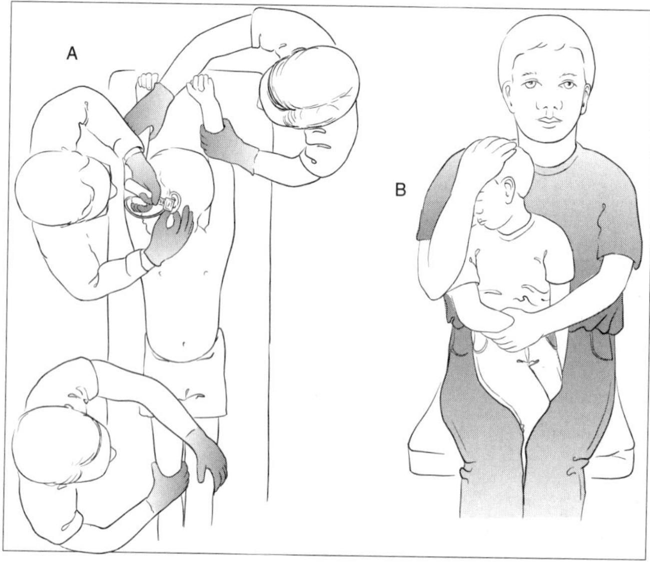

FIGURE 1.1 For brief restraint of an uncooperative infant or toddler, particularly to afford examination of ears or throat, parents or other assistants may be used to hold the child. **A:** In the supine position, an assistant at the head end of the table, holding both upper arms to the side of the head, can restrain the arms, head, and neck. Another assistant restrains the body and lower extremities by leaning over the legs while pressing on the knees. *In the prone position* (not illustrated), *the parent can hold the arms and body from the caudal end while leaning over the child. The clinician then stabilizes the head using the hand that holds the pinna of the ear.* **B:** *Toddlers may be able to be restrained in a sitting position on the parent's lap.* The child's legs are secured between the parent's legs. The arms and body are held tightly against the parent's chest using one arm while the other arm stabilizes the child's head against the parent's chest.

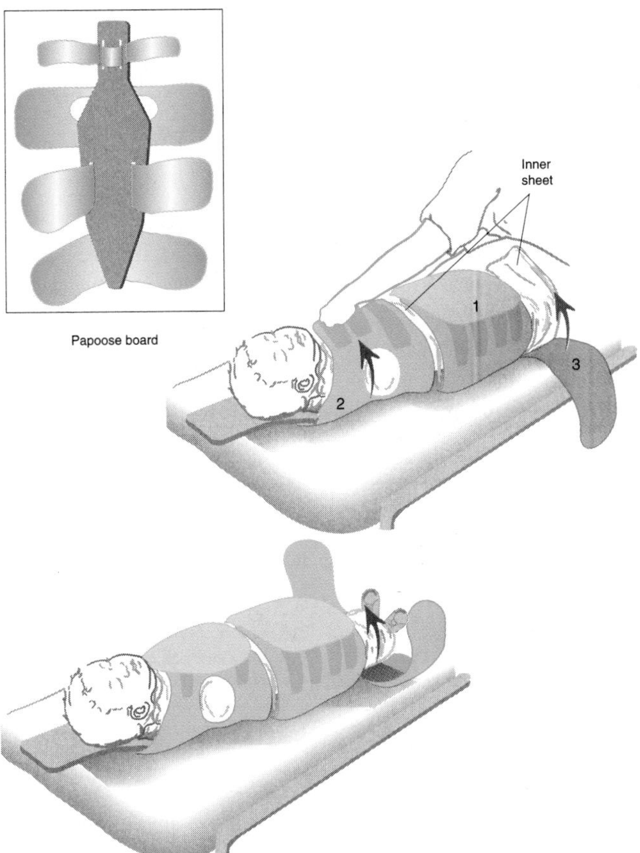

FIGURE 1.2 For long or complex procedures, immobilization of the child's whole body can be accomplished nontraumatically using a papoose board. An appropriate-sized papoose is selected and covered with a clean sheet. The child is placed supine on the sheet, which provides a hygienic barrier and prevents abrasions from the canvas/Velcro straps. The child is initially restrained across the mid-abdomen, followed by trunk and arms, and then by legs, as necessary.

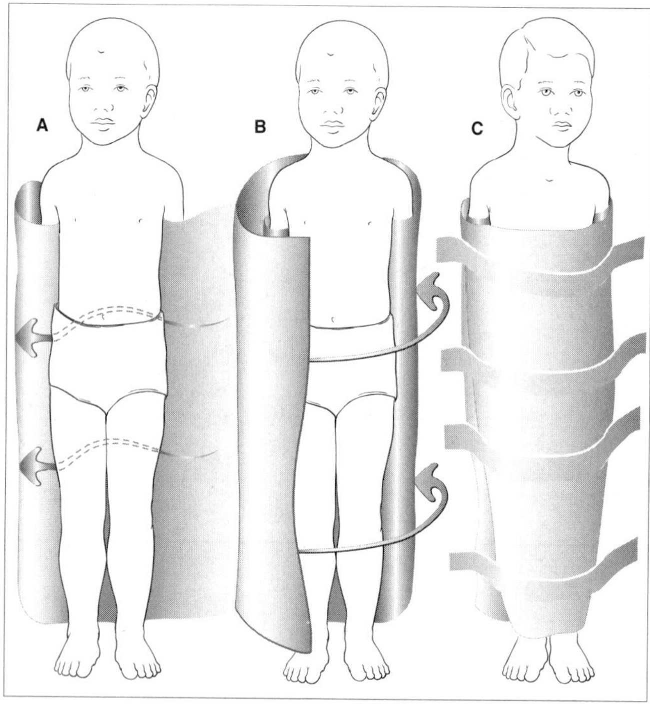

FIGURE 1.3 If a papoose board is not available, a folded sheet may be used to immobilize the child's arms and body. First the child stands on the stretcher. Next, the sheet is folded on itself along its length to a width that covers the child's trunk and legs. It is then initially placed behind the back, with the short end tucked under the right axilla and folded around the right arm, ending behind the back (**A**). The long end is tucked under the left axilla, wrapped around the left arm, then behind the back and around the chest to behind the back again (**B**). Now the child can be placed prone or supine, as desired, and secured with several strips of wide adhesive tape to the sides of the stretcher (**C**).

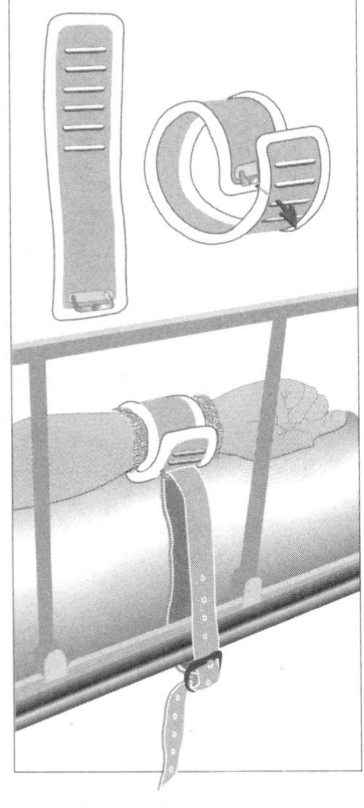

FIGURE 1.4 An uncooperative older child or adolescent who requires an emergency procedure, or one who is potentially violent, may require five-point restraint. The initial approach to a violent patient, and key points in effecting five-point restraint, are summarized in Tables 1.1 and 1.2. The most successful approach to this procedure involves a predesignated restraint team with well defined roles, directed by one person. Using a minimum of five people, one team member is assigned to immobilize each extremity, and the fifth member controls the head and airway. The placement of a Philadelphia collar or soft neck collar helps to prevent injury to the patient or team members from the patient's thrashing or biting. Extremities are best immobilized by holding down the large joints such as the shoulders, elbows, and knees. Leather restraints are first secured around the distal portion of each extremity and then secured to the stretcher as illustrated. These restraints should be tight enough to hold down the extremity without causing neurovascular compromise. Anxiolytic medications used in conjunction with physical restraint procedures can lessen the force necessary to restrain patients. Table 1.3 lists several such medications with dosing, indications, and side effects profiles.

TABLE 1.1 Approach to the Violent Patient

- Universal access to door
- Speak calmly but definitively
    - Request cooperation
    - Explain consequences
- Show of force
- Five-point restraint technique
- Weapons search

TABLE 1.2 Five-Point Restraint System

- Four persons for extremities, one for head
- Immobilize major joints
- Philadelphia collar or soft collar
- Secure restraints around extremity first, then tie down
- Tight enough to hold extremity without causing NV compromise

TABLE 1.3 Medications Used During Restraint Procedures

Drug Class	*Examples*	*Dose/Route*[a]	*Indications*	*Side Effects*
Anxiolytics	Diazepam (Valium) Lorazepam (Ativan) Midazolam (Versed)	0.05–0.1 mg/kg or 1–2 mg IV/IM q1–4 hr 0.05–0.1 mg/kg IV 0.2–0.4 mg/kg IN[c]	Ethanol withdrawal Drug intoxication/ withdrawal[b] Anger/aggression	Sedation Respiratory depression
Neuroleptics				
High potency	Haloperidol (Haldol)	0.1 mg/kg or 5–10 mg IM, PO q30–60 min	Hallucinations Delusions Violence	Extrapyramidal symptoms Sedation
Low potency	Chlorpromazine (Thorazine)	1–2 mg/kg or 100–200 mg q1 hr IM/IV		Sedation α-Adrenergic blockade Anticholinergic

IM, intramuscular; IN, intranasal; IV, intravenous; PO, oral.

[a] Dose suggested as mg/kg (for young children) or total mg (for adolescent/young adult). Route as indicated: note that diazepam is not well absorbed IM, and many practitioners advocate use of IV haloperidol, although such use is not Food and Drug Administration–approved.

[b] May need large doses for severe symptoms of acute toxicity due to amphetamine, phencyclidine, cocaine, and so forth.

[c] Maximum dose 6 mg.

CHAPTER 2 •

Basic Life Support Procedures

OVERVIEW

1. Determine responsiveness.
   A. Gently shake infant or child if no injury suspected.
   B. Speak loudly.
2. Call out for help.
3. Position infant or child.
   A. Place supine on firm surface.
   B. Keep neck immobilized if injury suspected.
4. Assess airway patency.
   A. Head tilt–chin lift
   B. Jaw thrust (if neck injury suspected)
5. Assess breathing.
   A. Watch for chest movement.
   B. Listen, feel for breaths.
6. Ventilate twice.
   A. Give two slow breaths.
   B. Watch for chest to rise.
   C. If no air movement, reposition and repeat.
   D. If still no air movement despite repositioning, perform airway obstruction maneuvers.
7. Check pulse.
   A. Use brachial or femoral in infant (<1 year).
   B. Use carotid in child (>1 year).
   C. Check for 3 to 5 seconds.
8. Perform chest compressions.
   A. Infant (<1 year)
      Position: one fingerbreadth below intermammary line
      Technique: third and fourth fingers on sternum
      Depth: one-third to one-half the depth of chest (0.5 to 1.0 inch)
      Rate: at least 100 times per minute
      Ratio: five compressions to one ventilation
   B. Child (1 to 8 years)
      Position: one fingerbreadth above xyphoid–sternal margin

Technique: heel of hand
Depth: 1.0 to 1.5 inches
Rate: 100 times per minute
Ratio: five compressions to one ventilation

C. Child (>8 years)
Position: two hands
Depth: 1.5 to 2.0 inches
Rate: 80 to 100 times per minute
Ratio: 5 compressions to 1 ventilation for one rescuer; 15 compressions to 2 ventilations for two rescuers

9. Activate emergency medical services (EMS).
   A. Call EMS after 1 minute of cardiopulmonary resuscitation (CPR).
10. Continue CPR.
11. Reassess airway, breathing, circulation.

CLINICAL TIPS

1. The head and neck should be immobilized at all times and the jaw thrust maneuver should be used to open the airway whenever a cervical spine injury is suspected.
2. Pressing too hard in the submental area or hyperextending the neck when performing airway maneuvers can cause upper airway obstruction.
3. The operator should ensure that a good seal is established and no air leak occurs when performing rescue breathing.
4. Breaths delivered slowly (while maintaining the proper overall rate) produce better ventilation and minimize gastric distention.
5. The head and neck should be repositioned to improve airway patency if the patient has inadequate chest wall excursions.
6. Chest compressions should be performed in a smooth and rhythmic fashion at a 1:1 compression-to-relaxation ratio.
7. If emesis occurs, the child's head should be turned to the side to clear the airway, maintaining immobilization of the neck as necessary.

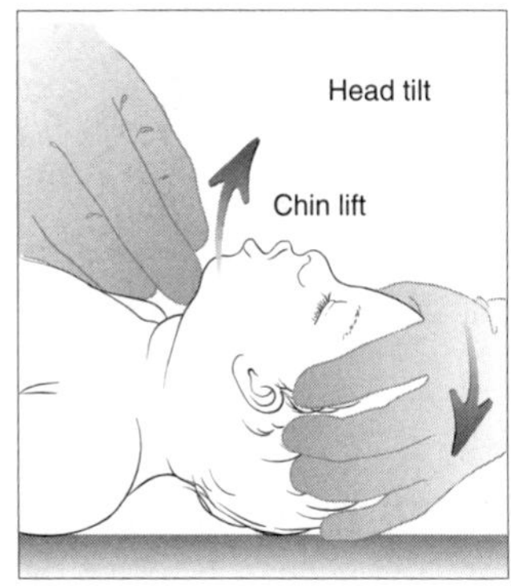

FIGURE 2.1 For nontraumatic arrests, airway patency is established using the head tilt–chin lift maneuver. One hand is placed on the patient's forehead while one or two fingers of the other hand are positioned along the lateral aspect of the chin. The patient's neck is extended by gently pushing the forehead while pulling upward on the mandible. It is important not to apply pressure to the submental area when performing this maneuver because this may produce airway obstruction.

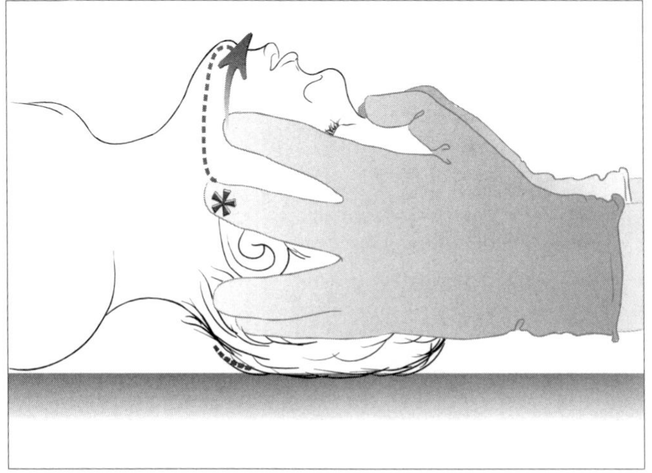

FIGURE 2.2 For traumatic arrests, the jaw thrust maneuver is performed rather than the head tilt–chin lift maneuver to minimize movement of the neck. The third or fourth fingers of both hands are hooked under the angle of the mandible as both thumbs are used to provide countertraction by pressing against the forehead. The mandible is lifted upward and outward with moderate force to open the mouth and displace the tongue anteriorly.

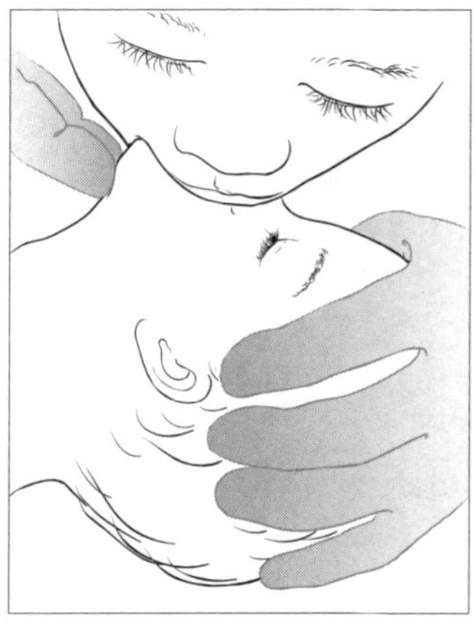

FIGURE 2.3 Rescue breathing for an infant is performed by placing the mouth over the patient's nose and mouth and forming a tight seal. Two initial breaths are delivered slowly (over approximately 1 to 2 seconds) with a pause between breaths. Rescue breaths are then given at a rate of 20 per minute.

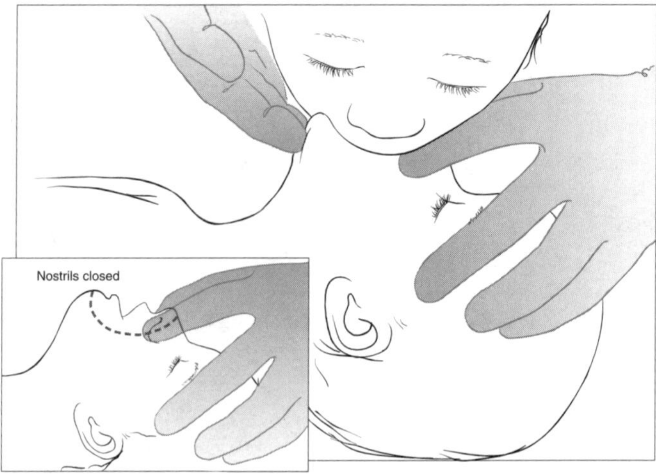

FIGURE 2.4 Rescue breathing for a child is performed by pinching the patient's nose closed and placing the mouth over the patient's mouth to form a tight seal. Two initial breaths are delivered slowly (over approximately 1 to 2 seconds) with a pause between breaths. Rescue breaths are then given at a rate of 20 per minute.

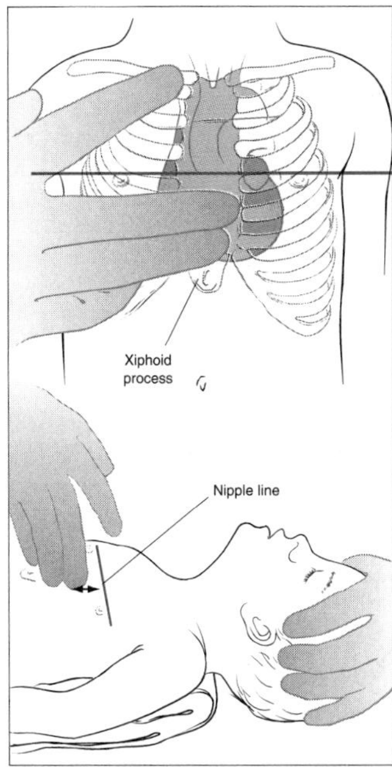

FIGURE 2.5 Chest compressions for an infant are performed by placing the third and fourth fingers one fingerbreadth below the intermammary line. The depth of compression is one-third to one-half the anteroposterior diameter of the chest (approximately 0.5 to 1 inch). The rate of compressions is at least 100 per minute, with a pause after each series of 5 compressions to deliver a rescue breath.

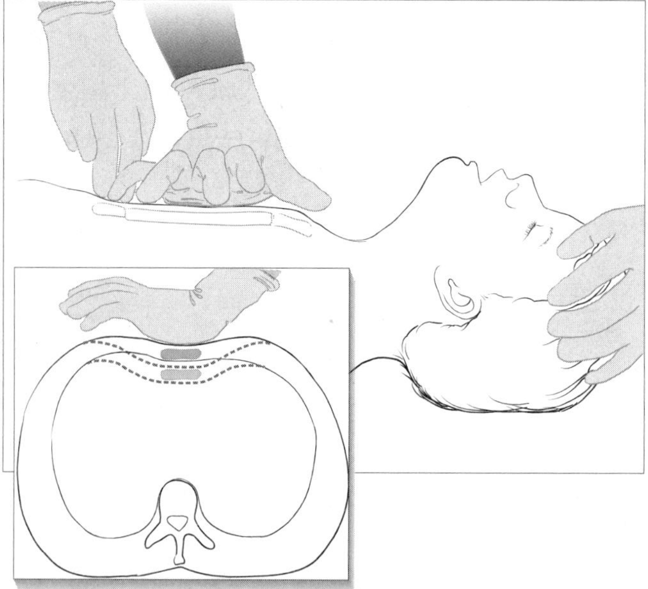

FIGURE 2.6 Chest compressions for a child are performed by placing the heel of the hand on the midline of the patient's sternum two fingerbreadths above the xiphoid–sternal margin. The depth of compression is one-third to one-half the anteroposterior diameter of the chest (approximately 1 to 1.5 inch). The rate of compressions is 80 to 100 per minute, with a pause after each series of 5 compressions to deliver a rescue breath (one rescuer) or a pause after each series of 15 compressions to deliver two rescue breaths (two rescuers).

CHAPTER 3

Suctioning the Upper Airway and Use of Airway Adjuncts

OVERVIEW

Suctioning the Airway

1. Perform suctioning under direct visualization in brief intervals not exceeding 30 seconds.
2. Provide supplemental oxygen during intervals between suctioning.
3. Use catheter-tip suction device for suctioning nasopharynx or for suctioning through an endotracheal tube or tracheostomy cannula.
4. Use dental-tip suction device for removing vomitus or particulate matter from pharynx.
5. Use tonsil-tip suction device for removing blood and blood clots from pharynx.

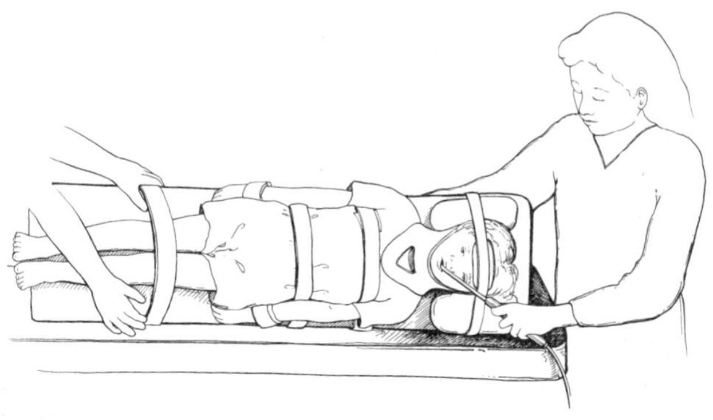

FIGURE 3.1 For the child with a possible cervical spine injury, the preferred method for suctioning vomitus from the oropharynx is to turn the patient to one side using a backboard. In this way, gravity helps clear the mouth and the child's neck remains immobilized.

OVERVIEW

Oropharyngeal Airway Insertion

1. Select oropharyngeal airway such that the tip reaches the angle of the mandible when the flange is at the central incisors.
2. Place patient supine, attach to cardiac monitor, and have dental tip suction device and self-inflating bag available.
3. Insert tongue blade to depress the tongue to achieve visualization of hypopharynx.
4. Under direct visualization, insert oral airway in the same orientation it will reside in hypopharynx (i.e., concave side facing inferiorly).
5. Assess patient's response to determine effectiveness of procedure. If respirations remain labored, replace airway with one more appropriately sized or take measures for definitive airway control.
6. If ventilation is improved and patient is tolerating airway, tape in place.

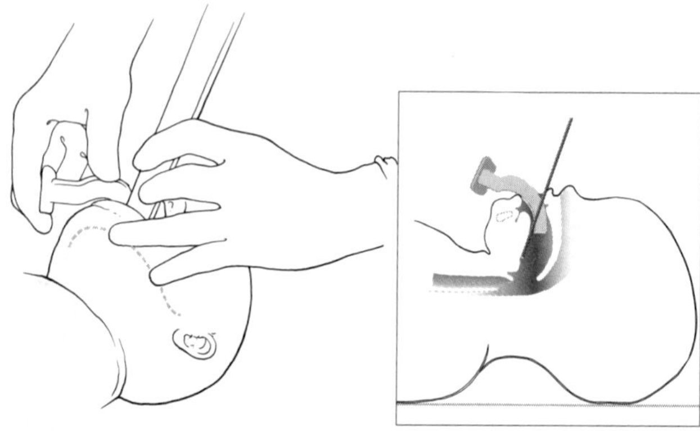

FIGURE 3.2 The preferred method for inserting an oropharyngeal airway is to use a tongue blade to place the airway under direct visualization. The airway should be inserted in the orientation in which it will reside (i.e., concave side facing inferiorly). Because it is rigid, inserting an oropharyngeal airway in the opposite orientation and then flipping it can cause soft tissue trauma and bleeding.

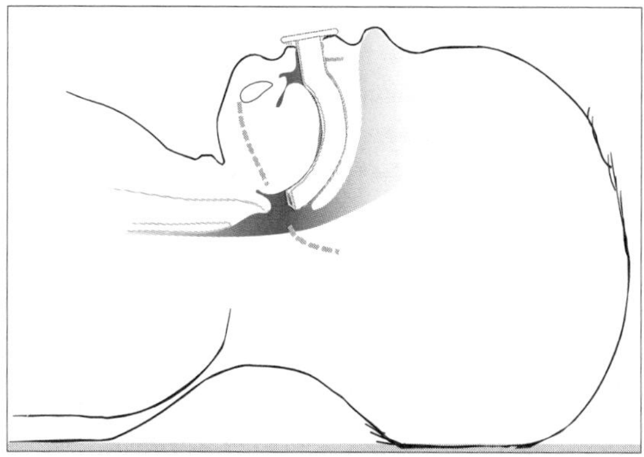

FIGURE 3.3 Proper position for an oropharyngeal airway.

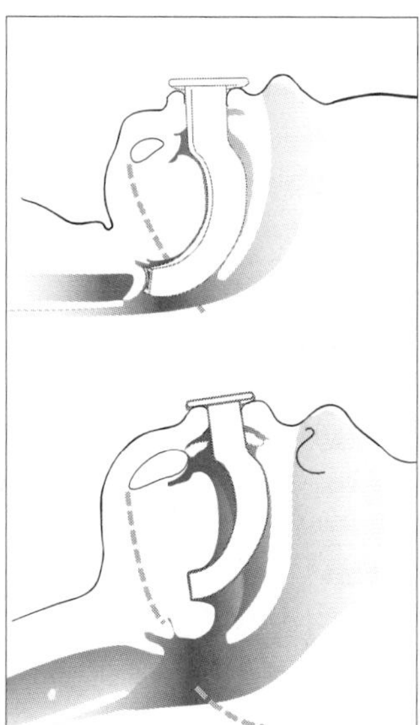

FIGURE 3.4 Insertion of an improperly sized oropharyngeal airway can worsen airway obstruction. Use of an airway that is too large can displace the epiglottis inferiorly over the glottic opening. An airway that is too small can impinge in the tongue, displacing it into the hypopharynx.

OVERVIEW

Nasopharyngeal Airway Insertion

1. Select nasopharyngeal airway such that the tip reaches the lobule of the ear when the opposite end touches the ipsilateral naris.
2. Place patient supine, attach to cardiac monitor, and have dental tip suction device and self-inflating bag available.
3. Before airway insertion, apply topical vasoconstrictor such as phenylephrine (Neo-Synephrine; Sanofi Winthrop Pharmaceuticals, New York, NY) to nares and lubricate nasal airway.
4. Occlude each nostril to determine which is more patent and use that side for insertion.
5. Insert nasopharyngeal airway so angled side faces nasal septum. If necessary, invert airway 180 degrees (i.e., with concave side facing superiorly) and then rotate it back to normal position after tip reaches posterior pharynx.
6. Assess patient's response to determine effectiveness of procedure. If respirations remain labored, replace airway with one more appropriately sized or take measures for definitive airway control.

CLINICAL TIPS

1. Stridor, snoring, poor aeration despite good chest wall movement, and cyanosis are signs of airway obstruction in children.
2. Deep suctioning of airway should be avoided to minimize risk of laryngospasm or vomiting.
3. When inserting an artificial airway, the patient should receive supplemental oxygen, appropriate monitoring should be performed, and a dental-tip

→

FIGURE 3.5 A nasopharyngeal airway can be sized properly by placing it adjacent to the child's face. The correct size matches the distance from the lobule of the ear to the nostril. A nasopharyngeal airway is always inserted so that the bevel faces the nasal septum. The usual method is to insert the airway with the concavity facing inferiorly. However, if the right nostril is occluded, the airway can be inverted 180 degrees (concavity facing superiorly) so that the bevel faces the septum with insertion on the left side. Once the tip is advanced beyond the nasal turbinates, the airway can then be rotated to the normal position. Because nasopharyngeal airways are soft and pliable, there is no risk of injury to the patient using this technique. After insertion, the tip of the airway should be positioned at the supraglottic region.

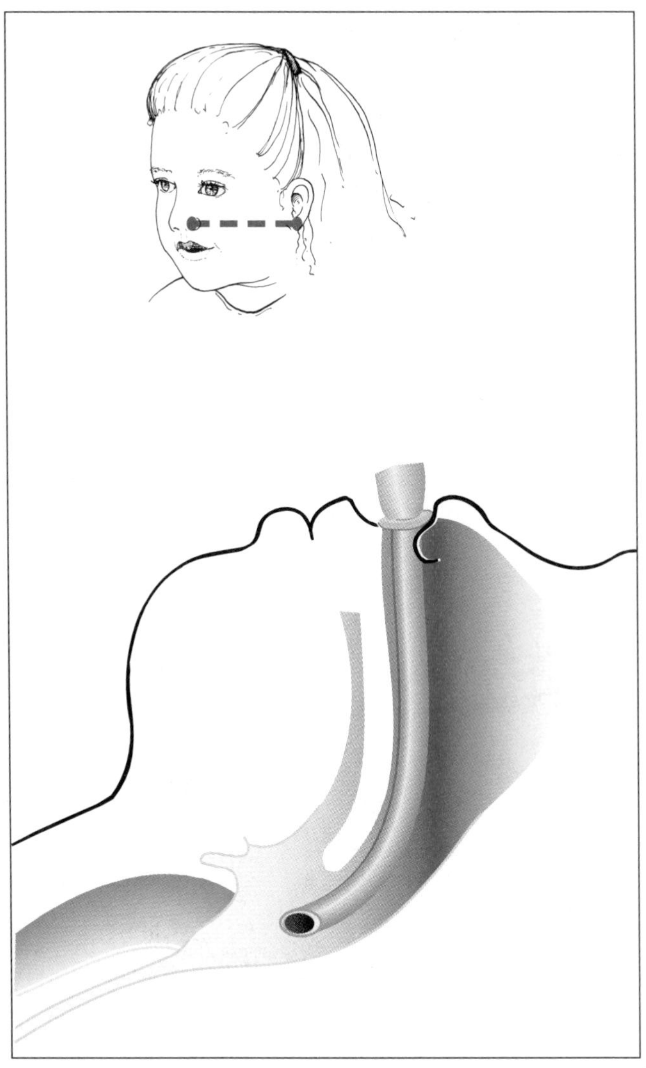

suction device and self-inflating bag-valve-mask circuit should be available.

4. An oropharyngeal airway is best suited to the management of a stuporous or unconscious child with an intact gag reflex.
5. A nasopharyngeal airway should be used for the conscious child with partial airway obstruction.

CHAPTER 4

Bag-Valve-Mask Ventilation

OVERVIEW

1. Assess patient—airway, breathing, circulation.
2. Establish airway patency.
   A. Chin lift (if no danger of cervical spine injury).
   B. Jaw thrust.
3. Select appropriate equipment sizes.
   A. Face mask should be the smallest size that completely covers the nose and mouth.
   B. Resuscitation bag should be large enough to ensure delivery of adequate tidal volume.
4. Apply mask to face with nondominant hand (or with both hands when two-person technique is used).
5. Compress resuscitation bag at appropriate rate with dominant hand (or with both hands as necessary when two-person technique is used).
6. Assess for mask leak.
7. Observe chest excursions and modify delivered tidal volume as needed.
8. Monitor patient response.

CLINICAL TIPS

1. A resuscitation bag that is one size too large always gives better results than one that is too small. This is especially true for apneic neonates, who initially require higher sustained peak inspiratory pressures for adequate ventilation. For these patients, an in-line pressure manometer should be used when available.
2. Chest excursions must be continually monitored during bag-mask-valve (BVM) ventilation; they should be similar to normal full respirations. Excursions that are too great may lead to gastric distention and possibly pneumothorax. Inadequate excursions result in delivery of an insufficient tidal volume.

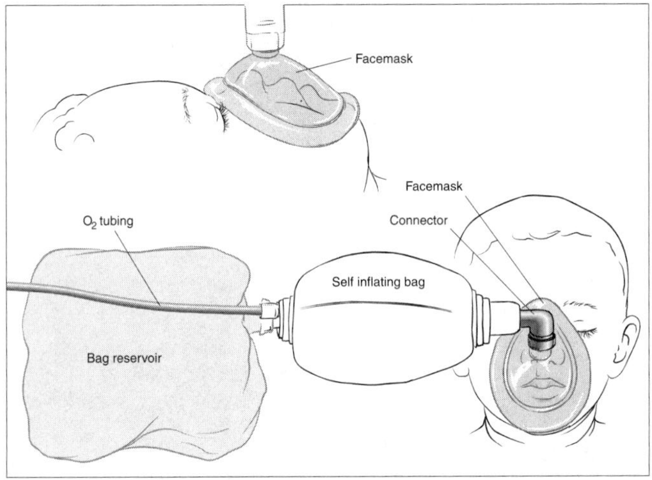

FIGURE 4.1 A bag-valve-mask setup incorporating a self-inflating bag is used most commonly in the emergency department because it is generally easier to use than an anesthesia bag system. When selecting a face mask, it is best to use the smallest mask that completely covers the nose and mouth. A bag that is too large can injure or compress the eyes (which may cause bradycardia). In addition, maintaining a mask seal adequate for delivering positive-pressure ventilation can be difficult with a mask that is too large or too small. It is often necessary to try more that one mask size before finding the proper fit.

TABLE 4.1 Oxygen Enrichment for Bag-Valve-Mask Ventilation

Device	*Oxygen Concentration Delivered*[a]
Oxygen line connected to bag	0.41
Corrugated tube reservoir	0.51–0.53
2.5-L bag reservoir	0.95–1.0

[a] Assumes an oxygen inflow rate of 15 L/min with self-inflating resuscitation bag. When used properly, a conventional anesthesia bag system reliably delivers an oxygen concentration of 1.0.

TABLE 4.2 Ventilatory Rates for Pediatric Patients

Infant	20–24 breaths/min
Child	16–20 breaths/min
Adolescent	12–16 breaths/min

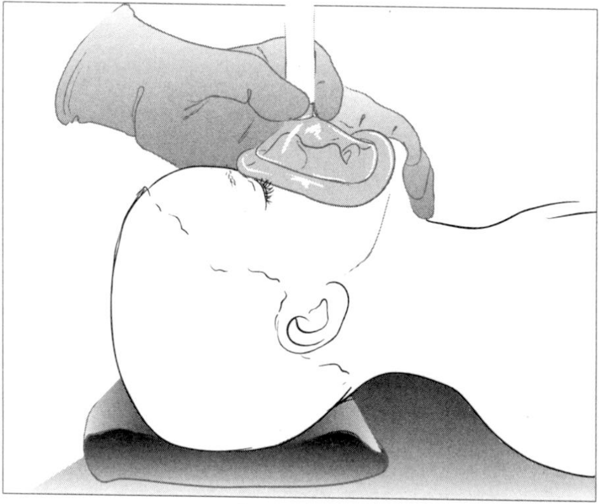

FIGURE 4.2 The head tilt–chin lift maneuver is commonly used to maintain airway patency and deliver positive-pressure ventilations in a nontraumatic arrest (see also Fig. 2.1). The thumb and index finger can be positioned as shown here or more widely spaced over the air-filled mask seal. The other fingers are used to pull upward along the lateral margin of the mandible, extending the neck slightly. It may be necessary to vary the position of the patient's head at times to find the most favorable alignment for airway patency.

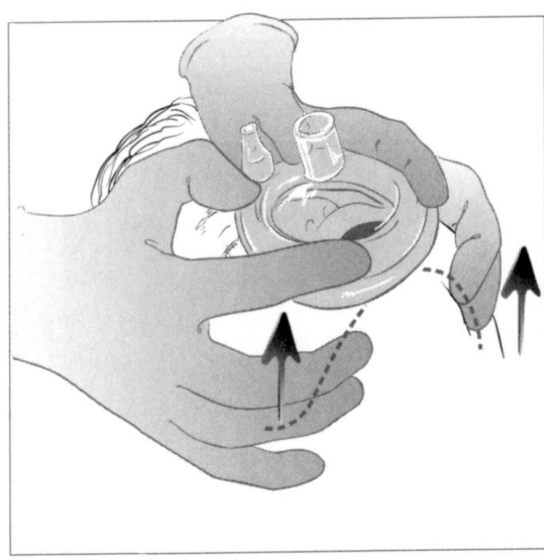

FIGURE 4.3 Securing the mask while maintaining the airway using the jaw thrust maneuver requires the use of both hands (see also Fig. 2.2). The thumb and index finger of each hand hold the mask in place while the other fingers are used to displace the mandible anteriorly. Although more difficult to perform successfully than the head tilt–chin lift maneuver, this method has the advantage of minimizing movement of the neck in a patient with a potential cervical spine injury.

3. Cricoid pressure (Sellick's maneuver) is effective in preventing both air entry into the stomach and regurgitation of gastric contents.
4. Pediatric patients with epiglottitis or other causes of significant supraglottic edema or swelling can often be managed successfully on a temporary basis with BVM ventilation alone. Immediate intubation may prove difficult or impossible with these patients. In such cases, greater attention to maintaining an adequate mask seal and higher ventilatory pressures (i.e., more forceful compression of the resuscitation bag) usually are necessary.

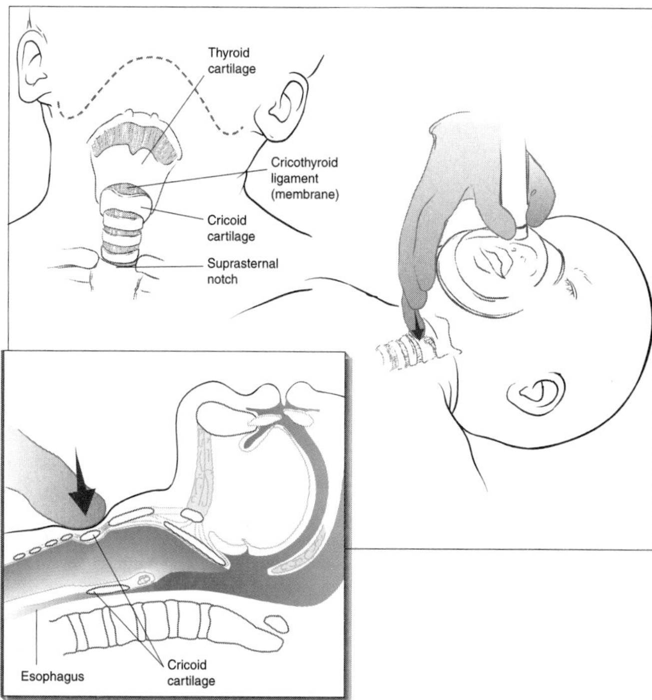

FIGURE 4.4 Cricoid pressure (Sellick's maneuver) tamponades the esophagus and thereby reduces the likelihood that positive-pressure ventilation will cause significant air entry into the stomach. For older children and adolescents, it is usually necessary to enlist the help of an assistant to perform this maneuver. With infants and younger children, it is often possible to simultaneously secure the mask with the index finger and thumb while applying cricoid pressure with the fifth finger.

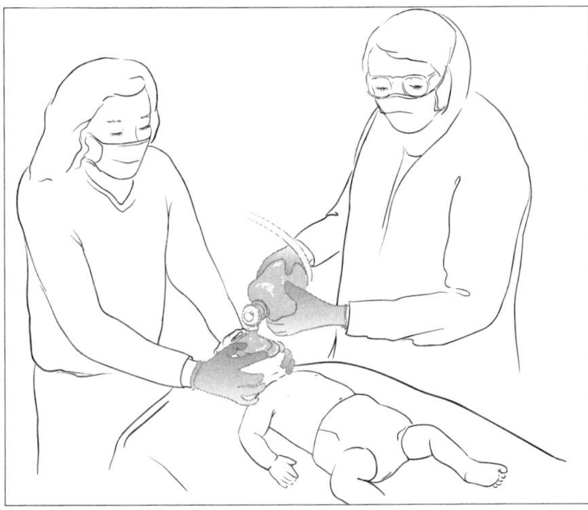

FIGURE 4.5 The two-person technique of performing bag-valve-mask ventilation is usually preferred whenever feasible. Using both hands to secure the mask and, when necessary, to compress the bag increases the likelihood of providing adequate ventilatory support. For most cases in the emergency department, delivery of the appropriate tidal volume is based on the patient's chest excursions; that is, the chest should rise and fall as in normal deep breathing.

CHAPTER 5

Emergent Endotracheal Intubation

OVERVIEW

Conventional Orotracheal Intubation

1. Prepare patient.
   A. Administer assisted or controlled bag-valve-mask (BVM) ventilation as needed.
   B. Attach patient to monitoring devices.
   C. Preoxygenate patient with 100% oxygen.
   D. Insert gastric tube to evacuate stomach contents as necessary.
2. Prepare and test necessary equipment.
   A. Check that light on laryngoscope blade is functioning properly.
   B. Inflate balloon on cuffed endotracheal tube (if used) to ensure there are no leaks.
   C. Insert stylet (if used) into endotracheal tube.
3. Position patient's head and neck; restrain patient appropriately as needed.
4. Perform direct laryngoscopy.
   A. Laryngoscopy using a straight blade (infants and children).
      1) Open patient's mouth.
      2) Insert blade from far right of oropharynx and sweep tongue to left; alternatively, insert blade over tongue just right of midline.
      3) Place tip of blade in vallecula.
      4) Pull upward at 45-degree angle.
      5) Identify anatomic landmarks.
      6) If epiglottis is not retracted, insert tip of blade posterior to epiglottis and lift upward.
   B. Laryngoscopy using curved blade (adolescents).
      1) Open patient's mouth.
      2) Insert blade over tongue just right of midline.
      3) Place tip of blade in vallecula.
      4) Pull upward at 45-degree angle.
      5) Identify anatomic landmarks.
      6) If epiglottis is not retracted, direct laryngoscopy should be attempted using straight blade.
5. Insert endotracheal tube.

6. Confirm tracheal placement (equal breath sounds, no sounds over stomach, capnography).
7. Position tube at midtracheal level.
   - A. Listen with stethoscope to left axilla.
   - B. Insert tube until breath sounds on left are diminished or absent (right endobronchial intubation).
   - C. Withdraw tube until breath sounds are first heard on left (tip at carina).
   - D. Withdraw tube an additional 1 to 3 cm as appropriate for age of patient.
8. Secure endotracheal tube.
9. Confirm proper tube position with chest radiograph.

CLINICAL TIPS

Conventional Orotracheal Intubation

1. A straight laryngoscope blade should be used for infants and children. A curved blade may be used for adolescents.
2. Using the teeth or alveolar ridge as a lever for the laryngoscope blade must be carefully avoided because this may cause tooth avulsion or gingival injury.
3. Inserting the tip of a straight blade into the vallecula of an infant or younger child and then lifting upward often exposes the glottic opening without causing trauma to the epiglottis. Making one such attempt with all intubations is recommended. If this fails, the standard method of directly retracting the epiglottis with the tip of the blade can then be performed.
4. In-line stabilization of the head and neck is necessary whenever conventional orotracheal intubation is performed for the patient who has a potentially unstable cervical spine.
5. If the vocal cords are not visible during direct laryngoscopy, the bright white reflection of the arytenoid cartilages may be used as a landmark. The glottic opening is anterior to these structures in the midline.
6. To identify the epiglottis during a difficult laryngoscopy, the operator may intentionally insert the laryngoscope blade into the esophagus and then gradually withdraw it until the epiglottis falls into view. This should not be performed routinely, however, because abrasion of the epiglottis can lead to swelling.
7. The endotracheal tube should be inserted so that the concavity is somewhat off the vertical plane rather than perfectly upright. The tube also should be

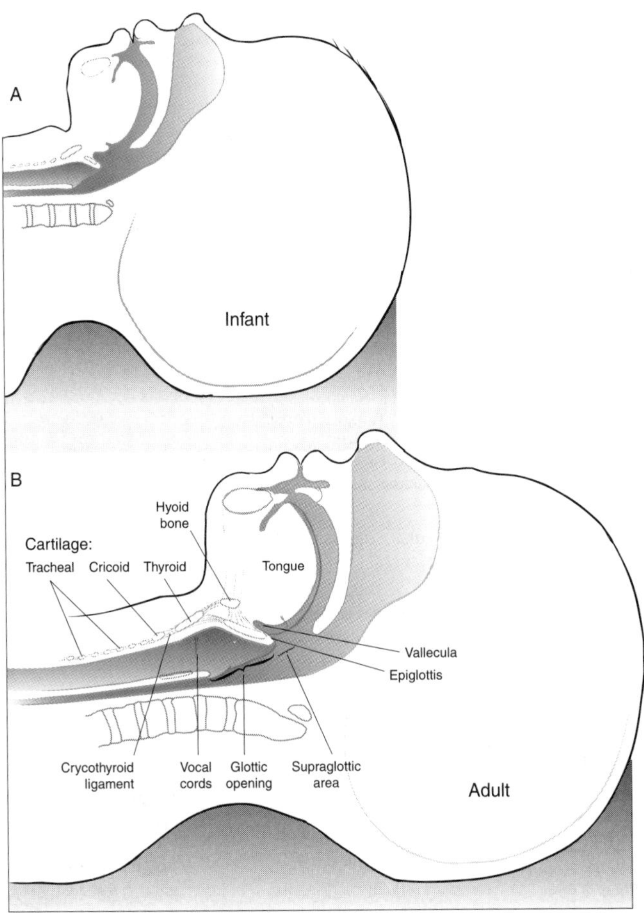

FIGURE 5.1 A comparison of infant (**A**) versus adult (**B**) airway anatomy reveals several clinically important differences: (a) the tongue of an infant is more rostral and larger relative to the size of the oropharynx, increasing the likelihood of obstruction and making retraction with a laryngoscope blade more difficult; (b) the epiglottis of an infant is larger relative to the size of the hypopharynx, less easily retracted by applying anterior traction to the vallecula and hyoepiglottic ligament, and more acutely angled over the glottic opening—all factors that make retraction of the epiglottis during direct laryngoscopy more difficult; and (c) the larynx of an infant is more rostral (opposite C3-4) compared with an adult larynx (opposite C4-5), making the angle of entry into the trachea for tube insertion more acute.

TABLE 5.1 Equipment Checklist: SOAPIM Mnemonic

Suction. Flexible catheter (for infants and children younger than 1 year) or Yankauer suction device (for older children and adolescents); suction tubing; functioning wall suction set on full (200 cm H_2O).

Oxygen and positive-pressure delivery system. Face masks; oxygen tubing; high-flow oxygen source (wall-mounted or tank oxygen); resuscitation bags.

Airway equipment. Laryngoscope handles and blades; endotracheal tubes; stylets; nasopharyngeal and oropharyngeal airways; equipment used for alternative approaches (e.g., fiberoptic laryngoscope, lighted stylet, extra-long guide wire for retrograde intubation).

Pharmacologic agents. Sedatives; analgesics; neuromuscular blocking agents; atropine.

Intravenous access. Peripheral or central venous catheters; intravenous tubing; intravenous fluids.

Monitors. Cardiac monitor; pulse oximetry; capnography.

TABLE 5.2 Formulas for Calculating Endotracheal Tube Sizes in Children[a]

Internal diameter (mm) = [16 + age (yr)]/4
OR
= [age (yr)]/4 + 4
OR
= [height (cm)]/20

[a] The internal diameter is also approximately equal to the size of the patient's fifth finger.

TABLE 5.3 Pediatric Endotracheal Tube Sizes

Weight/Age	*Internal Diameter (mm)*[a]	*Tube Marking at Lips (cm)*
Under 1,500 g	2.5 uncuffed	weight in kg + 6.0 cm
1,500–5,000 g	3.0 uncuffed	weight in kg + 6.0 cm
> 5,000 g–6 mo	3.5 uncuffed	12.0–13.0
6–18 mo	3.5–4.0 uncuffed	13.0–14.0
18 mo–3 yr	4.0–4.5 uncuffed	13.5–14.5
3–5 yr	4.5 uncuffed	14.5–15.5
5–6 yr	5.0 uncuffed	15.5–17.0
6–8 yr	5.5–6.0 uncuffed	17.0–19.0
8–10 yr	5.5–6.0 cuffed	19.0–20.0
10–12 yr	6.0–6.5 cuffed	20.0–21.0
12–14 yr	6.5–7.0 cuffed	21.0–22.0
14–16 yr	7.0–7.5 cuffed	22.0–23.0

[a] Two additional endotracheal tubes (one-half size larger and smaller) should also be readily available in case the initial estimation proves incorrect.

TABLE 5.4. Pediatric Laryngoscope Blade Sizes

Age/Weight	*Size (Type)*
2.5 kg	0 (straight)
0–3 mo	1.0 (straight)
3 mo–3 yr	1.5 (straight)
3–12 yr	2.0 (straight or curved)[a]
12–18 yr	3.0 (straight or curved)

[a] A curved blade may be used for older children, but a straight blade is usually preferred.

inserted from the right side of the oropharynx (an assistant can be enlisted to retract the cheek as necessary). These maneuvers prevent the tube from obscuring the operator's view of the glottic opening.

8. The operator should make certain to use both eyes when inserting the endotracheal type to preserve binocular vision and depth perception.

9. A plan should always be formulated for performing an alternative intubation approach if conventional orotracheal intubation is unsuccessful.

OVERVIEW

Blind Nasorotracheal Intubation

1. Prepare patient.
   A. Attach patient to monitoring devices.
   B. Apply topical anesthetic and topical vasoconstrictor to nasal mucosa.
   C. Administer mild sedative as needed.
   D. Position patient sitting upright with hands gently restrained as necessary.
   E. Preoxygenate patient with 100% oxygen.
2. Select an endotracheal tube and test balloon for any leaks.
3. Check nares for patency by occluding each one in turn.
4. If right nostril is patent, insert the tube on this side (concave downward) so that bevel faces nasal septum. If right nostril is not patent, insert the tube on left side by inverting it (concave upward). Once tip reaches posterior pharynx, rotate the tube back to normal position.
5. Insert tube until tip reaches supraglottic region; listen for breath sounds through tube and observe for fogging of tube with respirations.
6. Advance tube until breath sounds are lost (esophageal placement) and withdraw it a few centimeters so that tip is just proximal to glottis (optional).

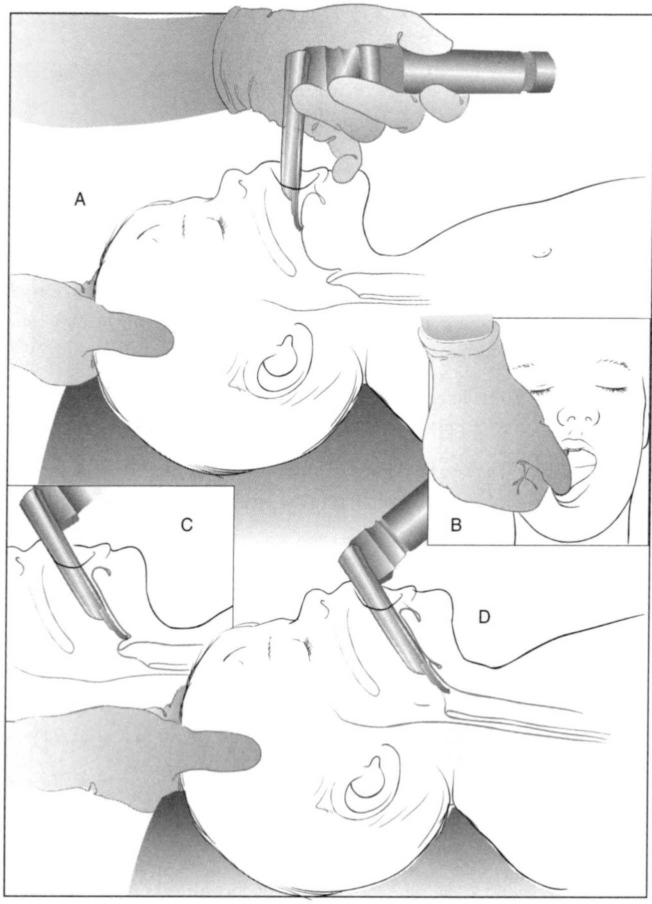

FIGURE 5.2 Direct laryngoscopy using a straight blade. **A:** The head is positioned with the right hand and the mouth is opened using the fifth finger of the left hand (if necessary). **B:** Alternatively, the mouth may be opened with the thumb and index finger of the right hand using a "scissors" technique. **C:** The laryngoscope blade is inserted under direct vision over the tongue and into the vallecula. One attempt may be made at this point to elevate the epiglottis by lifting upward on the laryngoscope handle at a 45-degree angle. **D:** If unsuccessful, the tip of the blade is used directly to retract the epiglottis, revealing the vocal cords and glottic opening.

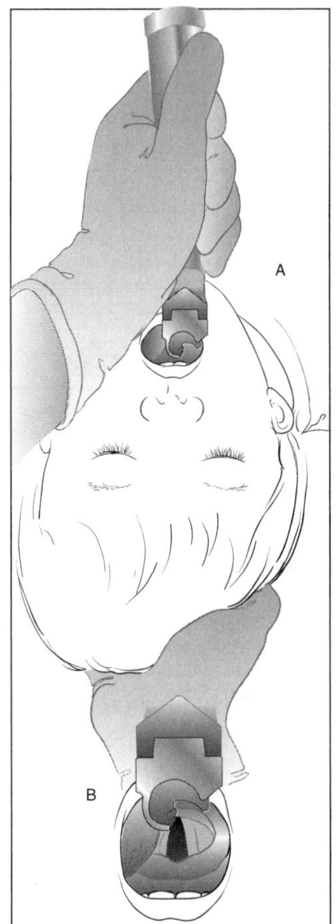

FIGURE 5.3 The novice practitioner is traditionally taught to insert a straight laryngoscope blade well to the right in the oropharynx (**A**) and then sweep the tongue to the left (**B**). However, inserting a straight blade just to the right of the midline is equally effective in most cases and usually a simpler technique.

7. Listen to breath sounds for a few seconds to get a sense of their rhythm.
8. Advance tube briskly at moment patient starts inspiration.
9. Any recognizable vocalizations (e.g., talking, moaning) indicate esophageal placement.
10. Confirm tracheal placement (equal breath sounds, no sounds over stomach, capnography).

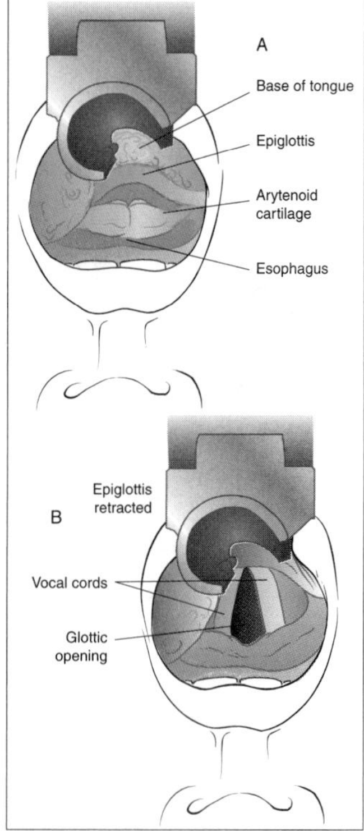

FIGURE 5.4 Anatomic landmarks for direct laryngoscopy. **A:** After initial retraction of the tongue with a straight blade, the epiglottis may remain draped posteriorly, partially or completely covering the glottic opening. **B:** Retraction of the epiglottis with the tip of the blade allows visualization of the glottis and surrounding structures.

11. After successful intubation, inflate balloon and secure tube.
12. Confirm proper tube position with chest radiograph.

CLINICAL TIPS

Blind Nasorotracheal Intubation

1. If blind nasotracheal intubation is unsuccessful after three or four attempts, an alternative method should be used.
2. This procedure is best suited for adolescents. Children are rarely, if ever, good candidates for blind nasotracheal intubation.
3. If the tip of the endotracheal tube gets caught in one of the pyriform sinuses, the operator will appreciate a bulge lateral to the midline on either

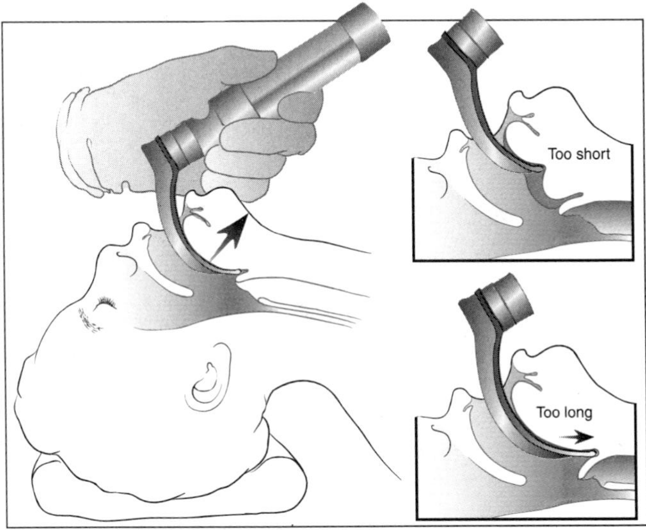

FIGURE 5.5 Direct laryngoscopy using a curved blade. The blade is inserted under direct vision until the tip is positioned in the vallecula. Pulling upward on the laryngoscope handle at a 45-degree angle retracts the tongue and at the same time elevates the epiglottis, revealing the vocal cords and glottis. Selection of the appropriate laryngoscope blade is especially important with this technique. A blade that is too small impinges on the midportion of the tongue, potentially obscuring the landmarks, whereas a blade that is too large can displace the epiglottis posteriorly over the glottic opening.

side of the neck. In such cases, the tube should be rotated back to a midline position before the next attempt at passage.

4. If the tip of the tube gets caught in the vallecula or anterior commissure of the vocal cords, the operator will appreciate a bulge in the submental region of the neck. In such cases, the patient's neck should be flexed somewhat before the next attempt at passage.
5. If the tube persistently enters the esophagus, the following may be effective: (a) using an Endotrol tube and pulling the ring to deflect the tip anteriorly, (b) applying cricoid pressure during insertion, and (c) extending the patient's neck.
6. If the ring of an Endotrol tube sits tightly against the nose after insertion, the ligature should be cut and the ring removed. Otherwise, tension on the ligature will cause the tube to exert continuous anterior pressure on the trachea.

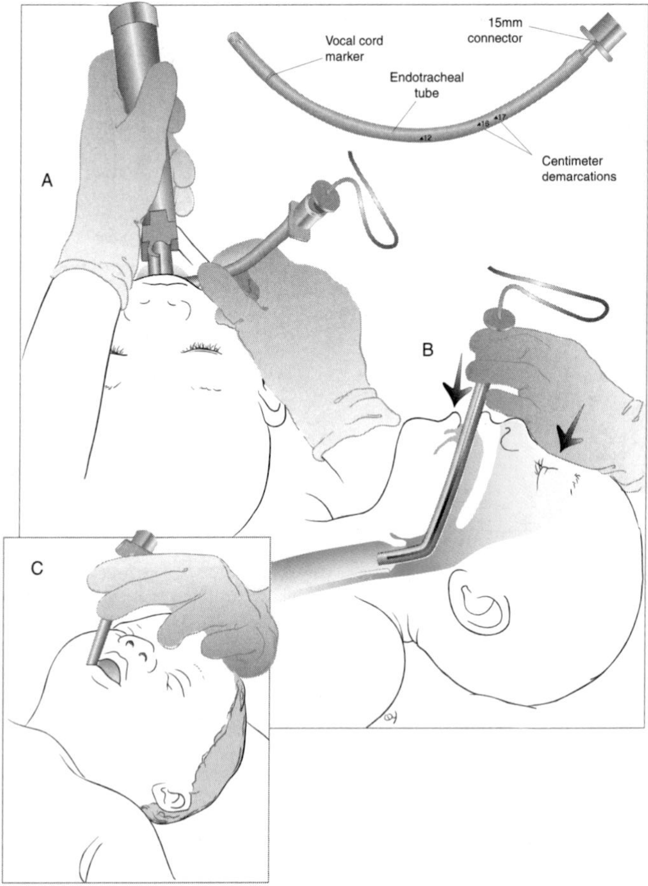

FIGURE 5.6 Insertion of the endotracheal tube. **A:** The tube is rotated somewhat laterally and inserted from the right of midline, so that the vocal cords can be kept in view at all times. **B:** The tube is inserted into the trachea and the laryngoscope blade is removed from the mouth. **C:** The stylet is removed and the tube held securely in place.

OVERVIEW

Lighted Stylet (Light Wand) Intubation

1. Prepare patient.
   A. Administer assisted or controlled BVM ventilation as needed.
   B. Attach patient to monitoring devices.

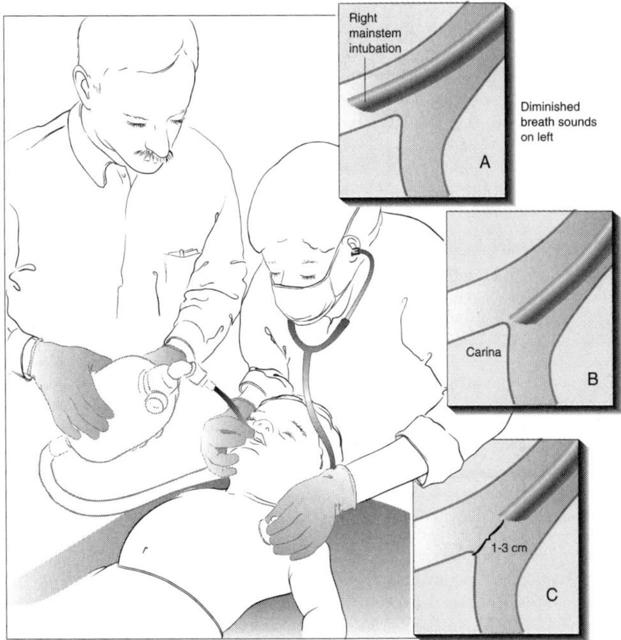

FIGURE 5.7 Confirming proper depth of tube insertion. **A:** While auscultating the left chest, the operator advances the endotracheal tube until breath sounds are diminished or absent (right mainstream intubation). **B:** The tube is then withdrawn until breath sounds are first heard again normally on the left, indicating the tip is just proximal to the carina. **C:** The tube is then withdrawn an additional 1 to 3 cm (depending on the age and size of the patient) to achieve proper midtracheal positioning of the tip.

C. Preoxygenate patient with 100% oxygen.
D. Insert gastric tube to evacuate stomach contents as necessary.

2. Prepare and test necessary equipment.
   A. Check intensity of light and fiberoptic element of lighted stylet.
   B. Inflate balloon on cuffed endotracheal tube (if used) to ensure there are no leaks.
   C. Lubricate stylet liberally and insert into tube; if necessary, cut segment from proximal end of tube or remove 15-mm connector.
   D. Bend styletted tube to 110-degree angle approximately 2 to 3 cm from distal end.

3. Grasp tongue and mandibular block with nondominant hand and pull outward to open mouth.

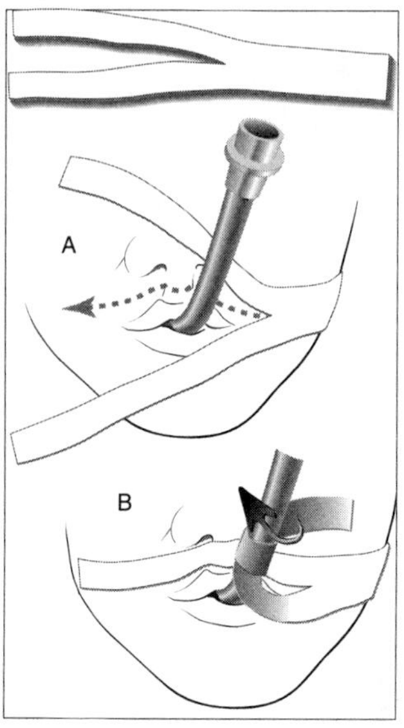

FIGURE 5.8 Securing the endotracheal tube. **A:** The tape is split into a "Y" and the base is applied to the cheek. **B:** One strip of tape is then applied to the skin above or below the lips while the other secures the tube. A second piece of tape may be applied from the other side in a similar manner for greater stability. Tincture of benzoin also may be used to increase adhesion.

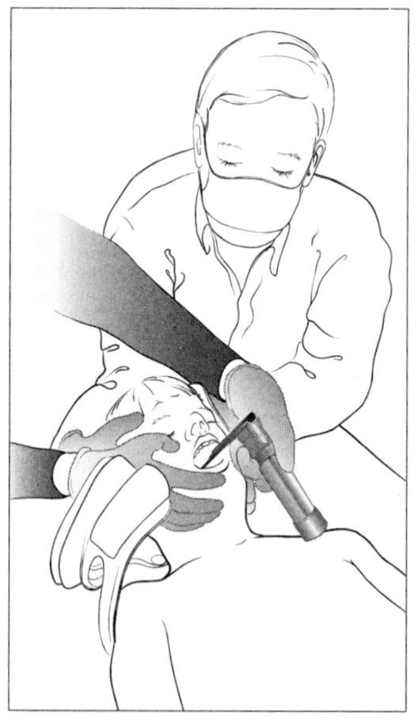

FIGURE 5.9 In-line stabilization of the head and neck should be performed during laryngoscopy and tube insertion whenever the patient is at risk for a cervical spine injury. The anterior portion of the cervical collar is removed as an assistant holds the patient's head and neck in a neutral position. As shown here, the assistant can stand above the head of the bed while crouching down to avoid interfering with intubation. If the patient is not fully immobilized with straps attached to a long board, a second assistant should hold the chest and shoulders in place to prevent movement of the torso.

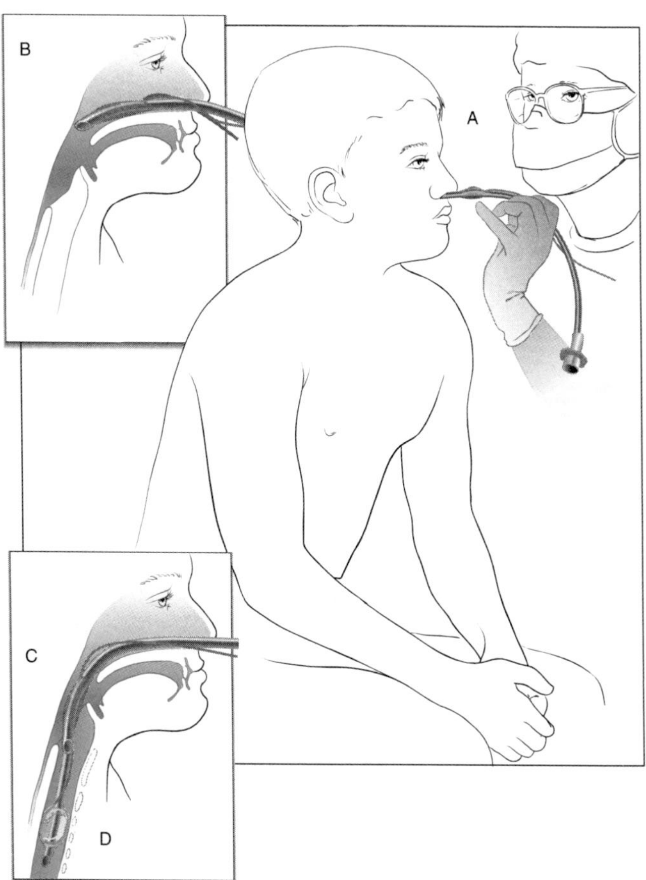

FIGURE 5.10 Blind nasotracheal intubation. **A:** The tube is inserted into the nostril with a "straight-in" orientation. **B:** After the tip passes the nasal turbinates, the angle at the posterior pharynx is carefully negotiated with steady pressure. Excessive force must be avoided to prevent formation of a traumatic false passage. **C:** The tube is positioned in the supraglottic region as indicated by breath sounds transmitted through the tube and fogging of the tube. **D:** At the onset of inspiration, the tube is briskly advanced into the trachea and the balloon is inflated.

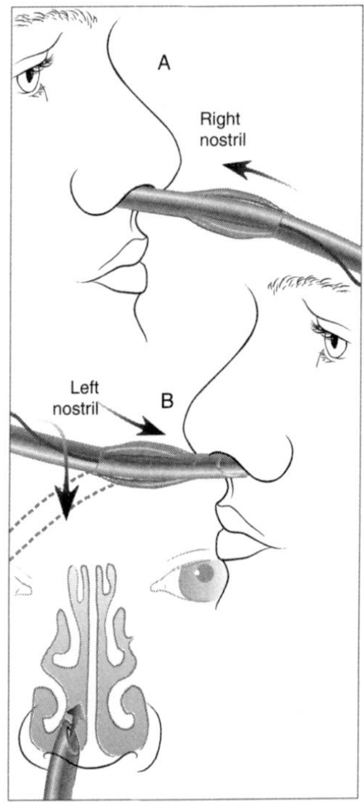

FIGURE 5.11 During blind nasotracheal intubation, the bevel of the endotracheal tube should face the septum to minimize the risk of injury to the nasal turbinates. **A:** With the tube concave downward (the standard initial approach), this necessitates insertion on the right side. **B:** If the right nostril is not adequately patent, the tube may be inserted on the left side by inverting it 180 degrees. The tube can then be rotated back to the normal position after the tip reaches the posterior pharynx.

4. Dim room lights as necessary.
5. Insert styletted endotracheal tube into patient's mouth along midline, following contour of tongue.
6. When tube reaches supraglottic region, direct it as far anteriorly as possible and continue to advance it until it passes through glottic opening into trachea.
7. Observe anterior neck to see characteristic focused, cherry-red glow at suprasternal notch ("jack-o-lantern" effect).
8. Carefully remove stylet.
9. Confirm tracheal placement (equal breath sounds, no sounds over stomach, capnography).
10. Position tube at midtracheal level.
11. Secure endotracheal tube.
12. Confirm proper tube position with chest radiograph.

CLINICAL TIPS

Lighted Stylet (Light Wand) Intubation

1. Lighted stylet intubation can often be performed with minimal movement of the patient's head and neck.
2. It may be necessary to dim the lights in a bright room to appreciate the appearance of the light from the lighted stylet on the patient's anterior neck. Whenever this is done, special attention must be given to the monitoring equipment during this time because visual cues regarding the patient's clinical condition (e.g., cyanosis) are not readily observed.
3. Esophageal intubation with a lighted stylet can be recognized by the characteristic dim, unfocused light seen on the anterior neck.
4. In the event of an esophageal intubation, the tube should be withdrawn to the hypopharynx before making another attempt. The operator often appreciates a subtle "pop" as the tube flips out of the esophagus and into the supraglottic region.
5. Because of the sharp bend in the styletted endotracheal tube, removal of the stylet may result in buckling of the tube and inadvertent extubation. For this reason, the tube should be held firmly in place against the patient's tongue as the stylet is carefully withdrawn with firm, steady pressure.
6. As with any stylet used during an endotracheal intubation, the tip should not extend beyond the distal end of the tube to avoid injury to the soft tissues.

OVERVIEW

Tactile (Digital) Intubation

1. Prepare patient.
   A. Administer assisted or controlled BVM ventilation as needed.
   B. Attach patient to monitoring devices.
   C. Preoxygenate patient with 100% oxygen.
   D. Insert gastric tube to evacuate stomach contents as necessary.
2. Select appropriate endotracheal tube and moisten tip to facilitate insertion.
3. Insert stylet (if used) into tube and bend styletted tube into gentle arc.
4. Insert index finger of nondominant hand into patient's mouth and palpate arytenoids.
5. Insert endotracheal tube with dominant hand, using index finger of nondominant hand as guide.

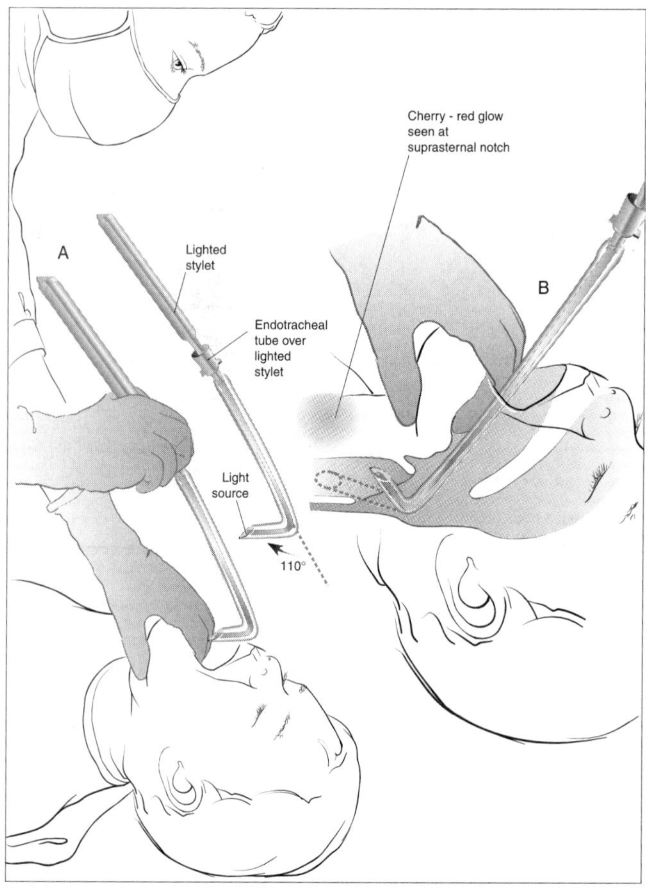

FIGURE 5.12 Lighted stylet (light wand) intubation. **A:** The mandibular block is grasped and pulled outward with the nondominant hand. **B:** The styletted endotracheal tube is inserted over the tongue along the midline until a focused, cherry-red glow is seen at the anterior neck proximal to the suprasternal notch. **C:** The tube is secured against the tongue with the index finger and the lighted stylet is carefully removed.

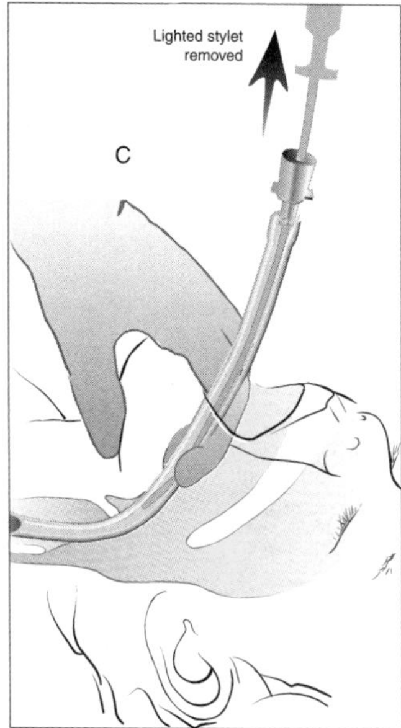

FIGURE 5.12 *(continued)*

6. Carefully remove stylet (if used).
7. Confirm tracheal placement (equal breath sounds, no sounds over stomach, capnography).
8. Position tube at midtracheal level (see Fig. 5.7).
9. Secure endotracheal tube.
10. Confirm proper tube position with chest radiograph.

CLINICAL TIPS

Tactile (Digital) Intubation

1. Tactile intubation is especially suited for neonates and small infants; they are edentulous and have a small upper airway.
2. It may be necessary manually to elevate the epiglottis to allow insertion of the endotracheal tube.
3. The thumb of the hand used to palpate the airway structures can also be used to apply cricoid pressure.

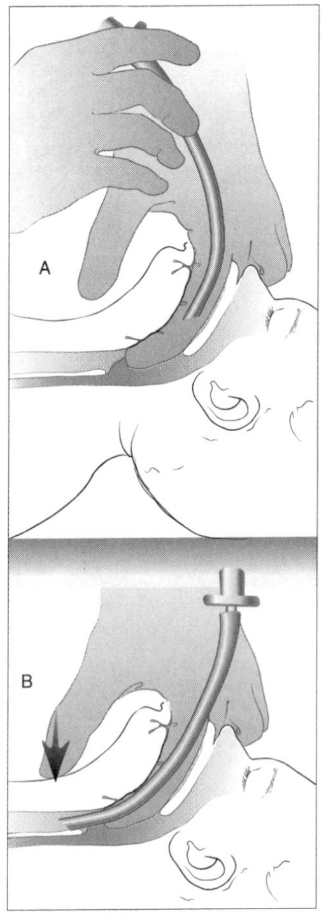

FIGURE 5.13 Tactile (digital) intubation. **A:** The index finger of the nondominant hand is used to palpate the arytenoids and retract the epiglottis. **B:** The tube is inserted using the index finger to guide the tip into the trachea. The thumb may be used to apply simultaneous cricoid pressure.

OVERVIEW

Retrograde Intubation

1. Prepare patient.
   A. Administer assisted or controlled BVM ventilation as needed.
   B. Attach patient to monitoring devices.
   C. Preoxygenate patient with 100% oxygen.
   D. Insert gastric tube to evacuate stomach contents as necessary.
   E. Prepare anterior neck aseptically and drape field.

F. Infiltrate skin and subcutaneous tissues overlying planned insertion site with local anesthetic.
G. Perform transtracheal instillation of lidocaine (optional).

2. Prepare and test necessary equipment.
   A. Attach standard 18-gauge intravenous catheter to fluid-filled syringe.
   B. Use extra-long, heavy-gauge wire.
   C. Inflate balloon on cuffed endotracheal tube (if used) to ensure there are no leaks.
3. Stabilize trachea with thumb and index finger of nondominant hand and locate cricothyroid membrane.
4. Insert needle using "straight in" (or slightly caudad) approach; apply negative pressure on syringe so that entry into trachea is indicated by appearance of bubbles in fluid.
5. As soon as needle enters trachea, rotate syringe so that needle points superiorly and advance catheter until hub rests against skin.
6. Remove needle syringe.
7. Insert guide wire until a sufficient length extends out nose or mouth of patient and then clamp wire at anterior neck.
8. Thread endotracheal tube over wire into nose or mouth of patient until tip of tube is in supraglottic region.
9. Pull wire taut and pass tube into trachea.
10. Remove clamp and withdraw tube through cephalad end of tube.
11. Confirm tracheal placement (equal breath sounds, no sounds over stomach, capnography).
12. Position tube at midtracheal level (see Fig. 5.7).
13. Secure endotracheal tube.
14. Confirm proper tube position with chest radiograph.

CLINICAL TIPS

Retrograde Intubation

1. With adolescents and some older children, the laryngeal prominence (thyroid cartilage) is the first landmark used in locating the cricothyroid membrane. The operator palpates inferiorly from this point until the second "bump" of the superior margin of the cricoid cartilage is felt. The cricothyroid membrane is just cephalad to this point.
2. The laryngeal prominence is not well developed in infants and younger children and can therefore not be used as a landmark for locating the

cricothyroid membrane. With these patients, it is necessary to palpate upward from the trachea until the more subtle prominence of the cricoid cartilage is located.

3. If the cricothyroid membrane cannot be located, a lower point of entry through an intercartilaginous space in the midline of the trachea can be used with additional risk to the patient.
4. The entry needle should be attached to a fluid-filled syringe so that entry into the trachea is indicated by the appearance of bubbles in the fluid.
5. It may be necessary to retrieve the guide wire from the hypopharynx using blunt forceps. If the wire is retrieved from the nose, a nasal intubation may be performed.

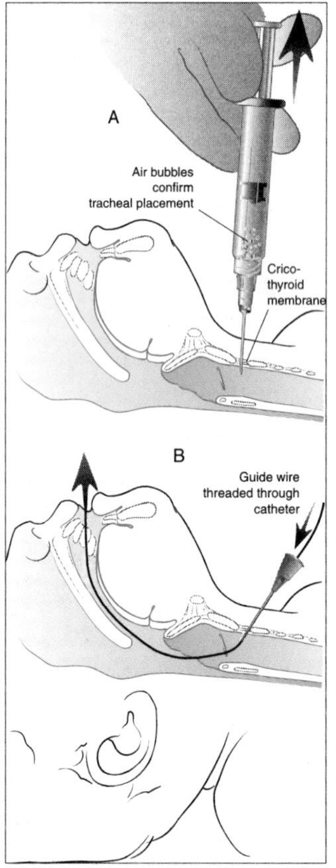

FIGURE 5.14 Retrograde intubation. **A:** The needle is inserted through the cricothyroid membrane with negative pressure on the fluid-filled syringe. Entry into the trachea is indicated by the appearance of bubbles in the fluid. **B:** The needle is directed anteriorly and the needle and syringe are removed as the catheter is advanced to its hub. The guide wire is inserted through the catheter until it can be retrieved from the nose or mouth. **C:** The endotracheal tube is threaded over the wire after the wire has been secured at the skin with a hemostat. The wire should be threaded through the Murphy side hole. **D:** The wire is pulled taut and the tube is advanced into the trachea over the wire. **E:** After successful intubation, the hemostat is removed, the wire is withdrawn through the proximal end of the tube, and the tube is advanced to the appropriate depth of insertion.

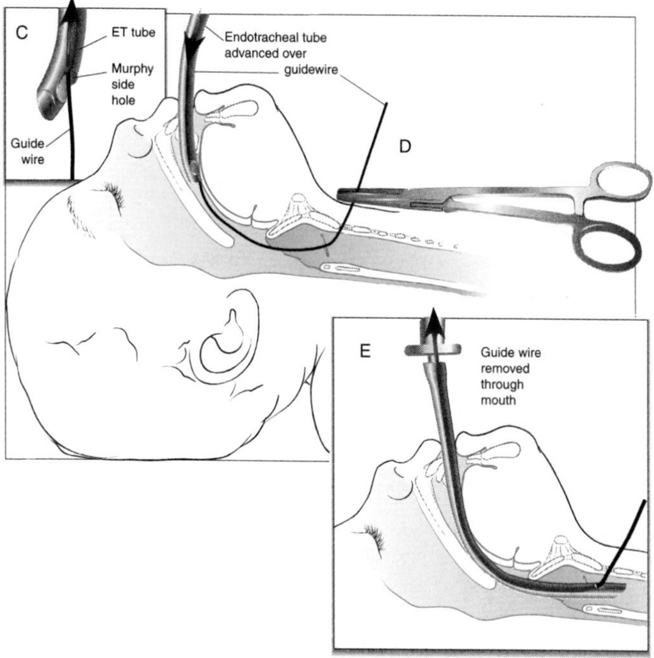

FIGURE 5.14 *(continued)*

6. If the tube cannot be passed easily into the trachea over the wire, the tube should be withdrawn somewhat as the tension in the wire is diminished. The wire should then be pulled taut again and another attempt made. In such instances, it may also be helpful to rotate the tube 90 degrees before reinsertion, or to use a smaller tube.
7. Failure to intubate the trachea after two or three attempts with the retrograde technique indicates that another method should be used.

OVERVIEW

Fiberoptic Nasotracheal Intubation

1. Prepare patient.
   A. Attach patient to monitoring devices.
   B. Preoxygenate patient with 100% oxygen.

C. Insert gastric tube to evacuate stomach contents as necessary.
D. Apply topical anesthetic and topical vasoconstrictors to nares.
E. Perform transtracheal instillation of lidocaine (optional).
F. Administer mild sedative as needed.

2. Prepare and test the necessary equipment.

   A. Check laryngoscope to see that fiberoptic tip can be manipulated through full range of positions.
   B. Check eyepiece to ensure good image resolution.
   C. Attach laryngoscope to wall suction or high-flow oxygen.
   D. Generously lubricate fiberoptic strand of laryngoscope.
   E. Select endotracheal tube and test balloon for any leaks.

3. Check nares for patency by occluding each one in turn; if patency is equal in both nares, then right side should be used for intubation.

4. Perform laryngoscopy.

   A. If nasal mucosa are adequately prepared with topical vasoconstrictor, the following method may be used.
      1) Insert endotracheal tube until tip reaches posterior hypopharynx.
      2) Pass fiberoptic filament of laryngoscope through endotracheal tube until it reaches supraglottic region.
      3) Deflect tip of fiberoptic filament and rotate laryngoscope back and forth to obtain panoramic view of supraglottic structures.
   B. If nasal mucosa cannot be adequately prepared, the following method must be used.
      1) Remove 15-mm connector from endotracheal tube if necessary.
      2) Slide endotracheal tube up entire length of fiberoptic laryngoscope.
      3) Insert fiberoptic filament through nose, around angle at posterior pharynx, and into supraglottic region.
      4) Deflect tip of fiberoptic filament and rotate laryngoscope back and forth to obtain a panoramic view of supraglottic structures.

5. Insert fiberoptic filament into trachea to level of carina.

6. Advance endotracheal tube into trachea.

7. Remove laryngoscope.

8. Confirm tracheal placement (equal breath sounds, no sounds over stomach, capnography).

9. Position tube at midtracheal level (see Fig. 5.7).

10. Secure endotracheal tube.

11. Confirm proper tube position with chest radiograph.

CLINICAL TIPS

Fiberoptic Nasotracheal Intubation

1. The nasal mucosa should be prepared with a topical vasoconstrictor whenever possible 2 to 4 minutes before laryngoscopy. Epistaxis is one of the primary causes of failure for this procedure.
2. Mild sedation may be necessary to facilitate a fiberoptic nasotracheal intubation. However, spontaneous respirations and normal airway reflexes should be preserved.
3. The suction port of a fiberoptic laryngoscope may be connected to high-flow oxygen. This port can then be used to blow secretions from the field of view while simultaneously delivering oxygen to the patient.

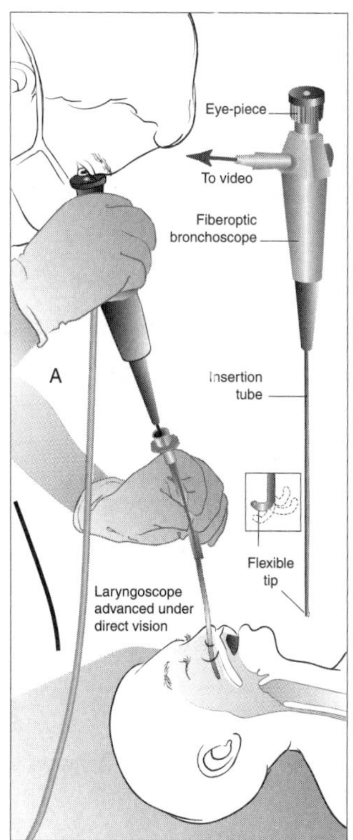

FIGURE 5.15 Fiberoptic nasotracheal intubation. **A:** The endotracheal tube is first threaded up the entire length of the fiberoptic strand. The fiberoptic laryngoscope is then inserted into the nose under direct visualization through the eyepiece. **B:** It is advanced beyond the angle at the posterior pharynx into the supraglottic area until the appropriate landmarks can be seen. Once the glottis is identified, the fiberoptic laryngoscope is further advanced into the trachea to the level of the carina. **C:** Using the fiberoptic laryngoscope as a guide, the endotracheal tube is inserted through the nose, into the hypopharynx, and through the glottic opening into the trachea. **D:** The laryngoscope is then carefully removed while the endotracheal tube is held securely in place. (*continued on next page*)

4. The laryngoscope should always be advanced under direct vision through the eyepiece because blind insertion leads to mucosal injury and bleeding.
5. If a patient has not been intubated within the first 3 minutes after initiating a fiberoptic nasotracheal intubation, the likelihood of success decreases significantly and another approach should be considered.

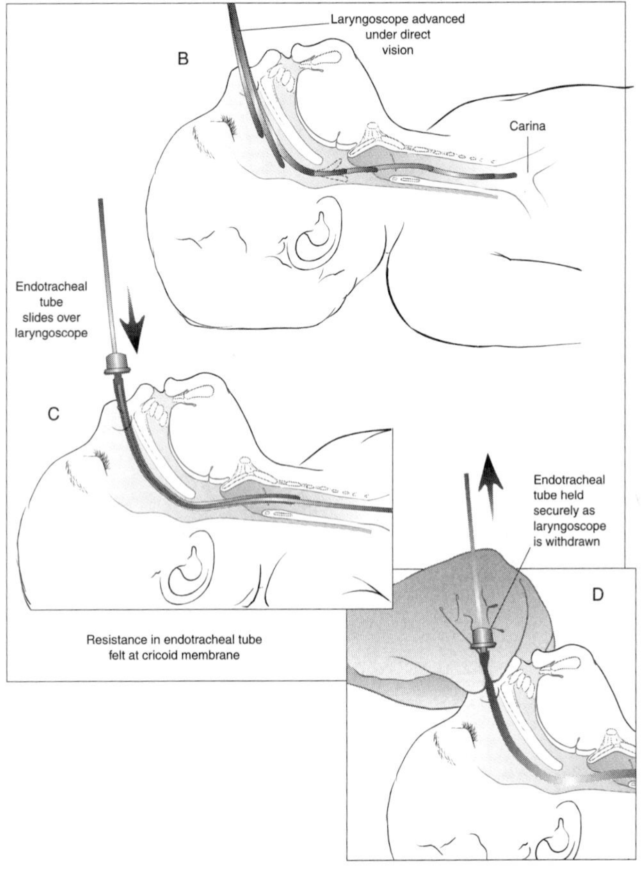

FIGURE 5.15 *(continued)*

CHAPTER 6

Obtaining a Percutaneous or Surgical Airway

OVERVIEW

Percutaneous Transtracheal Ventilation

1. Attach 3- to 5-mL syringe with a few milliliters of saline or lidocaine to needle and catheter.
2. Locate cricothyroid membrane, bound by thyroid cartilage superiorly and cricoid cartilage inferiorly.
3. Hold trachea in place and provide skin tension with thumb and middle finger of nondominant hand.
4. Place tip of needle at inferior midline of membrane, directing needle caudally at 30- to 45-degree angle.
5. Advance needle while pulling back on plunger of syringe. Appearance of air bubbles in syringe confirms intratracheal placement.
6. Slide catheter over needle until hub rests securely on skin surface.
7. Remove needle and syringe as a unit.
8. Connect high-pressure tubing and oxygen source to catheter.
9. Confirm correct placement with a few short bursts of oxygen.
10. Ventilate at appropriate rate by opening and closing permanent valve, or occluding side port, stopcock, or Y-connector.
11. Assess patient response.
12. Suture catheter securely in place.

CLINICAL TIPS

Percutaneous Transtracheal Ventilation

1. The laryngeal prominence does not fully develop until adolescence; the important landmarks are the hyoid bone and cricoid cartilage in young children.
2. If the cricothyroid membrane cannot be located, the catheter may be safely inserted in a lower intercartilaginous tracheal space.

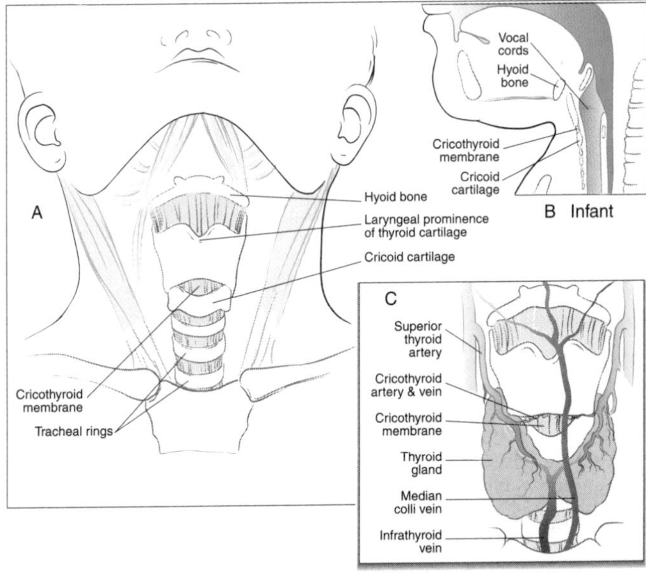

FIGURE 6.1 External anatomy of the upper airway. **A:** Cartilaginous skeleton of the extrathoracic airway. With older children and adolescents, the laryngeal prominence at the superior border of the thyroid cartilage can usually be palpated. The thyroid cartilage is followed inferiorly to locate the cricothyroid membrane. **B:** With infants and younger children, the laryngeal prominence is not developed. The rings of the tracheal cartilage are followed superiorly to locate the prominence of the cricoid cartilage. The cricothyroid membrane is just superior to the cricoid cartilage. **C:** A midline approach avoids the normal position of the cricothyroid artery.

3. The cricothyroid membrane should be punctured in the lower third to avoid the cricothyroid vessels.
4. One person should be assigned to hold the hub of the catheter in place until it is secured to prevent subcutaneous emphysema.
5. Regular mock codes with the equipment increase the likelihood of successful performance of the technique in emergency situations.

OVERVIEW

Surgical Cricothyrotomy

1. Identify landmarks in anterior neck by palpating hyoid bone, thyroid cartilage, and cricoid cartilage.

TABLE 6.1 **Equipment for Percutaneous Transtracheal Ventilation (PTV)**

1. High pressure oxygen source: 50 psi can be obtained directly from hospital wall outlet (used for adolescents and adults); 25 to 30 psi safely delivered through a standard regulator set at 10 to 12 L/min (used for younger children).
2. High pressure tubing.
3. Inline valve (permanent, side hole cut in distal end of tubing, Y-connector, or 3-way stopcock).
4. Syringe containing 2 to 3 mL of saline or lidocaine.
5. 16- or 18-gauge catheter.

2. When time permits, prepare skin with antiseptic solution and administer local infiltrative anesthesia.
3. Stabilize trachea with nonoperating hand.
4. Make vertical midline incision over cricoid membrane, attempting to avoid isthmus of thyroid gland.
5. While an assistant retracts skin and subcutaneous issue, bluntly dissect through sternohyoid muscle until cricothyroid membrane is visualized.

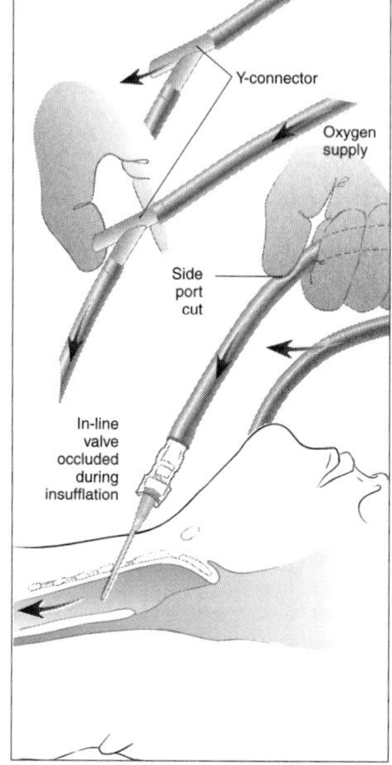

FIGURE 6.2 Percutaneous transtracheal ventilation is most effectively performed with pediatric patients using a permanent in-line valve system. Such systems provide a safer and more reliable means of delivering known oxygen pressure. However, percutaneous transtracheal ventilation can also be performed using other methods of delivering and venting gas, such as a Y-connector and two oxygen tubes or even a small hole cut in one side of a single oxygen tube.

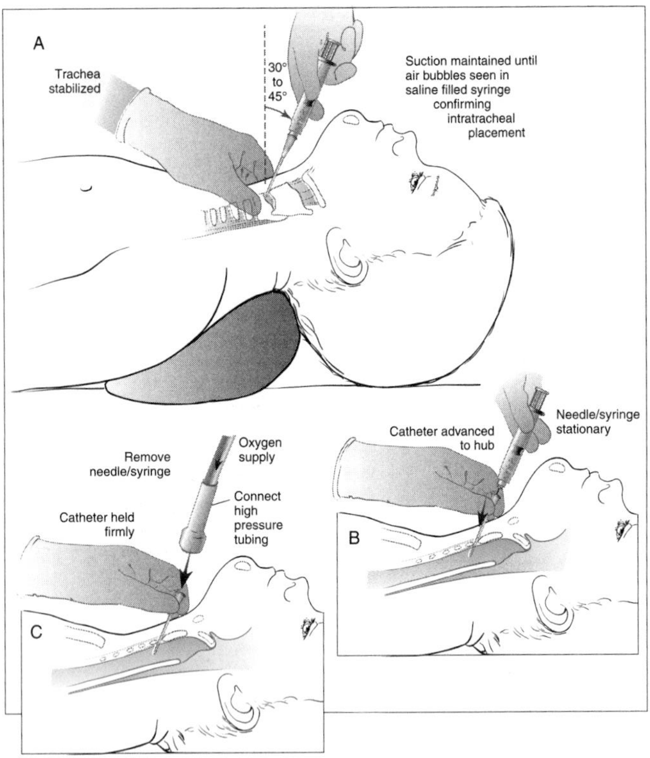

FIGURE 6.3 Performing percutaneous transtracheal ventilation. **A:** The needle is angled caudally at 30 to 45 degrees and inserted through the cricothyroid membrane until bubbles are seen in the fluid-filled syringe, indicating puncture of the trachea. **B:** The catheter is advanced to the hub as the needle and syringe are removed. **C:** The catheter is secured in place and connected to the oxygen delivery system.

6. Using no. 11 scalpel blade, make small incision near inferior border of membrane.
7. Insert pair of curved Mayo scissors or small curved hemostat into incision and spread jaws of scissors or hemostat to enlarge incision.
8. Maintain patency of incision either by keeping scissors or hemostats in place or by inserting trachea hook into inferior margin and gently lifting edge of incision anteriorly.

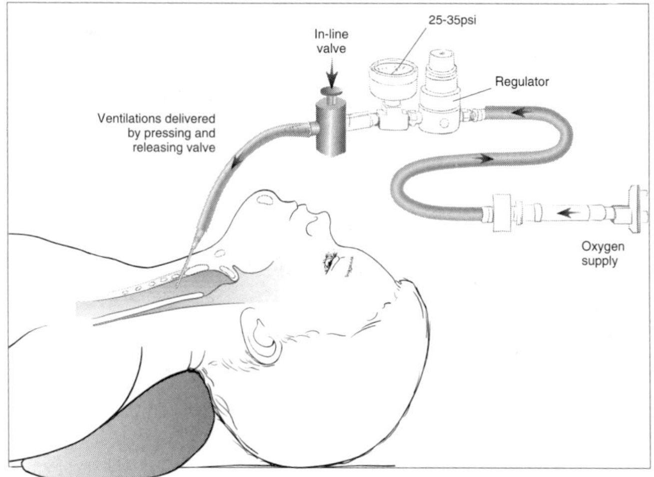

FIGURE 6.4 Positive-pressure ventilation is administered by pressing and releasing the inline valve (or opening and occluding the Y-connector or cut side port) using the inspiratory-to-expiratory ratios shown in Table 6.2.

9. Insert appropriately sized endotracheal tube or tracheostomy tube into incision and secure.
10. Assess adequacy of ventilation.

CLINICAL TIPS

Surgical Cricothyrotomy

1. Alternative means of airway control such as needle cricothyroidotomy or retrograde intubation should always be considered first, particularly if the patient is a young child.
2. The initial incision is made vertical and in the midline. This reduces the risk of damage to vascular structures.

TABLE 6.2 Ventilatory Rates for PTV (I:E RATIOS)

Standard	1:4 to 1:5 seconds
Elevated ICP	1:2 seconds
Airway obstruction	1:9 seconds

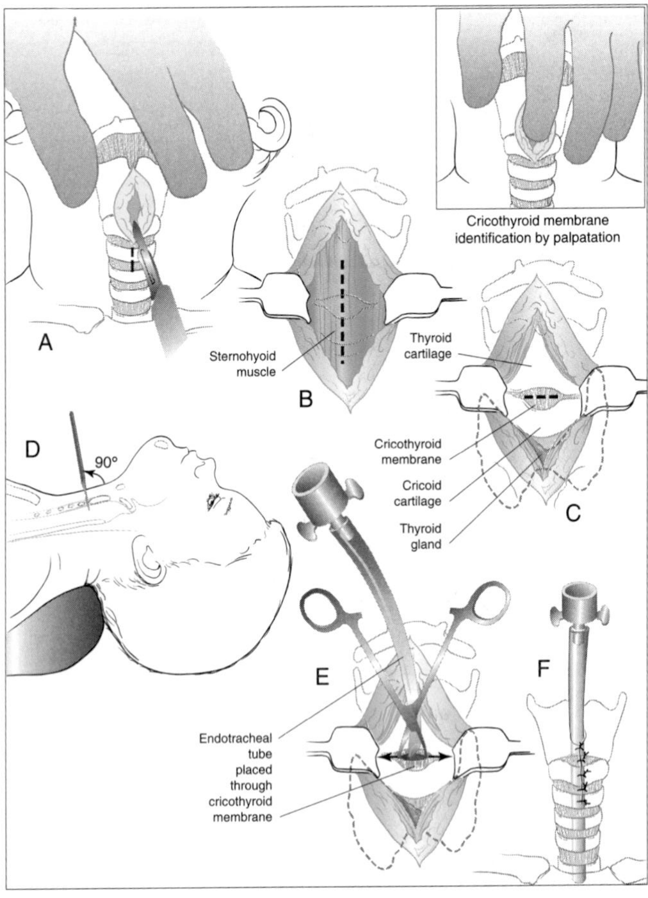

FIGURE 6.5 Surgical cricothyrotomy. **A:** Initial vertical incision with manual stabilization of the trachea. **B:** Skin retraction and exposure of the sternohyoid muscle. **C:** Retraction of the sternohyoid muscle and exposure of the cricothyroid membrane (note location of incision is indicated). **D:** Horizontal incision through the cricothyroid membrane with the scalpel perpendicular to the membrane. **E:** Hemostats or scissors used to maintain the opening in the membrane while a tracheal tube is passed through the incision and into the trachea. **F:** Tracheal tube secured in place.

3. In some cases, the cricothyroid membrane may not be easily visualized. In these instances, the membrane should be palpated with a fingertip. "Blind" incision is a technique of last resort because of the risk of damage to vascular structures in the area.
4. A tracheal hook or the blades of the scissors or hemostats should be used to keep the incision open and to maintain location of the incision.
5. If the incision is "lost," bubbles of exhaled air often identify its location. In the apneic patient, these may be produced by pressure on the anterior chest wall.
6. Even a small airway is better than none. If a small endotracheal or tracheostomy tube is all that will pass through the incision, then it should be used until more effective airway control can be established.

CHAPTER 7

Central Venous Access

OVERVIEW

1. Obtain consent, as appropriate.
2. Gather necessary equipment.
3. Attach monitors: cardiograph, pulse oximetry, blood pressure.
4. Select approach and position patient accordingly.
5. Prepare sterile field.
6. Infiltrate local anesthetic, as necessary.
7. Attach entry needle to small (3- or 5-mL) syringe and rinse with heparin.
8. Insert entry needle through skin and eject small volume of fluid to clear any skin plugs.
9. While applying negative pressure to syringe, insert needle until blood is aspirated from vein.
10. Advance needle an additional 1 to 2 mm, so tip is well within vessel lumen.
11. Carefully remove syringe from needle.
12. Insert guide wire, making sure proximal end is always secured.
13. Remove needle, leaving wire in place.
14. Enlarge skin puncture site by inserting no. 11 scalpel blade to its hub along wire.
15. Insert dilator to enlarge entry site (optional).
16. Insert venous catheter and aspirate blood to ensure proper placement.
17. Secure catheter in place with suture and apply dressing.
18. Obtain radiograph to confirm proper placement of catheter.
19. Document procedure in medical record.

CLINICAL TIPS

1. Ejecting a small volume of fluid from the entry needle after initial insertion through the skin clears any skin plugs and facilitates aspiration of blood.

2. The use of a small (3- to 5-mL) syringe initially to locate the vein prevents collapse of the vessel, even with a small, hypovolemic child.

3. If blood flow is not obtained after deep insertion of the entry needle, the needle should be slowly withdrawn while maintaining negative pressure on the syringe. If the vessel was inadvertently passed through, blood may be aspirated as the needle is withdrawn.

4. In locating the central vessel, the entry needle should be inserted and withdrawn in a slow, methodical pattern to prevent multiple vein lacerations.

5. Bright red blood or pulsatile flow indicate arterial puncture, although these findings may not be readily apparent when cardiac output is severely compromised. If there is any remaining question about whether the blood aspirated has a venous or arterial source, a specimen can be sent to the laboratory for blood gas analysis.

6. Use of a non–Luer-Lok syringe prevents accidental dislodgement of the needle on removal of the syringe before insertion of the guide wire.

7. After the syringe is removed from the entry needle, but before the guide wire is inserted, the hub of the needle should be occluded by a finger to prevent air embolus or blood loss.

8. The operator must always ensure that the proximal end of the guide wire is secured at all times to prevent entry of the wire into the central circulation.

9. If resistance is felt with removal of the guide wire through the needle, the wire and needle should be removed together to prevent shearing of the wire by the beveled tip of the needle

10. The catheter tip should not lie within the right atrium because this may result in erosion and perforation of the atrial wall.

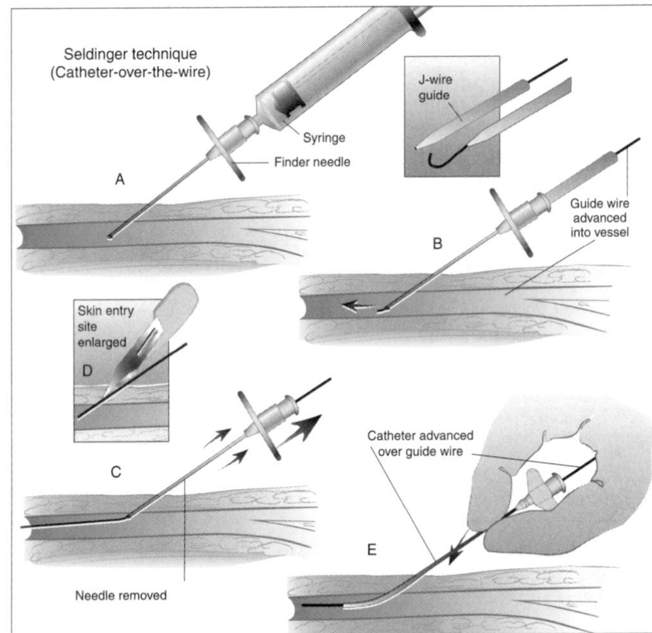

FIGURE 7.1 Catheter-over-the-wire (Seldinger) technique. **A:** The central vein is first punctured using a needle and syringe. **B:** The syringe is removed and the guide wire is inserted through the needle into the vein. **C:** The needle is removed and the wire is left in place. **D:** A small incision is made at the entry site to facilitate insertion of the catheter. **E:** The catheter is inserted over the guide wire and the wire is removed.

TABLE 7.1 Catheter Sizes for Pediatric Patients

			AVERAGE CATHETER LENGTH (CM)		
Age	*Average Weight (kg)*	*Average Height (cm)*	*Internal Jugular*	*Subclavian*	*Femoral*
1 mo	4.2	55	6.0	5.5	15.7
3 mo	5.8	61	6.6	6.0	17.3
6 mo	7.8	68	7.3	6.6	19.1
9 mo	9.2	72	7.6	6.9	20.1
1 yr	10.2	76	8.0	7.3	21.1
1.5 yr	11.5	83	8.7	7.9	22.9
2 yr	12.8	88	9.2	8.3	24.2
4 yr	16.5	103	10.6	9.6	28.1
6 yr	20.5	116	11.8	10.7	31.4
8 yr	26	127	12.9	11.7	34.2
10 yr	31	137	13.8	12.5	36.8
12 yr	39	149	15.0	13.5	39.9
14 yr	50	165	16.5	14.9	44.0
16 yr	62.5	174	17.3	15.7	46.3

TABLE 7.2 Catheter Diameters for Pediatric Patients

	Catheter diameter (French)		
Age	*Internal Jugular*	*Subclavian*[a]	*Femoral*
0–6 mo	3	3	3
6 mo–2 yr	3	3	3–4
3–6 yr	4	4	4
7–12 yr	4–5	4–5	4–5

[a] For infants and younger children, the subclavian approach should be performed only by highly experienced operators.

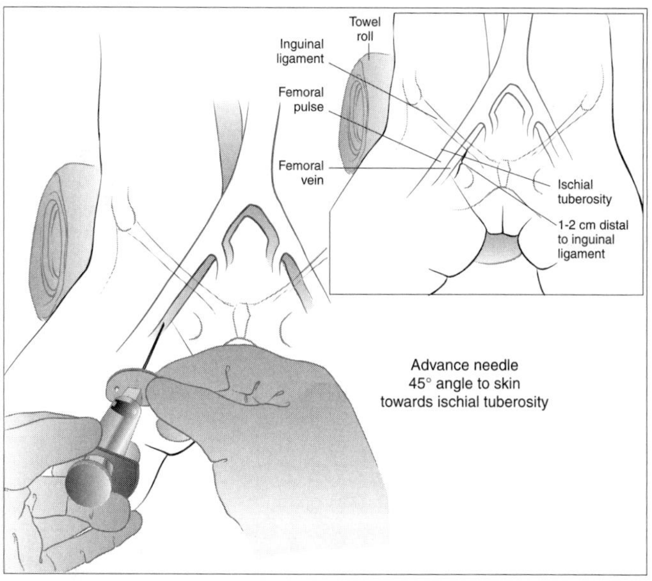

FIGURE 7.2 The entry site for femoral vein cannulation is located 1 to 2 cm medial to the femoral artery pulse (when palpable) and 1 to 2 cm inferior to the inguinal ligament. When the patient has weak or absent pulses, the entry site can be located by identifying the point halfway between the pubic tubercle and the anterior iliac spine and 1 to 2 cm inferior to the inguinal ligament.

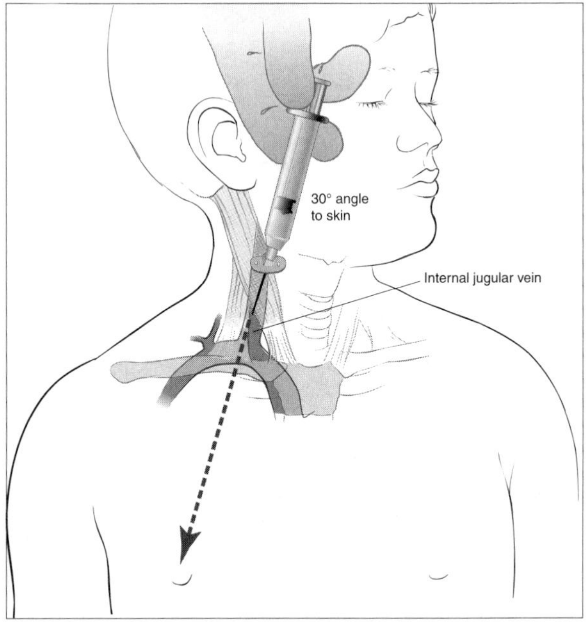

FIGURE 7.3 There are several possible sites for internal jugular vein cannulation. The entry site for the median approach, which is used most commonly, is located at the apex of the triangle formed by the two heads of the sternocleidomastoid muscle laterally and the clavicle inferiorly. The internal jugular vein is superficial and lateral to the carotid artery, which can be palpated just medial to the entry site.

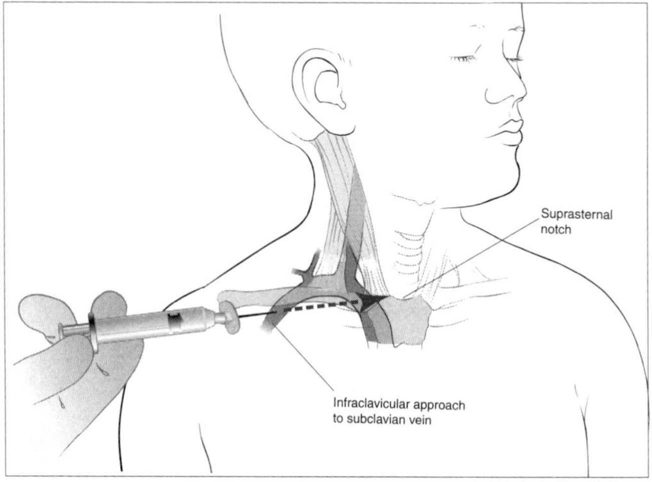

FIGURE 7.4 In pediatric patients, cannulation of the subclavian vein has the highest rate of complications (primarily pneumothorax and arterial puncture) among the methods used to obtain central venous access. For this reason, it is used least frequently and should be performed only by an experienced practitioner. The generally preferred method for subclavian vein cannulation is through an infraclavicular approach. The entry site for this method is just below the clavicle at the midclavicular line along a line that intersects the suprasternal notch.

TABLE 7.3 Advantages and Disadvantages of Specific Sites

Site	*Landmark*	*Advantage*	*Disadvantage*	*Complications*
Femoral vein	Femoral triangle, just medial to femoral artery pulse (if palpable)	Requires least operator experience, fastest, out of the way of resuscitation, anatomy exposed, available for direct compression	Risk of contamination, may be harder to secure, may be more uncomfortable for the patient, difficult in obese patients, need fluoroscopy to place Swan-Ganz catheter	Infection, bleeding, thrombosis
Internal jugular vein	Angle formed by the two heads of SCM muscle	Right side offers direct route to SVC, out of resuscitation field, anatomy exposed, available for direct compression	Requires operator experience, generally takes longer, more difficult in children <1 yr of age with short, fat necks, more difficult in patients with tracheostomy and those who are not intubated	Carotid artery puncture, PTX, on left side risk of thoracic duct injury, cardiac tamponade, multiple neuropathies, thrombosis, infection
External jugular vein	Visible in the neck crossing posteriorly over SCM muscle	Visible, superficial, available for direct compression, least complications	Difficult to cannulate central circulation from this site, if not visible cannot use this site	Hematoma
Subclavian vein	Supraclavicular: Lateral to clavicular head of SCM muscle above the clavicle Infraclavicular: Just beneath junction of middle and lateral thirds of the clavicle	Right side offers direct route to SVC, vein may be less collapsible	Requires operator experience, may be more difficult in patients <1 yr of age, no access to control bleeding	PTX, bleeding, tamponade, dysrhythmias, thoracic duct injury, catheter malposition, air embolism, neuropathies

SVC, superior vena cava; PTX, pneumothorax; SCM, sternocleidomastoid.

CHAPTER 8

Venous Cutdown Catheterization

OVERVIEW

Venous Cutdown Catheterization at the Distal Saphenous Vein

1. Scrub medial malleolus and surrounding area with aseptic solution.
2. Make 1- to 2-cm skin incision beginning 1 cm superior to medial malleolus and just posterior to anterior margin of bone.
3. Bluntly dissect subcutaneous tissue and fat with curved forceps.
4. Identify saphenous vein and gently separate it from surrounding tissue.
5. Insert loop of nonabsorbable suture around vessel and then cut loop so two ligatures are formed.
6. Tie off distal portion of vessel.
7. Lift proximal suture to elevate vessel and make small venotomy incision.
8. Cannulate vessel.
9. Tie proximal suture around catheter and vessel.
10. Close skin with nonabsorbable suture.
11. Stabilize cutdown site.

Venous Cutdown Catheterization at the Proximal Saphenous Vein

1. Begin 4- to 6-cm transverse incision at point where scrotal or labial fold meets thigh.
2. Use blunt dissection of adipose tissue to locate proximal saphenous vein just distal to its junction with femoral vein.
3. Isolate vein and perform venotomy and catheter insertion as described for distal saphenous vein cutdown.

CLINICAL TIPS

1. The most commonly used (and probably easiest) site for performing emergency venous cutdown catheterization is the distal saphenous vein at the ankle.

2. After making the initial skin incision, the remainder of the cutdown should normally be performed using blunt dissection to avoid injury to nerves and vessels.

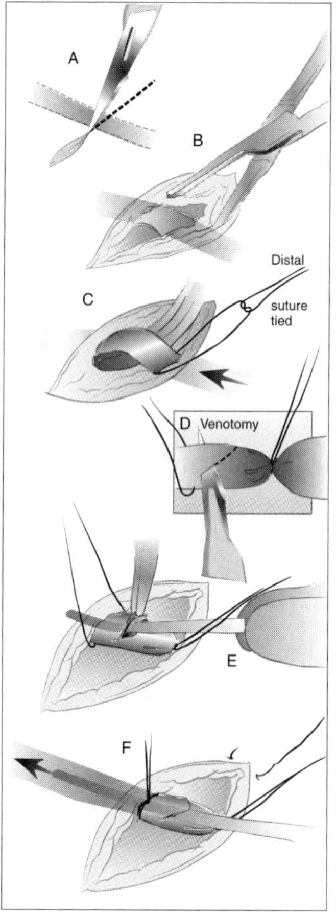

FIGURE 8.1 Procedure for venous cutdown catheterization. **A:** A transverse incision is made at the appropriate site. The incision should extend into the subcutaneous tissue but not deep enough potentially to lacerate the vein. **B:** The vein is isolated using blunt dissection. A suture is passed around the vein and cut to give two ligatures. **C:** The distal suture is tied and used to stabilize the vessel. **D:** Venotomy is performed to allow insertion of the catheter. Alternatively, the operator may choose to insert the catheter over a needle without performing a venotomy, in a manner similar to percutaneous catheterization. **E:** The catheter is inserted into the vein. Placement within the vessel is confirmed by aspirating blood or infusing fluid. **F:** The proximal suture is tied and the wound is closed and dressed.

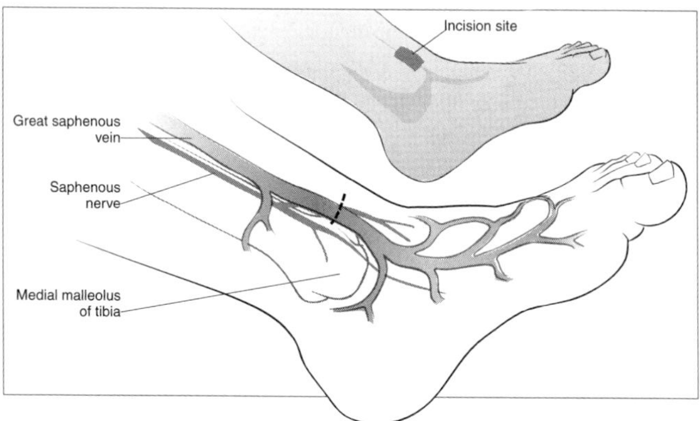

FIGURE 8.2 The most common site for venous cutdown catheterization is the distal saphenous vein at the ankle. The incision site is located just anterior and superior to the medial malleolus where the distal saphenous vein courses adjacent to the periosteum.

3. Slipping a loop of nonabsorbable suture (e.g., silk) around the vessel and then cutting the loop forms both ligatures needed to perform the procedure in a single step.
4. Once the ligatures are extended around the vessel, they can be used to manipulate the vessel more easily during venotomy and catheterization.
5. A larger-diameter catheter (16 or 18 gauge) should be used to maximize intravenous infusion.

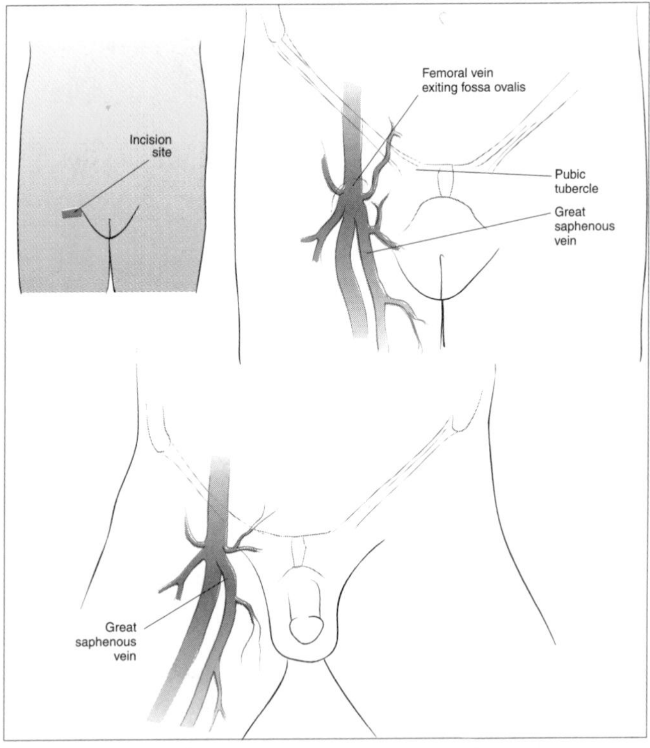

FIGURE 8.3 For patients requiring a large volume of fluid administered rapidly, the proximal saphenous vein at the groin is the preferred site for venous cutdown catheterization. However, this is a more technically difficult procedure with a higher rate of complications and should be performed only by an experienced practitioner. The incision site is located on the thigh at the lateral margin of the labial or scrotal fold (i.e., where the fold ends).

CHAPTER 9

Intraosseous Infusion

OVERVIEW

1. Restrain patient appropriately.
2. Prepare field aseptically.
3. Provide local anesthesia for awake patient.
4. Choose appropriate insertion site: proximal tibia for patients younger than 3 years, distal tibia for patients older than 3 years, or distal femur if failure to insert in tibia.
5. Insert needle perpendicular to bony cortex or angled slightly away from the joint space.
6. Use steady, back-and-forth rotational movement rather than "rocking" needle from side to side.
7. Aspirate marrow to confirm needle placement or infuse small amount of saline and aspirate, looking for pink fluid.
8. Attach to intravenous infusion setup and secure line.
9. Monitor for extravasation and swelling of tissue.

CLINICAL TIPS

1. The needle should not be angled into the joint space to avoid injuring the growth plate of the bone.
2. Excessive or sudden force should not be used, because this often results in puncture of both cortices.
3. If marrow or blood is not aspirated, it may be helpful to insert a few milliliters of saline and reaspirate; obtaining pink-tinged fluid indicates likely placement in the marrow cavity.
4. All standard life support medications can be safely injected through an intraosseous line.

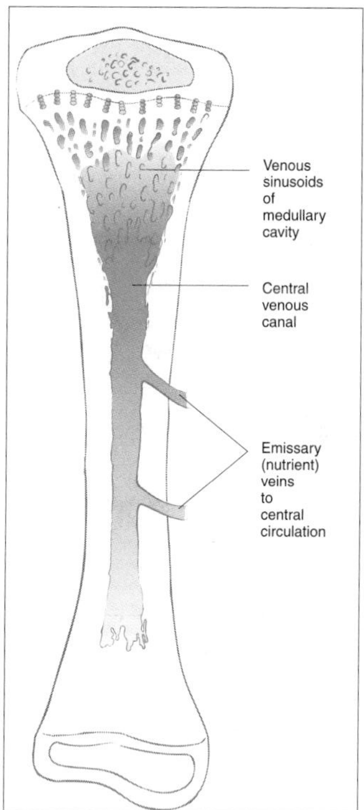

FIGURE 9.1 The marrow space of the long bones functions essentially as a noncollapsible vein. Blood flows from the venous sinusoids of the medullary cavity of the long bones to drain into a central venous canal. From the central canal, blood drains by nutrient or emissary veins into the central circulation.

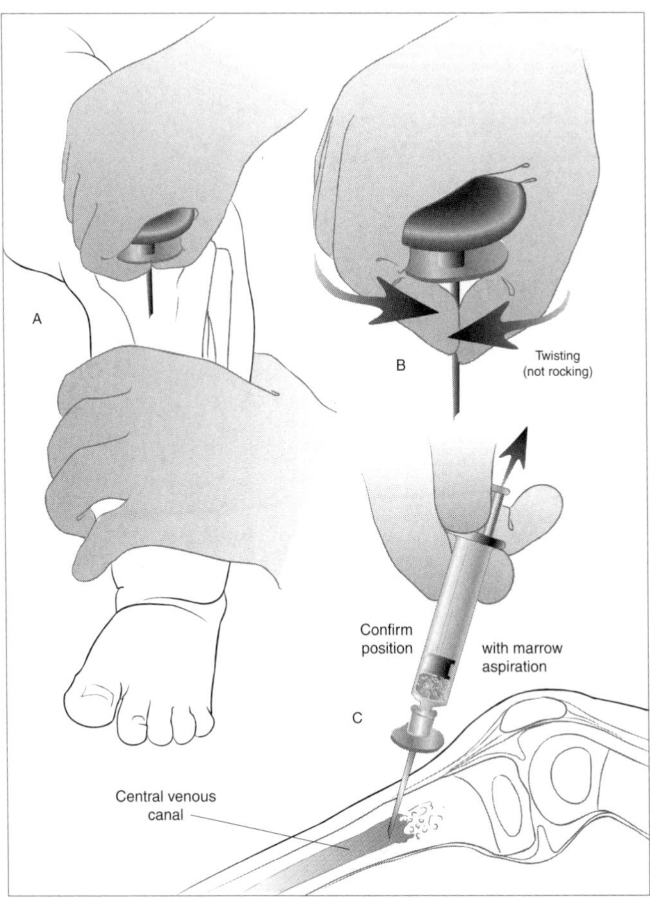

FIGURE 9.2 Procedure for intraosseous infusion. **A:** The needle is angled slightly away from the joint space or, as some more recent sources have recommended, perpendicular to the bone. **B:** A back-and-forth "screwing" motion is used to insert the needle. "Rocking" the needle from side to side results in enlargement of the puncture site and extravasation of infused fluid. **C:** Intramedullary placement is confirmed by aspirating marrow.

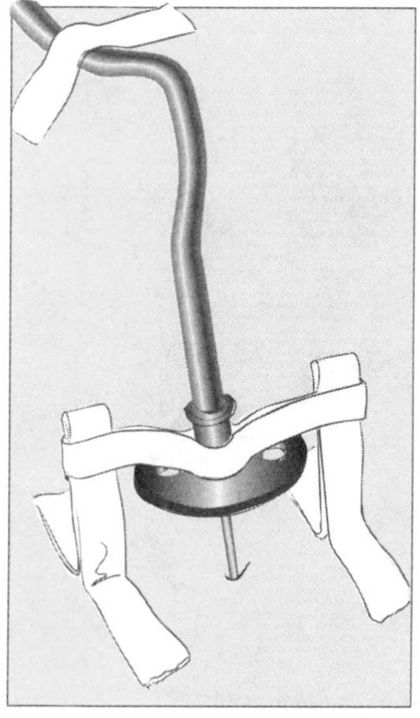

FIGURE 9.3 Securing an intraosseous line.

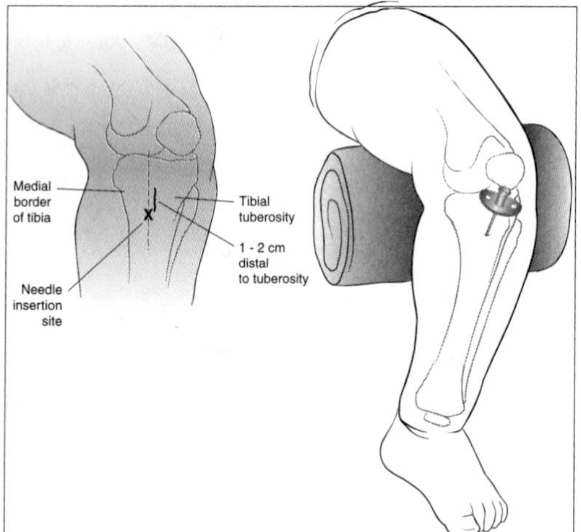

FIGURE 9.4 The entry site at the proximal tibia for intraosseous line insertion is located 1 to 2 cm distal to the tibial tuberosity in the middle of the anteromedial ("flat") surface of the tibia. This is the preferred site for patients up to 3 to 4 years of age.

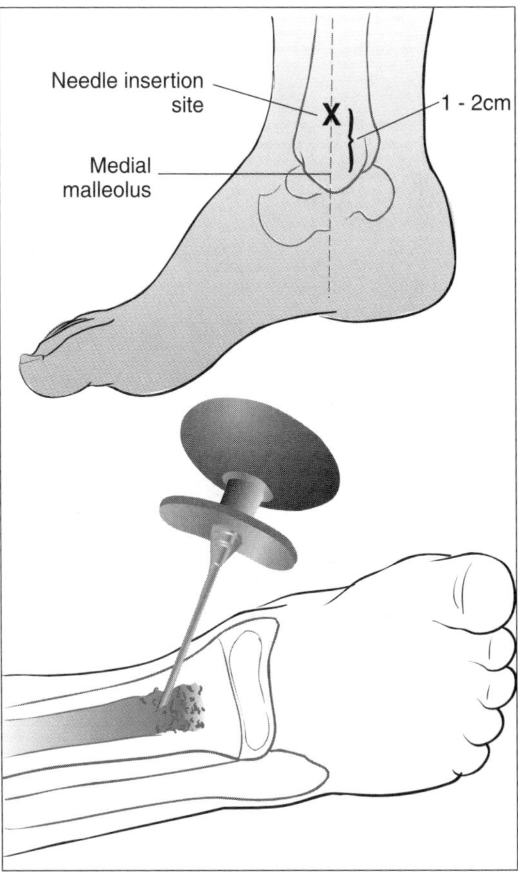

FIGURE 9.5 The entry site at the distal tibia for intraosseous line insertion is located 1 to 2 cm proximal to the medial malleolus halfway between the anterior and posterior borders of the bone. This site is used for older children.

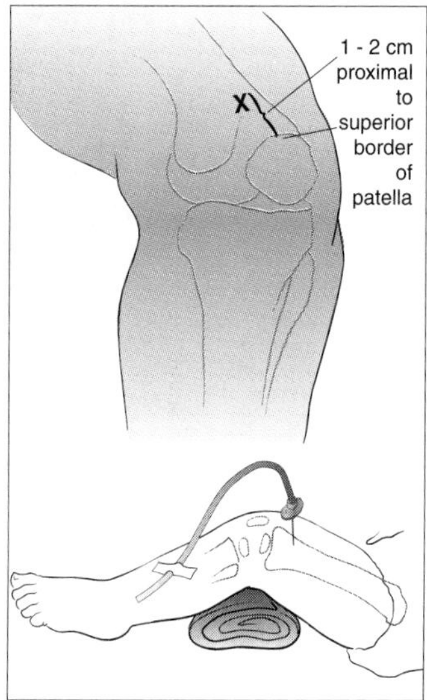

FIGURE 9.6 The entry site at the distal femur for intraosseous line insertion is located in the midline 1 to 2 cm proximal to the superior border of the patella. This site is used as a secondary site in infants or when the operator fails to enter the tibia.

CHAPTER 10

Cardiac Pacing

OVERVIEW

Transvenous Pacing Using Electrocardiographic Guidance

1. Establish central venous access.
2. Attach patient to electrocardiograph (ECG) machine using limb leads.
3. Insert first 10 cm of pacer wire into catheter sheath.
4. Connect negative pole of pacer wire to a V lead of ECG machine by an insulated wire with an alligator clip at each end.
5. Turn on ECG machine to read appropriate V lead.
6. Advance wire and, if a floating wire is used, inflate balloon when tip has entered vena cava.
7. Follow changing patterns of P waves and QRS complexes as wire is advanced through central vessel into right ventricle.
8. Once tip of wire is in right ventricle, deflate balloon and further advance until a current of injury (ST segment elevation) is shown on ECG.
9. Disconnect from ECG machine and connect to pacemaker.
10. Set output to 5 mA, full demand mode, rate appropriate for age, and turn pacer on.
11. If capture does not occur, turn off pacemaker and reposition wire.
12. Once 100% capture is attained, turn output down until capture is lost. Set output for two to three times this value (pacing threshold).
13. Check sensor function by turning rate down until below patient's intrinsic rate. If it is sensing appropriately, pacing should stop. Reset at desired minimum heart rate.
14. Suture pacer wire in place.
15. Check chest radiograph and ECG for proper placement. The ECG should show left bundle branch block pattern.

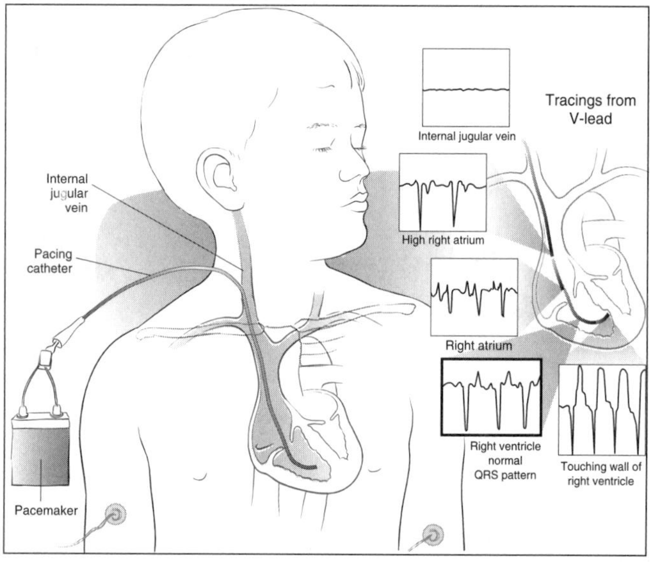

FIGURE 10.1 Transvenous pacemaker placement can be performed through the right internal jugular vein in older children and adolescents (see also Chapter 7). For most younger children, the femoral vein is the easiest and safest approach, assuming there is sufficient forward flow of blood that a flow-directed (balloon) catheter can be used. A continuous tracing is obtained by attaching the proximal end of the wire to the V lead of an ECG machine. This provides information about the position of the wire tip as it is advanced through the central circulation to the heart. *It is important to remember that the ECG machine must be well grounded (i.e., with a properly functioning, three-pronged plug) to minimize the possibility of inducing ventricular fibrillation.*

OVERVIEW

Transcutaneous Pacing

1. Sedate patient as indicated.
2. Apply adhesive electrodes to anterior and posterior chest walls.
3. Connect patient to monitoring system of pacing module.
4. Set rate just above patient's rate.
5. Set system on demand mode if patient has an intermittently acceptable intrinsic rate; otherwise set system on asynchronous mode.
6. Set output to lowest value.

7. Turn on pacer.
8. Gradually increase output until capture is noted.
9. Set output just above pacer threshold.
10. Set rate to minimum desired rate.
11. Make plans for transvenous pacing.

CLINICAL TIPS

Transvenous Pacing

1. The natural curve of the pacer wire should be used to aid in positioning the tip in the right ventricle (i.e., curving toward the left side of the chest).
2. The operator should ensure that the catheter sheath is larger than the pacer wire before beginning the procedure.
3. If no evidence of capture exists or if capture is intermittent, the pacemaker should be turned off and the pacer wire repositioned. Often a clockwise or counterclockwise twist of the catheter is helpful in this situation.

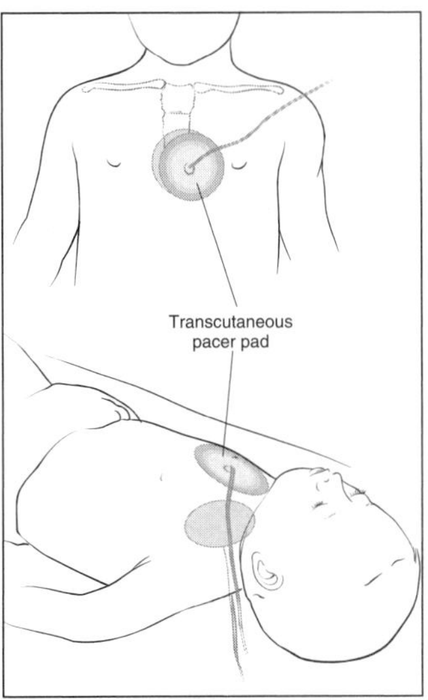

FIGURE 10.2 Transcutaneous pacing electrodes are easily applied to the anterior and posterior chest walls using self-adhesive strips. The normal location of the V3 lead of the ECG is an ideal anterior position, whereas the posterior lead should be placed on the upper back between the scapula. If capture does not occur in these positions, the posterior lead can be moved to a more lateral or even axillary location. If possible, the leads should not be placed over bony structures such as the scapula.

4. If ventricular ectopy develops, the catheter should be withdrawn until this ceases. If ectopy is frequent, administration of intravenous lidocaine may be necessary before continuing with the procedure.
5. The pacer wire should be coiled at the skin surface after suturing to decrease the likelihood of dislodgement.
6. The on/off switch on the pacemaker should be covered at all times to avoid accidental power loss.

CLINICAL TIPS

Transcutaneous Pacing

1. If possible, the pacer electrodes should not be placed over bony structures such as the scapula.
2. The two pacer electrodes should not touch one another, to prevent a short circuit, which could result in a loss of delivered current.
3. It may be necessary to trim the adhesive strips on the pacer electrodes to decrease the size of the pads with infants and small children.

CHAPTER 11

Cardioversion and Defibrillation

OVERVIEW

Synchronized Cardioversion

1. Assess patient.
   A. For patients who are hemodynamically unstable, perform cardioversion before establishing intravenous access or securing definitive airway.
   B. For patients who are stable, administer supplemental oxygen and intravenous sedation and analgesia before performing cardioversion.
2. Turn cardioverter on.
3. Attach electrocardiogram leads to patient (if stable).
4. Select lead that displays tallest R wave.
5. Set machine on synchronous mode.
6. Apply electrode paste or gel to paddles.
7. Select energy and charge unit (0.5 J/kg for initial attempt; then double the dose for subsequent attempts).
8. Place paddles firmly on chest in appropriate positions.
9. Ensure that operator is not contacting patient and that patient is not contacting any metal parts of stretcher.
10. Clear area ("All clear!").
11. Apply current by depressing discharge buttons simultaneously and holding paddles in place for several moments.
12. If dysrhythmia persists, double energy level, recharge unit, and apply current after 2- to 3-minute interval (if patient's clinical condition permits).
13. If postcardioversion dysrhythmia develops in the patient, treat appropriately.
14. After patient is stabilized, address other management issues (e.g., administration of antiarrhythmic agents, correction of metabolic abnormalities).

Defibrillation

1. Perform defibrillation when indicated before establishing intravenous access or securing definitive airway.

2. Apply electrode paste or gel to paddles.
3. Turn machine on.
4. Select "quick look" paddle leads to assess rhythm.
5. Apply paddles firmly to appropriate position on chest.
6. If monitor waveform appears to be asystole, rotate paddles 90 degrees to assess rhythm in another plane because true rhythm may be fine ventricular fibrillation (VF).
7. Select energy and charge unit (2 J/kg for the initial attempt; then 4 J/kg for the second and third attempts).
8. Ensure that operator is not contacting patient and that patient is not contacting any metal parts of stretcher.
9. Clear area ("All clear!").
10. Apply current by depressing discharge buttons simultaneously.
11. If dysrhythmia persists, double energy level, recharge unit, and reapply current.
12. After three unsuccessful attempts, focus on correcting underlying process that is lowering fibrillation threshold.

CLINICAL TIPS

1. Hemodynamic instability is indicated by hypotension, signs of inadequate cerebral or peripheral perfusion (e.g., lethargy, agitation, weak pulses, mottling), or heart failure.
2. Before assuming that a dysrhythmia is asystole rather than fine VF, the operator must turn to another lead on the unit or rotate the monitoring electrode paddles 90 degrees.
3. For infants and younger children weighing less than 10 kg, 4.5-cm diameter paddles are recommended. For children over 10 kg, 8-cm (adult) paddles should be used.
4. Commercial pastes and gels lower the transthoracic impedance more than saline pads; alcohol pads and sonographic gel are contraindicated as paddle/chest interface materials.
5. The synchronous mode must be set for direct cardioversion. The asynchronous mode must be set for defibrillation.

6. With extreme tachycardia, the cardioverter may not be able to deliver a synchronous shock. Depending on the patient's condition, it may be necessary to set the machine on asynchronous mode to administer an electrical discharge.
7. If pediatric paddles are unavailable, adult-size paddles usually can be used effectively for infants and younger children with the anteroposterior placement method.
8. Defibrillation is not indicated for the treatment of asystole.
9. Precautions during synchronized cardioversion that minimize the risk of injury to operator and patient include:
   A. Sedation and analgesia (when appropriate).
   B. Selecting proper paddle size.
   C. Liberal application of electrode paste or gel.
   D. Using the lowest recommended energy level initially.
   E. Allowing 2 to 3 minutes between successive cardioversion attempts.

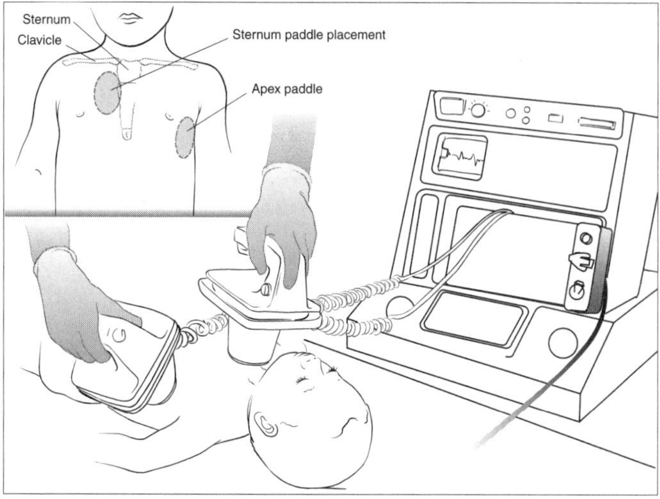

FIGURE 11.1 When pediatric paddles are used to perform cardioversion or defibrillation, the paddle labeled *apex* should be placed over the fourth and fifth intercostal spaces lateral to the nipple, whereas the paddle labeled *sternum* should be placed just below the right clavicle lateral to the sternum.

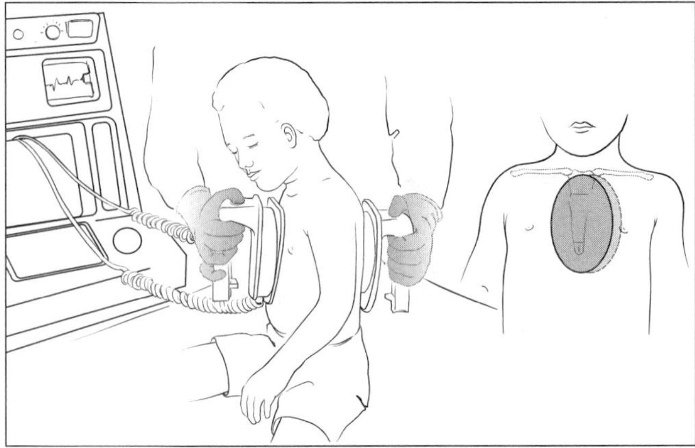

FIGURE 11.2 If pediatric paddles are unavailable, adult-sized paddles can be used for pediatric patients by using an anteroposterior placement. With the patient upright or lying on one side, the sternum paddle is applied directly over the sternum and the apex paddle is placed on the back between the scapulae. This method decreases the likelihood that the larger paddles will contact one another during delivery of the current.

CHAPTER 12

Cervical Spine Immobilization

OVERVIEW

1. Assess any prior immobilization and correct or modify as necessary.
2. Stabilize head and neck in neutral position using in-line immobilization.
3. Apply cervical collar (best as two-person procedure).
   A. Check collar size.
   B. Assemble collar (if necessary).
   C. Slide collar behind neck.
   D. Slide chin piece up chest wall.
   E. Fasten Velcro on collar.
   F. Recheck neutral alignment.
4. Position patient on supine board.
   A. If patient is supine:
      1) Logroll child, maintaining in-line manual immobilization.
      2) Place long spine board under child.
      3) Roll child as a unit onto board.
   B. If patient is seated:
      1) Position short spine board behind child.
      2) Secure child to short board.
      3) Place long spine board alongside child.
      4) Pivot and lower child onto long board (knees/hips bent).
      5) Lower child's legs to long board.
5. Secure patient to spine board.
   A. Place soft spacing devices on both sides of head and neck.
   B. Apply forehead strap.
   C. Apply chin support strap.
   D. Apply shoulder and pelvis straps.
6. Evaluate effectiveness of procedure.
   A. Maintain head and neck in neutral position.
   B. Assess for respiratory/airway compromise.
   C. Ensure immobilization prevents any significant movement of head and neck.

7. Reassess ABCs (airway, breathing, circulation).
8. Repeat neurologic examination.

CLINICAL TIPS

1. Cervical injury should always be suspected with any patient with blunt trauma.
2. The most important initial goals in a trauma resuscitation are to stabilize the primary injury and to prevent secondary injury.
3. Adequate cervical immobilization will be achieved only if the appropriate equipment and proper sizes are used.
4. Effectiveness of cervical immobilization should be reassessed frequently.
5. Neurosurgical consultation should be sought early when indicated.
6. Cervical immobilization should not be removed until clinical and (if necessary) radiographic "clearing" are completed and normal results from a neurologic examination obtained.

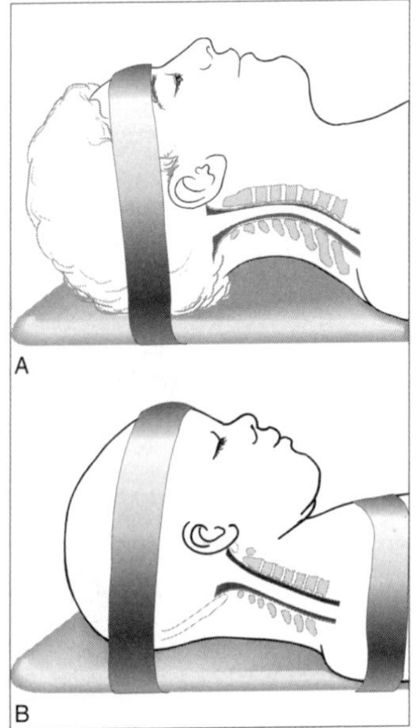

FIGURE 12.1 A: When an adult lies supine on a hard spine board, the neck is maintained in an essentially neutral position. B: Because the occiput of younger children is relatively large compared with an adult's, the neck tends to be slightly flexed when these patients are immobilized on a spine board. This characteristic is present until approximately 8 years of age. Consequently, when immobilizing a young child, it is often necessary to place a small pad or towel roll under the shoulders (elevating the torso slightly) to maintain the neck in a neutral position.

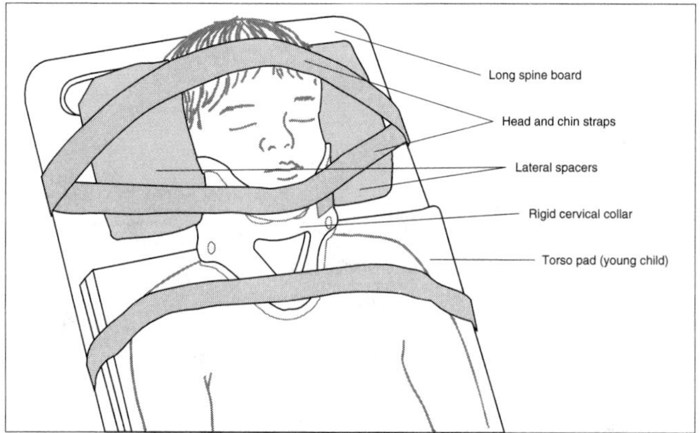

FIGURE 12.2 Ideal immobilization, including long spine board, spacer to elevate torso, hard collar, soft lateral spacers, and forehead and chin straps.

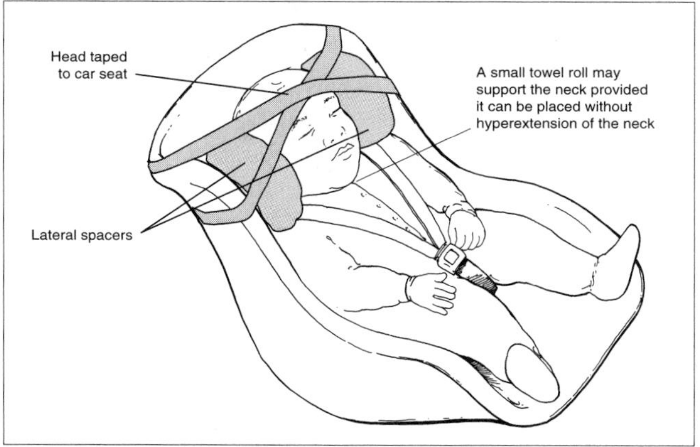

FIGURE 12.3 Young infants can sometimes be effectively immobilized using a car seat. This technique is especially useful when appropriate equipment (e.g., torso spacer, small cervical collar) is not readily available. This method should not be used for an infant who has multiple injuries, hemodynamic instability, or airway compromise.

Flexion
Hyperextension
Collar too short
Collar too tall
Neutral position maintained with correct collar size
A

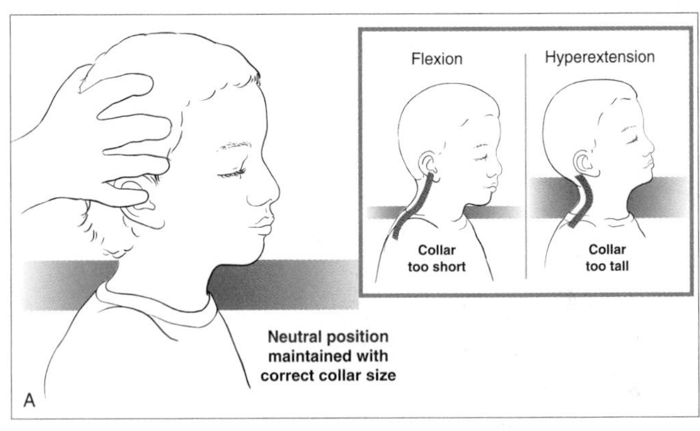

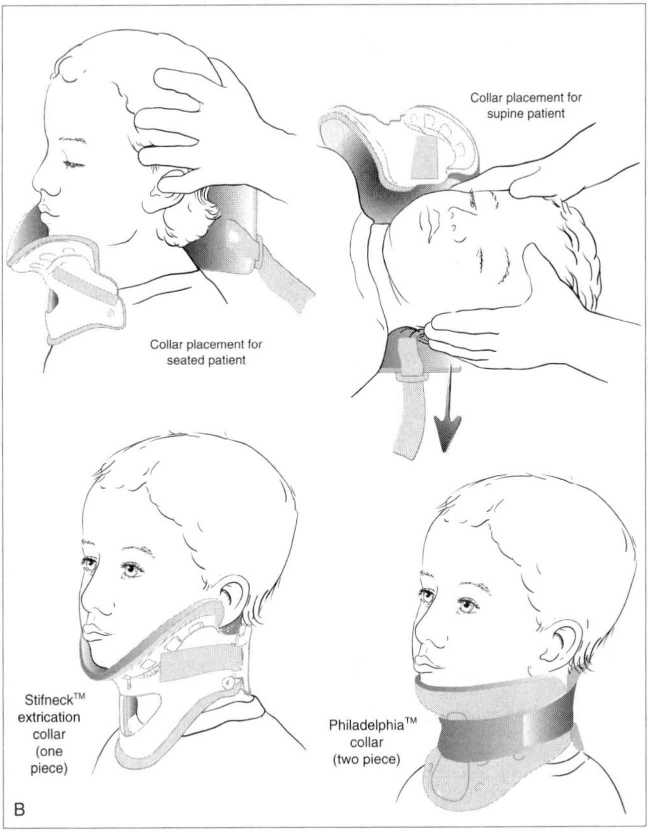

Collar placement for supine patient
Collar placement for seated patient
Stifneck™ extrication collar (one piece)
Philadelphia™ collar (two piece)
B

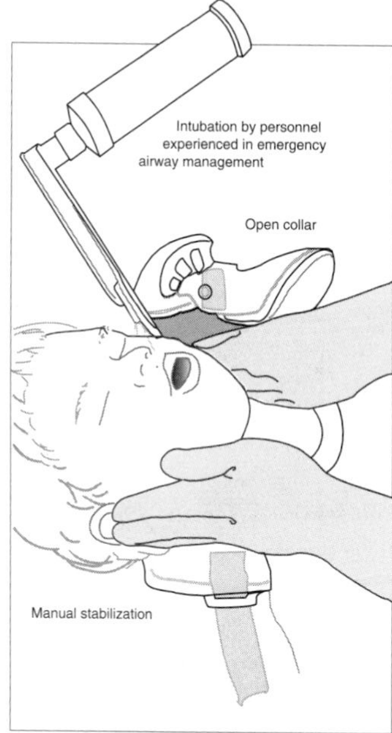

FIGURE 12.5 Manual in-line stabilization of the cervical spine can be performed during endotracheal intubation by holding both sides of the patient's head and using the forearms to prevent movement of the patient's shoulders and torso. In this way, a single person can adequately immobilize the patient's neck without impeding maneuvers necessary to secure the airway (see also Chapter 5).

FIGURE 12.4 A: The collar selected for a pediatric patient should maintain the neck in a neutral position. A collar that is too short allows flexion of the neck, whereas a collar that is too tall causes hyperextension of the neck. **B:** Application of a cervical collar should ideally be performed by two people. While one person immobilizes the patient's cervical spine, the other person carefully applies the collar and secures the straps without moving the patient's head, neck, or torso.

CHAPTER 13

Helmet Removal

OVERVIEW

One-person Technique

1. Untie straps.
2. Stand at cephalad end of patient.
3. Place hands on each side of helmet at ears and spread if possible.
4. Maintain in-line stabilization and begin to slide off.
5. Tilt backward to clear nose.
6. Return to neutral when nose is cleared.
7. When occiput is cleared, walk hands with slow, progressive movements to position where hands are encircling the occiput while heels of hands are on helmet rim.
8. Gradually push off helmet with heels of hands in slow, progressive movements.
9. Maintain in-line stabilization until able to stabilize.

Two-person Technique

1. Untie straps.
2. Person in caudad position places hands on occiput and jaw.
3. Second person in cephalad position maintains in-line stabilization while spreading sides of helmet over ears.
4. Tilt backward to clear nose and return to neutral position.
5. Slide off.
6. Second person maintains in-line stabilization.
7. First person applies collar, tape, and foam pads.

Bivalve Technique

1. One person maintains stability with hands on jaw and occiput.
2. Helmet is cut in coronal plane at ear level using cast saw.
3. Ties are cut and foam is cut.
4. Anterior portion is removed.
5. Posterior is slid off.
6. Collar, tape, foam pads are applied.

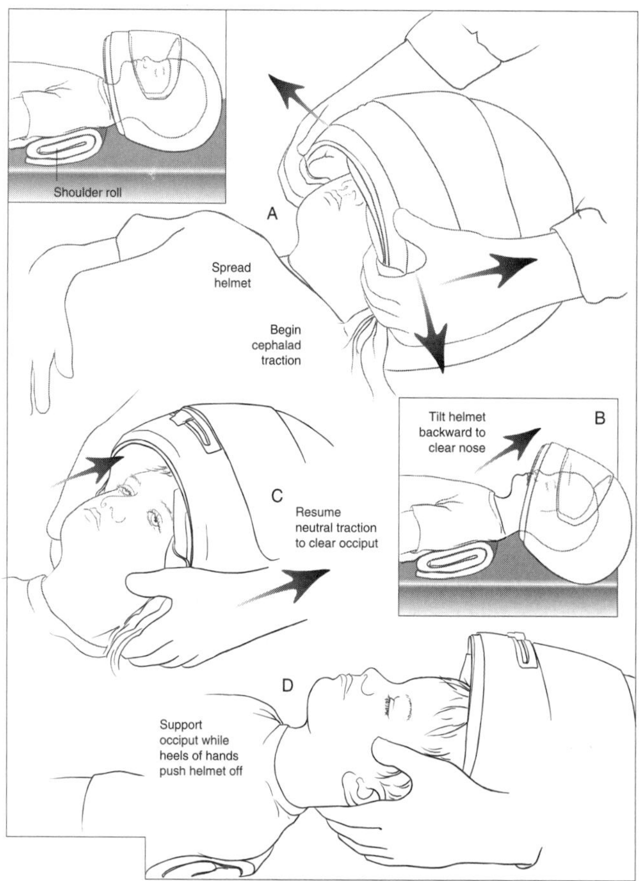

FIGURE 13.1 One-person technique. Although unlikely in the emergency department, it is sometimes necessary for a single person to remove a helmet without assistance (e.g., a rescue situation). Before removal, a small pad or towel roll should be placed under the patient's shoulders so that the neck is in a neutral position, and the helmet straps should be released or cut. **A:** The operator grasps the helmet at ear level from a cephalad position and spreads it laterally using both hands. The helmet is carefully pulled cephalad while in-line stabilization is maintained. **B:** In older children, it is necessary to tilt the helmet gently backward while removing it to clear the patient's nose. **C:** Once the nose is cleared, the helmet should be rotated back to its normal orientation and pulled further cephalad. **D:** As the helmet begins to clear the occiput, the clinician should walk both hands to the occiput in slow, progressive movements. The patient's head and neck are maintained in a neutral position as the heels of both hands are used to push the helmet off completely. In-line stabilization should then be maintained until immobilization can be appropriately secured.

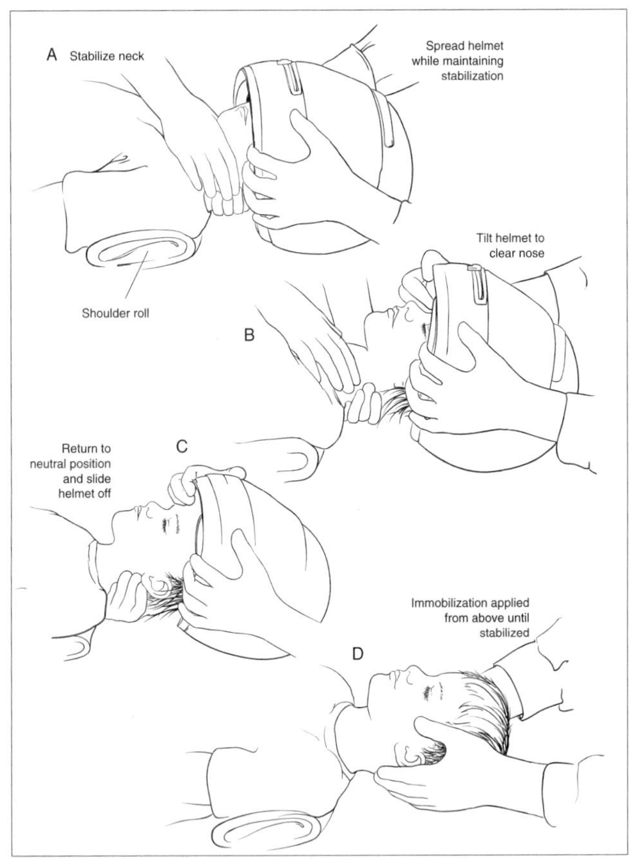

FIGURE 13.2 Two-person technique. This method is used most commonly in the emergency department. **A:** As with the one-person technique, a small towel roll or pad should be placed under the shoulders to maintain the head and neck in a neutral position. One person stands above the patient (cephalad) initially holding the helmet, and one person stands beside the patient (caudad). **B:** The operator in the caudad position releases or cuts the helmet straps and then immobilizes the head and neck. This is done by putting one hand behind the patient's occiput while the other hand stabilizes the mandible (i.e., with the thumb on one side of the mandible and the index and middle fingers on the other side). When doing this, care must be taken not to obstruct the airway. The operator in the cephalad position then spreads the helmet and pulls carefully until it begins to slide off. As it is being removed, the helmet should be tilted slightly backward to clear the nose. The operator in the caudad position should ensure that the patient's head does not tilt with the helmet. **C:** Once the nose is cleared, the helmet should be rotated back to its normal orientation and removed. **D:** The operator in the cephalad position then assumes responsibility for maintaining in-line stabilization until appropriate immobilization can be established.

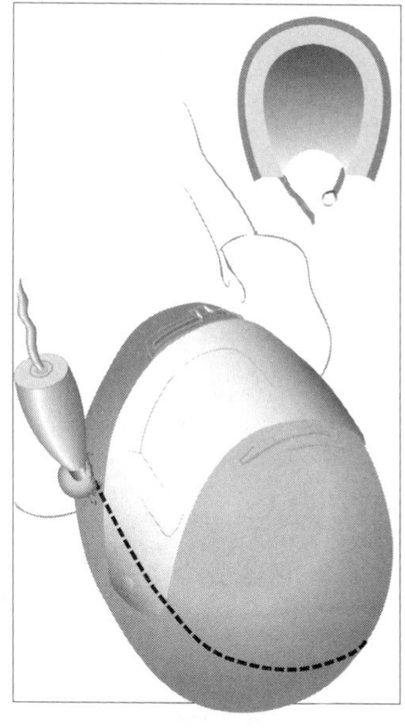

FIGURE 13.3 The bivalve technique, which is the safest method for the patient known to have a cervical spine injury, involves cutting the helmet with a cast saw in a coronal plane. One operator is designated to stabilize the neck from a caudad position as described for the two-person technique. The helmet should be cut at ear level in the coronal plane. The anterior half of the helmet is removed by cutting the straps and the foam padding. The posterior half is gently pulled out cephalad as the person at the caudad position stabilizes the head and neck.

CLINICAL TIPS

1. The clinician should make no attempt to spread a rigid, full-faced motorcycle helmet. The foam lining of the interior yields to gentle pulling.
2. The helmet should be tilted backward before the level of the nose to avoid injury.
3. Shoulders should be elevated because all helmets cause cervical flexion.
4. Metallic strips should be removed before taking the lateral spine radiograph.

CHAPTER 14

Diagnostic Peritoneal Lavage

OVERVIEW

1. Prepare patient by using sedation and restraint as necessary; insert nasogastric or orogastric tube and bladder catheter.
2. Sterilely prepare abdomen and apply sterile drapes, exposing approximately 4 cm around umbilicus.
3. Select infraumbilical or supraumbilical approach as indicated, then infiltrate selected site with lidocaine with epinephrine.
4. Using 18-gauge angiocatheter, 19-gauge needle, or equipment provided in a commercial kit, enter peritoneal cavity.
5. Pass soft end of guide wire through catheter or needle into peritoneal cavity.
6. Using a no. 11 scalpel blade, incise skin where guide wire enters, enlarging hole.
7. Thread lavage catheter onto wire and then, directing it caudally, into peritoneal cavity.
8. Attempt to aspirate fluid from peritoneal cavity; if any frank blood is recovered in a young child, this is deemed to be a positive result and procedure can be terminated.
9. If no frank blood is recovered, instill 10 to 15 mL/kg of normal saline or Ringer's lactate rapidly by gravity.
10. When all fluid is in peritoneal cavity, patient may be rocked from side to side; bag is then dropped to a level below abdomen.
11. Fluid recovered in bag should be sent to laboratory for analysis.

CLINICAL TIPS

1. Alternative imaging techniques should be considered based on availability and patient condition.
2. Surgical consultation should be obtained early in the management of the patient.

3. Adequate restraint and conscious sedation should be used as needed to minimize risk of injury.
4. A gastric tube and bladder catheter should be inserted to reduce risk of inadvertent puncture of the stomach or bladder.
5. Local anesthetic containing epinephrine should be used to decrease bleeding around the site of insertion of the lavage catheter. This helps to reduce the possibility of a false-positive result.
6. The supraumbilical approach should be used for young infants and small children and for those patients who are pregnant, have pelvic fractures, or who have local irritation or skin infection in the infraumbilical area. For patients who have had previous abdominal surgeries, the site farthest from the previous incision is used. The infraumbilical approach is indicated for all others.
7. The needle should be directed slightly caudad. A lateral trajectory of the needle (off the midline) must always be avoided.
8. The guide wire should advance very smoothly. If it does not, then both the wire and the insertion needle should be removed.
9. The lavage catheter should be directed caudally during insertion.
10. Infusion of saline or Ringer's lactate into the peritoneal cavity should be limited to 10 to 15 mL/kg to avoid interference with respiratory function.
11. If the clinical condition permits, the patient should be rolled from side to side to allow the lavage fluid to wash over the peritoneal cavity.
12. It is necessary to recover only 3 to 5 mL/kg of fluid. If less fluid is recovered, the patient can be rolled from side to side or the blunt lavage catheter can be repositioned or replaced.

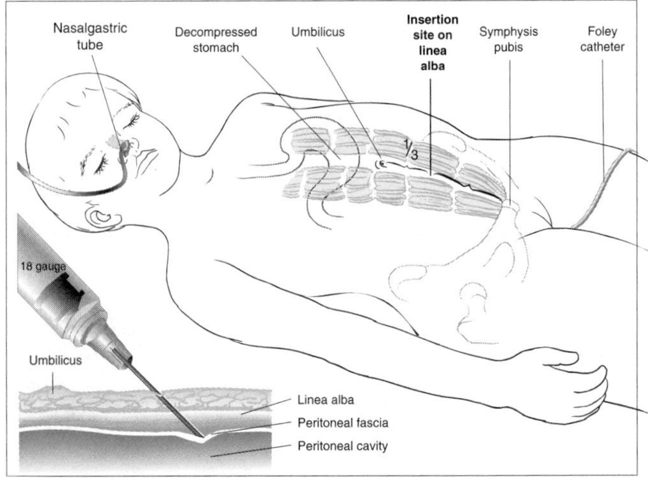

FIGURE 14.1 For most pediatric patients, the infraumbilical site of entry should be used. This is located in the midline inferior to the umbilicus approximately one-third the distance from the umbilicus to the pubic symphysis. Because the bladder of infants and small children may extend well into the abdominal cavity, a supraumbilical site of entry should be used for these patients (not shown). This is located in the midline superior to the umbilicus at approximately the same distance used for the infraumbilical approach (usually 1 to 2 cm). The needle and catheter are directed caudally on insertion. Two distinct pops should be felt—one as the needle penetrates the linea alba and the one as the peritoneal fascia is penetrated. An initial attempt to aspirate blood is made. For the child younger than 8 years of age, any significant blood return should be considered positive. For an older child or adolescent, 5 to 10 mL of aspirated blood is a positive result. If no blood return is obtained, the catheter should be advanced and the needle removed. Of note, blood inadvertently aspirated from an abdominal wall vessel clots; blood obtained from the peritoneal cavity should not clot.

TABLE 14.1 Indications for Diagnostic Peritoneal Lavage

A. General:
   1. Other imaging modalities unavailable or yield equivocal results.
   2. US unavailable and patient condition prevents transport to CT scanner.
   3. Monitoring difficult or impossible outside of ED as a result of inadequate staffing or available equipment.
   4. Surgical backup availability greater than 15 to 30 minutes.
B. Significant blunt abdominal trauma with (assumes other imaging modalities unavailable or inappropriate, see above):
   1. Obtundation.
   2. Equivocal physical examination.
   3. Patient age or developmental level preventing accurate physical examination.
   4. Unexplained hypotension.
C. Stab wounds (controversial):
   1. Abdominal stab wound without obvious evidence of intraabdominal injury, after local exploration of the wound.

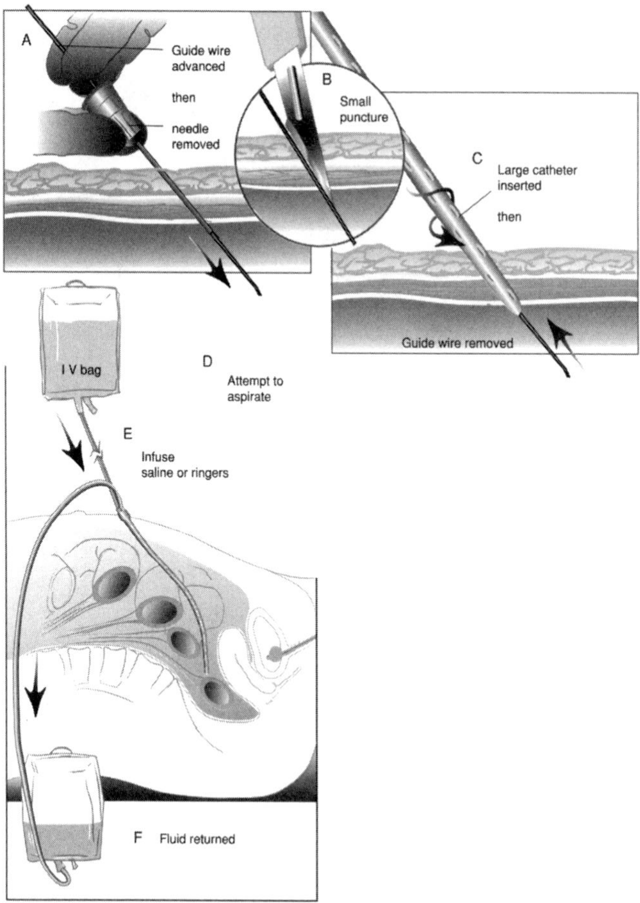

FIGURE 14.2 A: Guide wire advanced through needle. B: Small puncture with scalpel. C: Lavage catheter advanced into the peritoneal cavity over the guide wire. D: An initial attempt is made to aspirate blood from the peritoneal cavity. E: Ten to 15 mL/kg normal saline or Ringer's lactate is infused through the lavage catheter. F: The bag is dropped to a level below the abdomen and the fluid is recovered by gravity.

TABLE 14.2 Criteria for Diagnostic Peritoneal Lavage to be Considered Positive

1. Gross blood aspirated from the peritoneal cavity.
2. Greater than 100,000 RBCs per mm^3 in returned lavage fluid (blunt trauma).
3. Greater than 5000 RBCs per mm^3 in return lavage fluid (stab wound).
4. Greater than 500 WBCs per mm^3.
5. Fecal material in returned lavage fluid.

TABLE 14.3 Criteria for a Diagnostic Peritoneal Lavage to be Considered Equivocal

1. 50,000 to 100,000 RBCs per mm^3 in return lavage fluid.
2. 100 to 500 WBCs per mm^3 in return lavage fluid.

CHAPTER 15

Tube Thoracostomy and Needle Decompression of the Chest

OVERVIEW

Needle Decompression

1. Assemble equipment and assign duties to personnel.
2. Explain procedure and obtain consent (as indicated).
3. Position patient, and prepare and anesthetize (as time allows) skin and subcutaneous structures.
4. Advance needle over superior aspect of rib while maintaining negative pressure in syringe.
5. When air returns, advance catheter into pleural cavity.
6. Remove needle and attach three-way stopcock and large syringe.
7. Evacuate pneumothorax.
8. Obtain chest radiograph.

Tube Thoracostomy

1. Assemble equipment and assign duties to personnel.
2. Explain procedure and obtain consent (as indicated).
3. Position patient, and prepare and anesthetize (as time allows) skin and subcutaneous structures.
4. Incise skin over rib below interspace of intended tube placement.
5. Bluntly dissect subcutaneously and superiorly.
6. Enter pleural space with clamp tips closed and confirm location by exploration with finger.
7. Insert chest tube, directing tube superiorly and posteriorly.
8. Attach to water seal and suction.
9. Secure chest tube with suture, gauze, and tape.
10. Obtain chest radiograph.

CLINICAL TIPS

1. All necessary equipment should be assembled and tube size(s) should be checked before starting.
2. Adequate sedation and analgesia must be provided for the conscious patient.
3. For tube thoracostomy, the incision should be made directly over the rib.
4. Passage of the chest tube should not be attempted through too small an incision.
5. A probing finger should be used whenever possible to verify that the pleural space has been entered and to identify the diaphragm and any adhesions.
6. For needle decompression of a pneumothorax, a saline-filled syringe is used to detect bubbles.

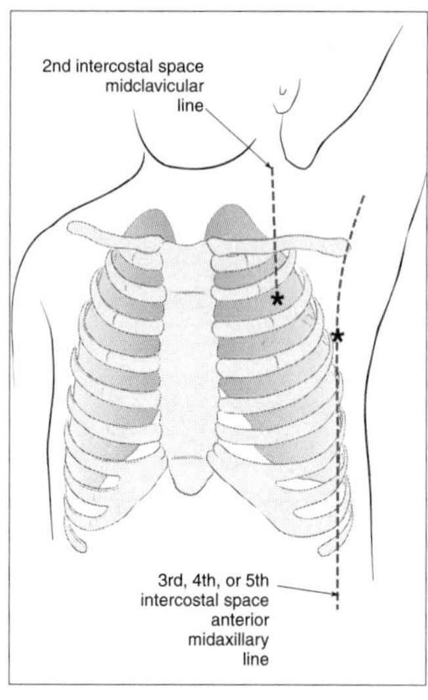

FIGURE 15.1 The most common sites for inserting a needle, catheter, or chest tube are (*a*) the second intercostal space at the midclavicular line (anterior) and (*b*) the third, fourth, or fifth intercostal space at the anterior midaxillary line (lateral). Although commonly used in the past for chest tube placement, the anterior site is now used almost exclusively for needle decompression of a tension pneumothorax. The lateral site is recommended for most patients who require evacuation of air or fluid from the chest. It can also be used to decompress a tension pneumothorax, if necessary. The point of entry for the lateral approach is at the fourth or fifth intercostal space for children and adolescents. The third intercostal space is preferred for newborn infants. A reasonable approximation of the appropriate entry site for most patients is directly lateral to the nipple. Insertion at this point usually avoids injury to the spleen or liver, even with a patient who has an elevated hemidiaphragm.

TABLE 15.1 Chest Tube Size

Age (50th Percentile Weight)	*Tube Size (French)*
Premature (1–2.5 kg)	10–14
Neonate (2.5–4.0 kg)	12–18
6 mo (6–8 kg)	14–20
1–2 yr (10–12 kg)	14–24
5 yr (16–18 kg)	20–32
8–10 yr (24–30 kg)	28–38

Adapted from *Textbook of Pediatric Advanced Life Support,* American Heart Association, 1994.

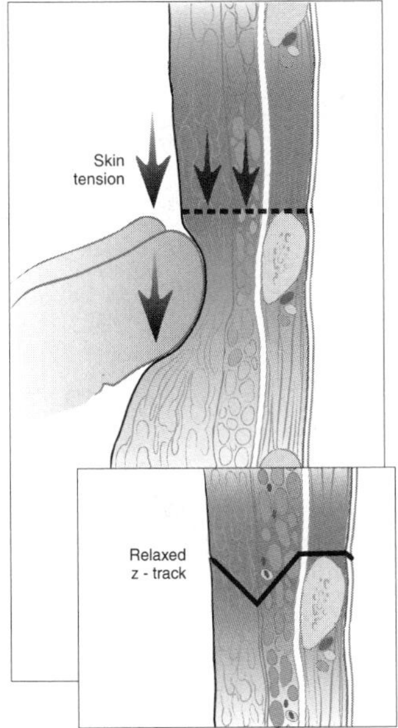

FIGURE 15.2 Z-track method for insertion of a needle or catheter. Before the catheter is advanced, the patient's skin and subcutaneous tissues are stretched 1 to 2 cm inferior to the proposed point of insertion. This tension is maintained while the needle or catheter is inserted and advanced. Once the tension is released and the needle or catheter is removed, the tract will be discontinuous through the tissue planes.

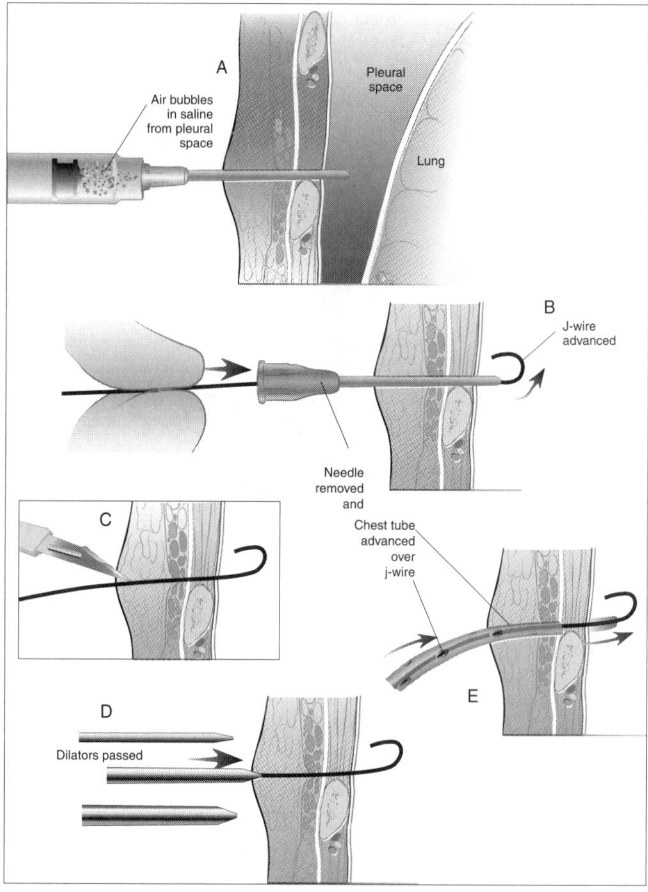

FIGURE 15.3 The modified Seldinger technique is used most often to place a small catheter ("pigtail") into the pleural space. A needle attached to a partially saline-filled syringe is advanced over the rib at the appropriate site of insertion (**A**). Air bubbles are aspirated when the needle enters the pleural space. A J-tipped guide wire is advanced through the needle into the pleural space (**B**). A small incision is made to allow insertion of the catheter over the wire into the pleural space (**C**). The operator may also use progressively larger dilators (**D**) to allow insertion of a small chest tube (**E**).

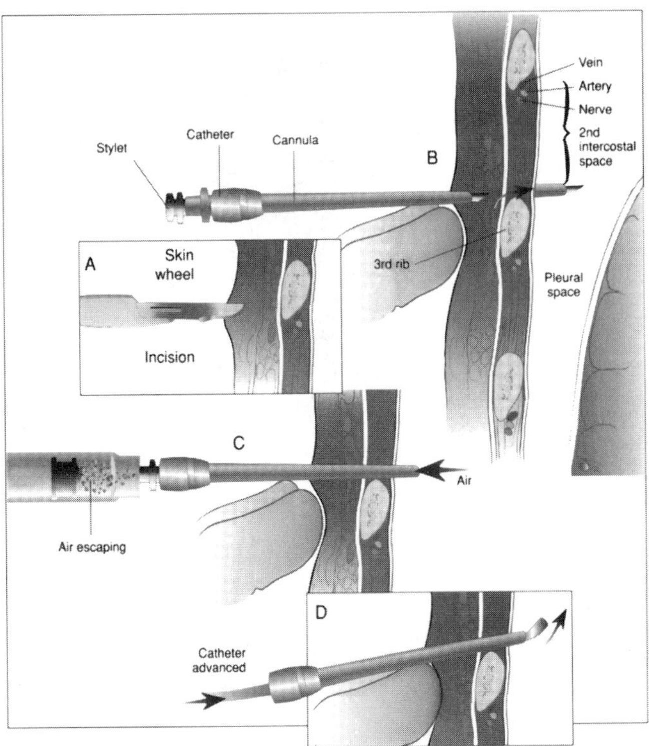

FIGURE 15.4 As an alternative to the modified Seldinger technique, the trocar method can also be used to insert a catheter into the pleural space. This should be distinguished from the trocar method of inserting a chest tube, which is not commonly used for pediatric patients. In this case, a small trocar with a surrounding cannula is used to enter the pleural space. **A:** After appropriate local anesthesia, an incision is made at the point of entry. **B:** While the skin is retracted inferiorly, the trocar/cannula assembly is advanced over the rib and into the pleural space. **C:** After removal of the trocar, aspiration of air bubbles using a partially saline-filled syringe confirms intrapleural placement. **D:** A small catheter is introduced through the cannula into the pleural space. The cannula can then be removed.

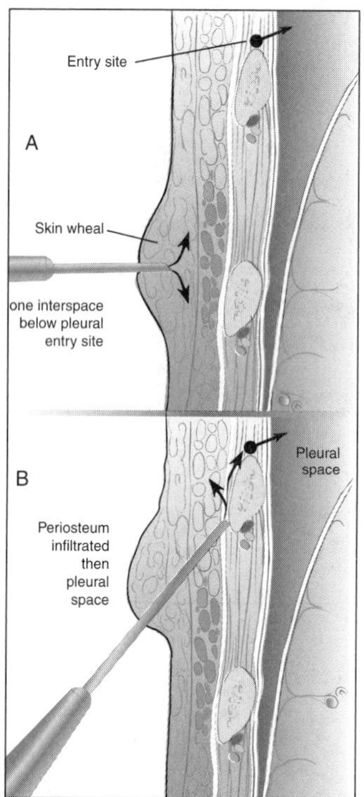

FIGURE 15.5 When possible, the area of the chest where tube thoracostomy will be performed should be well anesthetized. The total amount of lidocaine used for local anesthesia, however, should not exceed 5 mg/kg to avoid systemic toxicity. Local anesthesia is not performed if the patient's clinical condition does not allow sufficient time. **A:** A skin wheal is raised one interspace below the planned insertion site. This can be done with a smaller-gauge needle to minimize pain. **B:** A larger needle is then inserted through the anesthetized skin, and lidocaine is infiltrated into the subcutaneous tissue and muscle along the path of entry into the pleural space. The operator advances the needle while alternating injection of lidocaine with aspiration to ensure that the needle has not entered a blood vessel. When the superior aspect of the rib is reached, the periosteum is infiltrated. Entry into the pleural space is indicated by a loss of resistance and easy aspiration of either fluid or air.

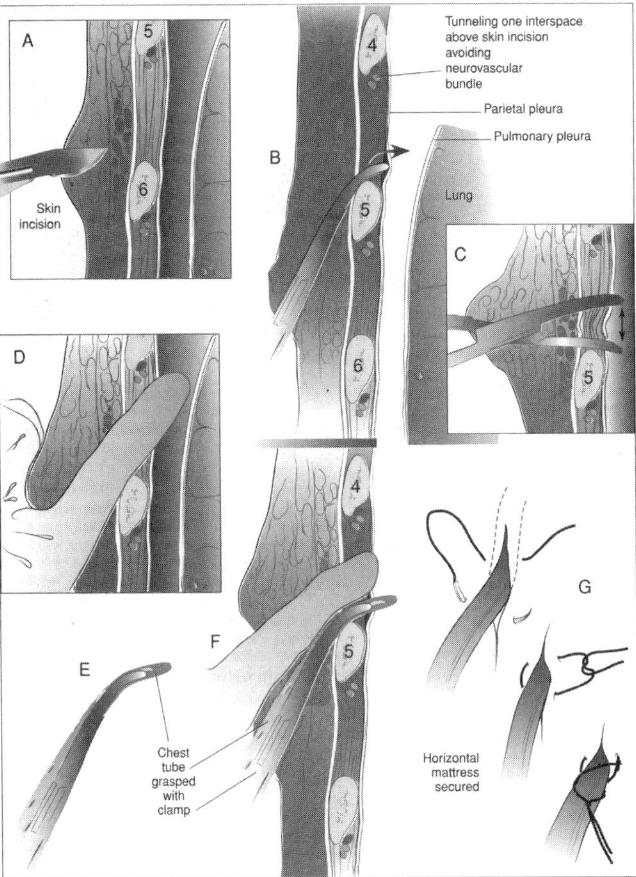

FIGURE 15.6 Blunt dissection technique for thoracostomy. **A:** Incision is made one interspace inferior to proposed point of thoracostomy tube insertion. **B:** Blunt dissection through the subcutaneous tissue using a clamp. **C:** Clamp spread after entering pleural space. **D:** Probing finger inserted to confirm pleural placement and identify the diaphragm and any adhesions. **E, F:** Chest tube grasped with clamp and inserted with the finger as a guide. **G:** Tube sutured firmly in place.

CHAPTER 16

Emergency Thoracotomy

OVERVIEW

1. Rapidly apply sterile povidone–iodine solution to chest wall.
2. Make incision at fourth or fifth costal interspace from sternum, along rib margin to posterior axillary line, cutting through skin and muscles of chest wall.
3. Cut through intercostal muscles with heavy scissors along upper rib margin.
4. Insert Finichetto's chest wall retractor with bar extending into axilla and use ratchet handle to open ribs.
5. Using suction, remove any blood obstructing a clear view of heart; remember that blood can be saved for autotransfusion.
6. Open pericardium anterior to phrenic nerve. Remove any blood or clots and explore myocardium for injuries; keep heart as warm as possible using warm saline or heat lamps.
7. Apply direct pressure to any sites of hemorrhage from heart—pressure should be maintained until injury can be definitively repaired.
8. Repair any myocardial injuries, if possible. Be careful to avoid damage to coronary arteries or phrenic nerve. Atrial lacerations may be repaired with a simple running stitch and ventricular lacerations with interrupted stitches reinforced with Teflon pledgets.
9. If no myocardial injury is found, retract left lung out of chest anteriorly and superiorly. Identify aorta, separate it from esophagus and prevertebral fascia, and occlude it using fingers, a vascular camp, vascular tape, or an aortic tamponade device.
10. Explore thoracic cavity for other sources of bleeding and apply pressure to any bleeding site identified; vessels that can be exposed may be cross-clamped.
11. If heart is beating spontaneously, continue resuscitation with fluids and blood. If not, begin open cardiac massage and then defibrillate using internal paddles.

CLINICAL TIPS

1. The clinician must be familiar with the indications for emergency thoracotomy and apply this technique selectively.

2. When indicated, thoracotomy should be performed promptly. Survival is more likely in patients who have evidence of cardiac activity.
3. Work quickly—in this situation, seconds count.
4. Insert Finichetto's retractor with the bar and ratchet handle extending into the axilla (upside down and backward). This places the bar at the base of the incision, allowing extension of the incision into the right side of the chest, if needed.
5. In most cases, the pericardium should be opened. Tamponade can be difficult to diagnose on clinical grounds alone.
6. When the pericardium is opened it should be opened widely. This prevents accidental herniation of the heart through a small opening, which may result in further restriction of cardiac function.
7. When a ventricular injury is identified, it can usually be closed with simple interrupted sutures. These may have to be reinforced with Teflon pledgets. If the injury is near a coronary artery or the phrenic nerve, it should be closed with a mattress stitch.
8. When cardiac compressions are required, a two-handed technique is preferred.

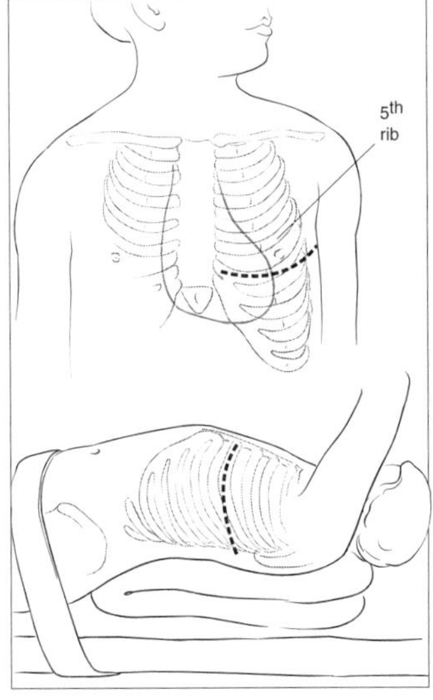

FIGURE 16.1 The incision for an emergency thoracotomy is made at the left fourth or fifth intercostal space from the sternal border to the posterior axillary line. The correct line of incision passes just below the left nipple and follows the curve of the rib. In women, breast tissue should be spared by manually retracting the breast superiorly, if necessary. In the girl, the clinician should avoid cutting the breast bud. The initial skin incision is extended through the underlying adipose and muscle tissue down to the rib. The intercostal muscle tissue is then cut using Mayo scissors along the upper border of the rib so as not to damage the neurovascular bundle, which runs along the lower rib margin.

Incision may be
extended medially
Finichetto
rib spreader
Rachet handle

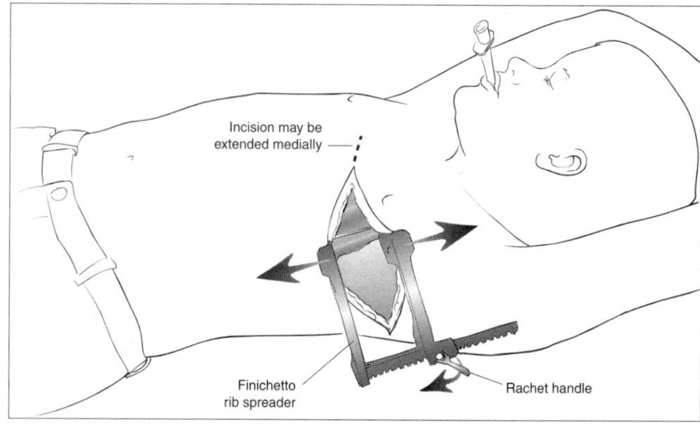

FIGURE 16.2 Once the chest wall is open, the chest wall retractor (rib spreader) is placed into the incision. Finichetto's device is used most commonly in the emergency department. Proper placement of the chest wall retractor is critical to the success of this procedure. The bar and ratchet handle should be placed so that they are perpendicular to the base of the incision, with the bar extending into the axilla. Insertion in this fashion allows extension of the incision into the right chest, if necessary. Once the chest wall retractor is in place, the ratchet handle is used to open the ribs.

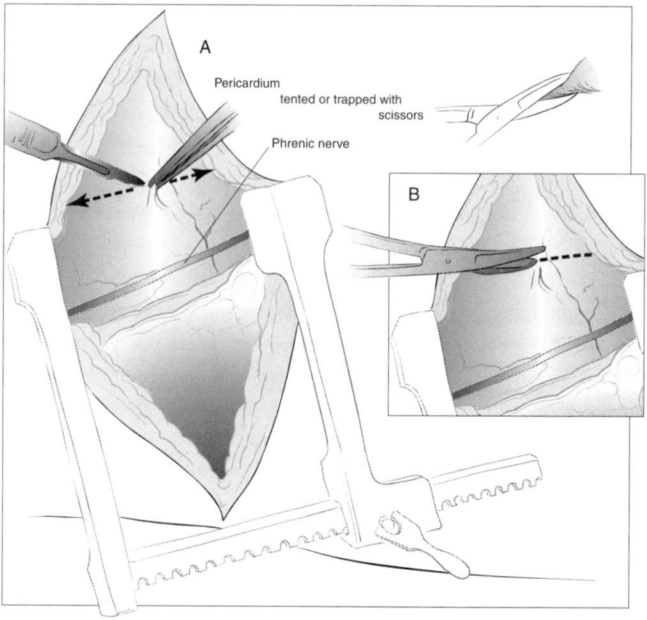

A
Pericardium
tented or trapped with
scissors
Phrenic nerve
B

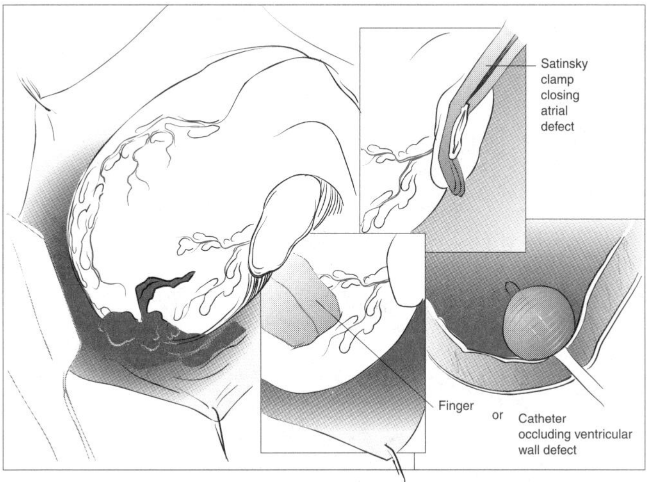

FIGURE 16.4 If opening the pericardium relieves a tamponade, all clots should be removed from the pericardial space and the myocardium should be quickly explored to identify the source of bleeding, usually an atrial or ventricular laceration. When such a laceration is found, it should be occluded to prevent further hemorrhage. For a ventricular injury, the first method to use is to place a fingertip over the bleeding site and apply direct pressure. Another rapid method is to pass a Foley catheter through the hole, inflate the balloon, and apply gentle traction to the catheter so that the balloon occludes the hole. It is important not to apply excessive traction because the balloon often pulls completely through the hole. Fluids can also be rapidly administered through the Foley catheter when using this technique. In the case of an atrial laceration, a vascular (Satinsky) clamp may be used temporarily to close the defect.

FIGURE 16.3 After the ribs are retracted open, the next task is to control obvious hemorrhage. If an obvious site of bleeding can be readily identified, direct pressure should be used to stop it if possible. If, on opening the chest, no bleeding occurs, the pericardium should be examined and in most cases opened. The pericardium should be opened by an initial incision made anterior to the phrenic nerve. Once the pericardium is open, the incision should be extended widely, which allows for easy exploration of the myocardium and prevents herniation of the heart through a small opening. **A:** The pericardium may be grasped with a pair of forceps and then nicked with a scalpel. **B:** When pericardial tamponade is present, the pericardial sac may be so tense that it cannot be grasped with forceps. In such cases, the pericardium may be trapped between the blades of a pair of Mayo scissors and then cut.

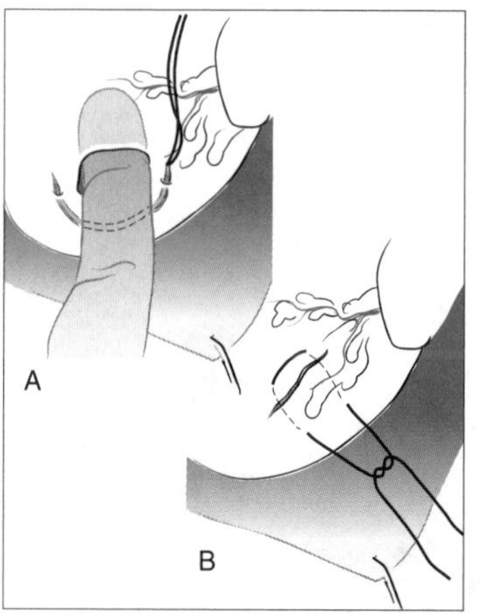

FIGURE 16.5 Definitive closure of a cardiac injury can usually be accomplished with simple running (atrial) or interrupted (ventricular) 3-0 nonabsorbable sutures. If the laceration is close to a coronary artery or to the phrenic nerve, a mattress should be used to avoid ligating the artery or nerve. The needle is passed beneath the occluding finger or around the Foley catheter. With a Foley catheter, care must be taken not to puncture the balloon. Ventricular wall, like all muscle tissue, separates easily, making suturing somewhat difficult. It may be helpful to place Teflon pledgets on either side of the laceration to reinforce the tissues. If the heart is beating, it may be impossible immediately to repair the cardiac defect. In such cases, temporizing measures should be continued until the patient can be taken to the operating room and placed on cardiopulmonary bypass.

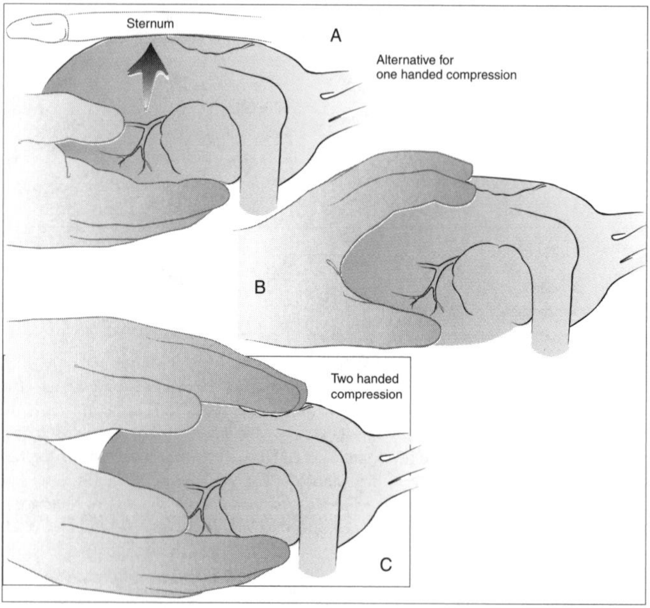

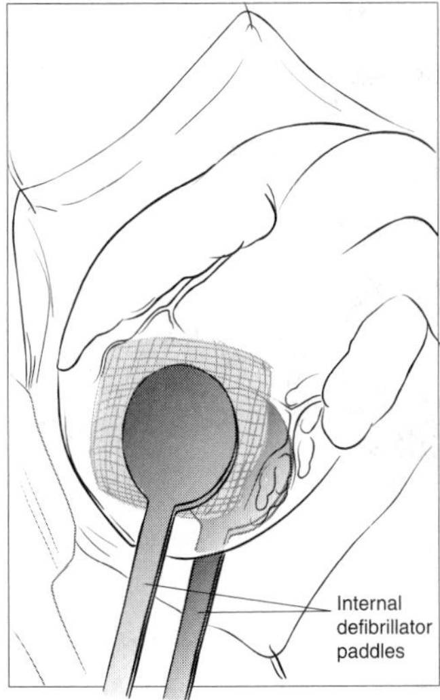

FIGURE 16.7 If the heart does not resume beating after the previously described measures, internal defibrillation should be performed. Using saline-soaked pads as conductive material, one paddle is placed posteriorly, usually behind the left ventricle, and the other is placed anteriorly, over the right ventricle. The paddle size for an adolescent is 6 cm, for a child 4 cm, and for an infant 2 cm. The ideal defibrillator charge for a child is unknown; however, it has been suggested that starting doses should be in the range of 5 J and proceed to 20 J. The starting dose of electricity for an adolescent is 20 J with subsequent doses of 40 and 60 J, if necessary.

FIGURE 16.6 After pericardial tamponade has been relieved, the heart may resume spontaneous activity. If not, direct compressions should be initiated after any cardiac defects are repaired. Pressure should be applied progressing from the apex of the heart to the base to maximize forward flow of blood. The rate of compressions should be 100 beats per minute. **A:** Direct cardiac compressions can be performed with one hand by pressing the heart against the sternum. **B:** Alternatively, the heart may be compressed between the thumb and fingers of one hand. **C:** The one-handed methods carry a small risk of cardiac perforation, and compression against the relatively plastic sternum of a child may be less effective than in an adult. Consequently, the two-handed technique is preferred when possible. One hand is placed beneath the heart and one above it. Starting at the heels of the hands, pressure is progressively applied through the palm and to the fingertips.

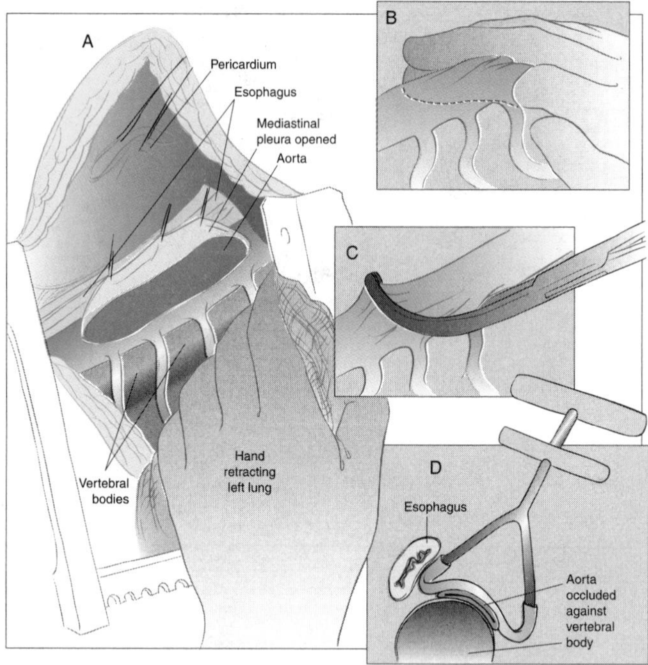

FIGURE 16.8 If significant bleeding into the abdomen is suspected, the aorta should be identified and occluded to improve perfusion to the brain and myocardium. This is best accomplished by first rotating the left lung superiorly out of the chest. The operator can then palpate along the posterior portion of the ribs until the vertebral bodies are encountered. The aorta lies just anterior to the vertebral bodies. **A:** After the aorta is visualized, the mediastinal pleura is incised and, using blunt dissection, the aorta is freed from its anterior attachment to the esophagus and its posterior attachment to the prevertebral fascia. **B:** The initial technique for aortic occlusion is to trap the aorta between two fingers. If an extended period of aortic occlusion is anticipated, however, a more definitive measure should be performed. **C:** Aortic occlusion using a vascular clamp. **D:** Aortic occlusion by compression against the vertebral bodies using a specially designed occlusion device.

CHAPTER 17

Regional Anesthesia

OVERVIEW

Regional Anesthesia

1. Regional anesthesia is indicated in several situations where local infiltration anesthesia is impractical or excessively painful, such as nailbed laceration repair; complex procedures for paronychial drainage; manipulation of foreskin tightly entrapped in a zipper; excision of ingrown toenail; and repair of large laceration of palm or sole.
2. Before regional anesthesia, a careful examination for perfusion, sensation, and motor nerve function of the affected extremity is performed and documented.
3. Skin preparation is accomplished with povidone–iodine.
4. One percent lidocaine *without epinephrine* is injected with a 25- to 27-gauge needle (0.5- to 1.0-inch for upper extremity, and 1.0- to 1.5-inch for lower extremity; other local anesthetics are listed for comparison in Table 17.1).
5. The needle is directed for each specific block as noted. Paresthesia (tingling or jolts in nerve distribution) may occur if the needle mechanically stimulates the nerve fibers. If paresthesia is elicited, the needle should be withdrawn slightly to avoid intraneuronal injection.
6. Before anesthetic injection, aspiration for blood is always done to avoid intravascular injection.
7. In general, a slightly smaller volume of anesthetic is injected if a paresthesia was elicited and the needle has to be repositioned.
8. Optimal anesthesia may take up to 10 to 20 minutes.

CLINICAL TIPS

Nerve Block Anesthesia

1. An anesthetic solution containing epinephrine should never be used for nerve blocks of the fingers, toes, or penis.
2. Nerve blocks are often preferable over local infiltration anesthesia for procedures involving the hands or feet because insertion of the needle at the appropriate sites for a nerve block is usually much less painful than through the highly innervated skin of the palm of the hand or sole of the foot.

TABLE 17.1 Characteristics of Commonly Used Local Anesthetics

		Physiochemical properties				Maximum allowable dose	
Infiltration Anesthetic	*Concentration*	*Lipid Solubility*	*Relative Potency*	*Onset of Action (min)*	*Duration (min)*	*mg/kg*	*mL/kg*
Procaine (Novocaine)	1%	0.6	1	5–10	60–90	7–10	0.7–1
Lidocaine (Xylocaine)							
Without epinephrine	1%	2.9	2	2–5	50–120	4–5	0.4–0.5
With epinephrine (1:200,000)	1%	2.9	2	2–5	60–180	5–7	0.5–0.7
Nepivacaine (Carbacaine)	1%	0.8	2	2–5	90–180	5	0.5
Bupivacaine[a] (Marcaine)	0.25%	27.5	8	5–10	240–480	2	0.8

[a] Some authorities do not recommend bupivacaine for use in children younger than 12 years of age.

3. For certain procedures (e.g., nailbed repairs, replacing a minor fingertip avulsion, or incision and drainage of a paronychia), a digital block of the finger or toe is always the anesthetic method of choice.
4. When repairing injuries, the sensory and motor function of distal structures should be first tested if possible (depending on the child's age) so that no confusion occurs over whether any neurologic damage resulted from the initial injury or the nerve block.
5. To obtain adequate anesthesia of the hand or foot, it is sometimes necessary to combine two or more nerve blocks.

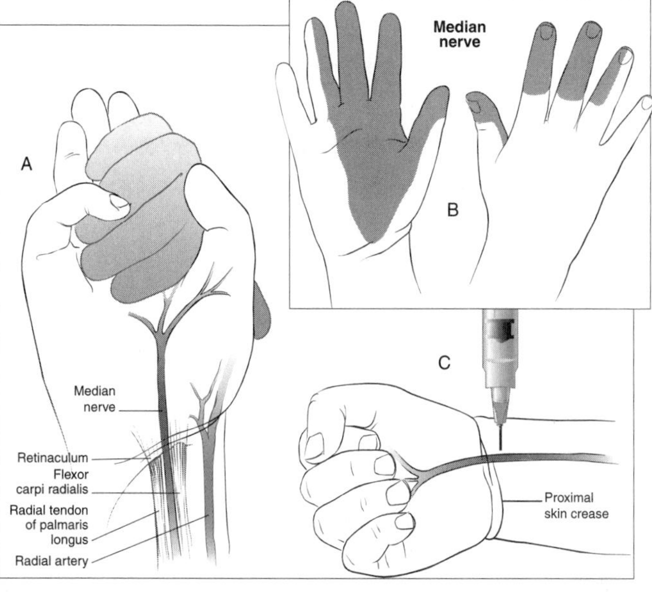

FIGURE 17.1 Median nerve block. **A:** The median nerve lies between the more medial palmaris longus tendon and the more radial flexor carpi radialis. These tendons are visualized by having the patient make a fist and then flexing the wrist against resistance. **B:** A median nerve block is used to provide anesthesia to the palmar aspect of the thumb, index and middle fingers, and the radial aspect of the fourth digit. **C:** After skin preparation, the needle is inserted perpendicularly, just radial to the palmaris longus tendon at the level of the proximal skin crease. A pop may be felt as the retinaculum is pierced. The appropriate depth is usually 0.5 to 1.0 cm in children. If no paresthesia is elicited, 3 to 5 mL of anesthetic is injected. If paresthesia does occur, after reposition a slightly smaller volume, 2 to 3 mL, is sufficient. Optimal anesthesia may take up to 10 to 20 minutes.

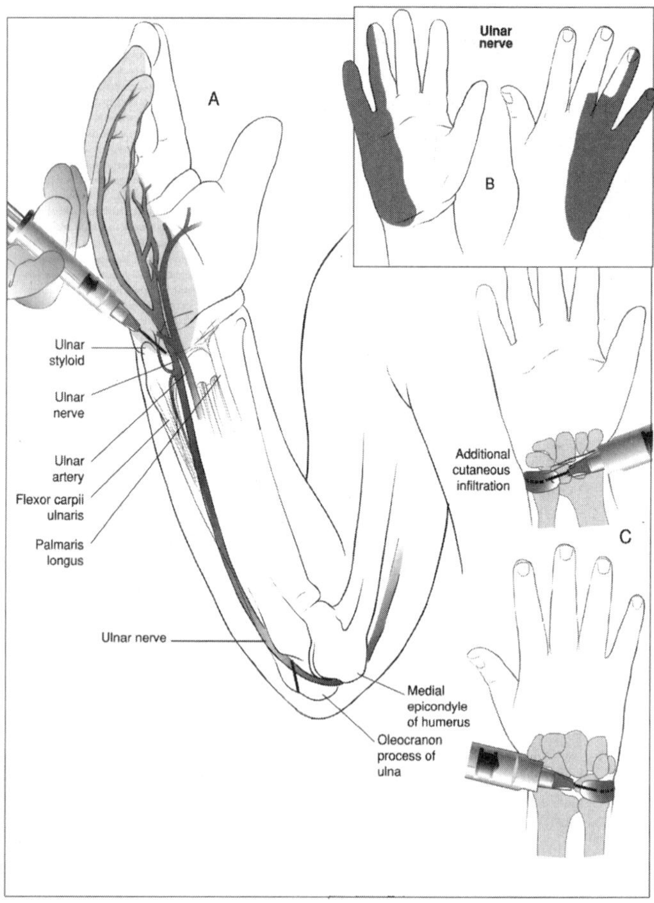

FIGURE 17.2 Ulnar nerve block. At the elbow, the ulnar nerve lies between the medial epicondyle and the olecranon. At the wrist, it is between the flexor carpi ulnaris tendon and the ulnar artery (**A**). An ulnar block may be used to anesthetize dorsal and palmer aspects of the of the ulnar side of the hand, fifth finger, and ulnar side of the fourth finger (**B**). The nerve is located by having the patient flex the wrist against resistance, making the flexor carpi ulnaris tendon prominent. The wrist insertion site is just radial to the tendon, between the tendon and arterial pulse, at the proximal skin crease (**A**). After skin preparation, a small wheal is raised by injecting anesthetic at this site, then the needle is directed perpendicular to the skin surface to a depth of approximately 0.5 cm (just deep to the tendon). If paresthesia is elicited, the needle is repositioned and 1 to 3 mL of anesthetic is injected. If no paresthesia is noted, a larger volume, 3 to 5 mL, may be used. Additional skin infiltration may be necessary for the dorsal cutaneous branch (**C**).

6. Unlike infiltration anesthesia, when performing a nerve block it usually is necessary to wait at least 15 minutes after injection to obtain the full anesthetic effect.

7. If the patient reports numbness and tingling (paresthesias) on insertion of the needle, the needle should be withdrawn 1 to 2 mm before injecting the

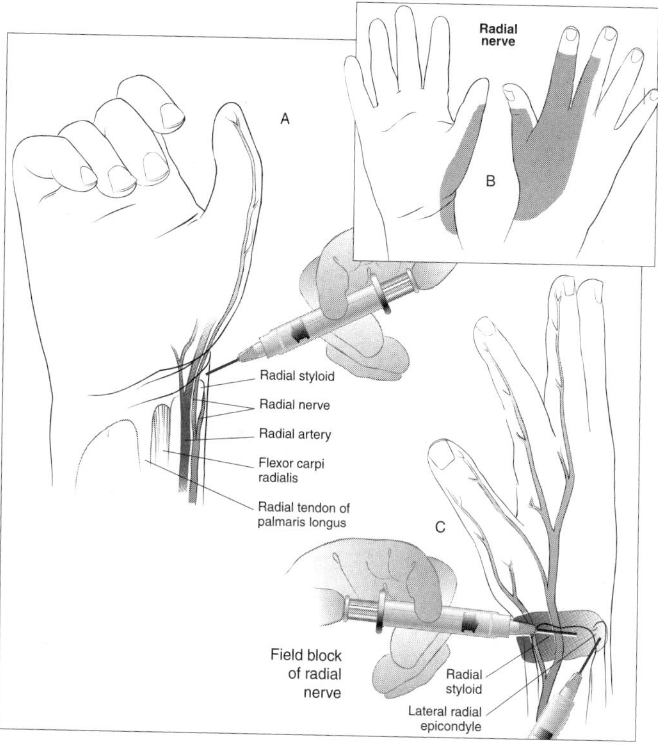

FIGURE 17.3 Radial nerve block. The radial nerve divides into several branches proximal to the wrist, but a major branch lies lateral to the flexor carpi radialis tendon close to the radial artery (**A**). Radial nerve block is used to provide anesthesia for the radial portion of the thenar eminence, dorsal surfaces of the thumb, and proximal two thirds of the index, middle, and radial aspect of the fourth finger (**B**). To anesthetize the major peripheral branch of the radial nerve, the needle is inserted just lateral to the radial artery, at the proximal palmar wrist crease, to the level of the artery. After careful avoidance of intravascular injection by aspiration, the area is injected with 2 to 4 mL of anesthetic. Subsequently, the dorsal cutaneous branches may be anesthetized with a field block, injecting up to 5 mL of anesthetic in a cuff-like distribution of the dorsoradial skin (**C**).

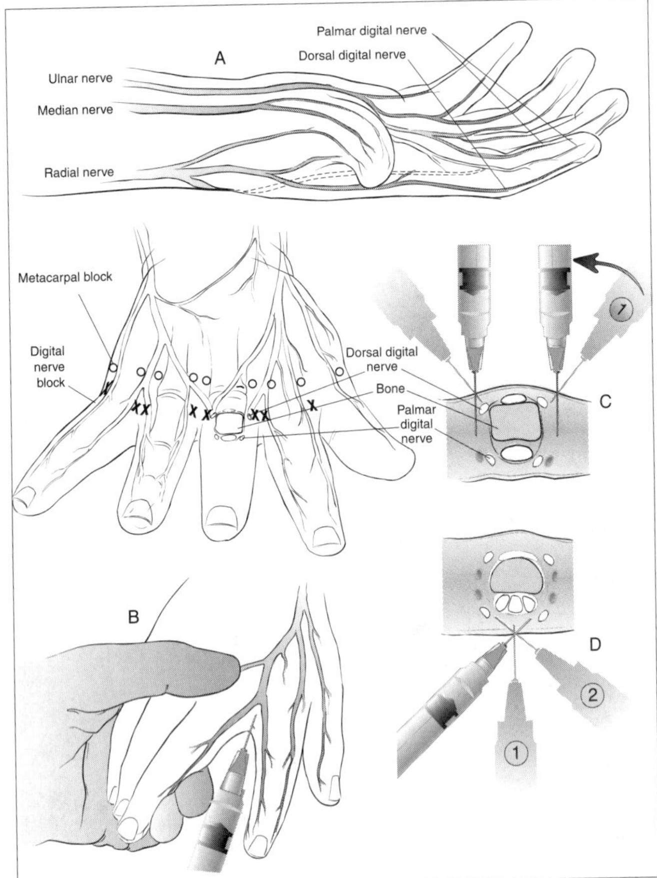
A
Palmar digital nerve
Dorsal digital nerve
Ulnar nerve
Median nerve
Radial nerve
Metacarpal block
Digital nerve block
Dorsal digital nerve
Bone
Palmar digital nerve
C
B
D
1
2

anesthetic solution so that intraneuronal injection does not occur. With younger children, the occurrence of paresthesias may be difficult to distinguish from the pain of the injection.

8. Aspiration of blood should always be performed before injecting the anesthetic solution to prevent intravascular injection.

OVERVIEW

Dorsal Penile Nerve Block

1. Cleanse base of penis with povidone–iodine or other antiseptic solution.
2. For neonates, use 0.8 mL 1% lidocaine *without epinephrine* in a 1-mL syringe. For older children, use 1 to 5 mL of lidocaine *without epinephrine*. For

FIGURE 17.4 Digital nerve blocks. Each digit of the hand is supplied by four nerves that branch off from the ulnar, median, and radial nerves (**A**). In cross-sectional view, the two dorsal digital nerves lie along the phalanx at 2 and 10 o'clock positions, and the two palmar digital nerves lie at 4 and 8 o'clock positions. Both dorsal and palmar fingertip sensation is supplied by the palmar digital nerves for the middle three fingers, and thus anesthesia of the palmar nerves alone is sufficient for distal anesthesia in these digits. For the thumb and fifth fingers, all four nerves must be blocked to obtain adequate distal anesthesia.

In all techniques, the fingers are examined carefully before nerve block for perfusion, sensation, and nerve function. For distal digital nerve block (**B**), after skin preparation, a 25- to 27-gauge needle is inserted into the dorsal aspect of the interdigital web space distal to the metacarpophalangeal joint [*x* marks in (**C**)]. The needle is advanced toward the bone, and after aspiration to insure against intravascular injection, 0.5 to 1.0 mL of anesthetic is injected. The needle is then directed volarly and an additional 0.5 to 1.0 mL of anesthetic is injected, after aspiration, near the volar surface of the finger, close to bone [similar to the illustration for metacarpal block shown in (**C**)]. The procedure is then repeated on the other side. Adequate anesthesia is usually achieved in 5 to 10 minutes.

Proximal block of the common (palmar) digital nerves may be accomplished by a dorsal (**C**) or palmar (**D**) approach. The dorsal approach begins by raising a skin wheal with anesthetic (**C**, *1*) between the metacarpal bones on the dorsum of the hand 1 to 2 cm proximal to the web space [*o* marks in (**C**)]. The needle is then directed toward the palmar side, advancing to just under the skin, and, after aspiration, 2 to 3 mL of anesthetic is deposited. The procedure is then repeated on the other side of the metacarpal to ensure that both sides of the involved digit are anesthetized. For the palmar technique, the needle is inserted at the distal palmar crease, over the center of the metacarpal head (**D**, *1*). Anesthetic solution is injected as the needle advances toward the bone. The needle is withdrawn slightly and redirected toward the radial aspect of the metacarpal head, advanced a few millimeters, and, after aspiration, 1.0 to 1.5 mL of anesthetic is injected (**D**, *2*). The needle is withdrawn slightly and angled toward the ulnar aspect of the metacarpal head, advanced again, and, after aspiration, an additional 1.0 to 1.5 mL anesthetic injected. Anesthesia is usually effective in 10 to 15 minutes.

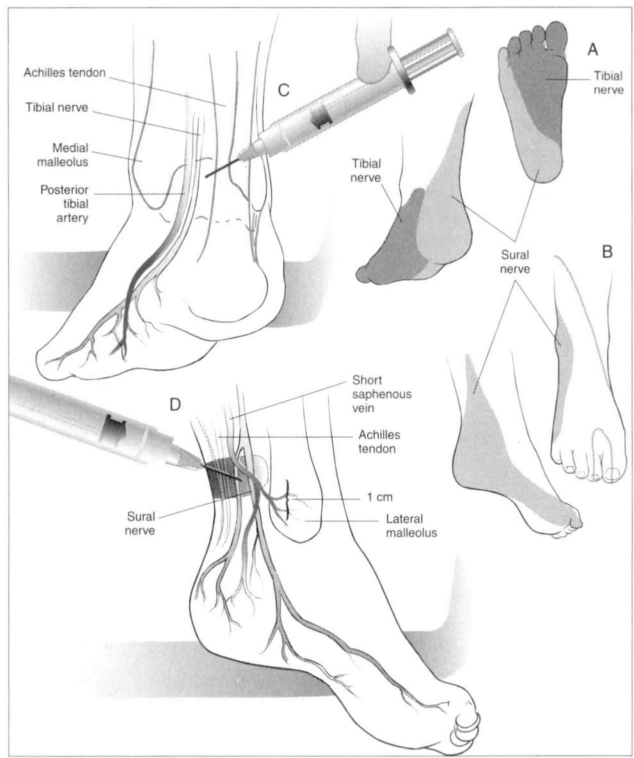

FIGURE 17.5 Posterior tibial and sural nerve blocks. The posterior tibial and sural nerves supply sensory innervation to the entire sole and heel of the foot (**A**, **B**). These areas are difficult to anesthetize with infiltrative anesthesia, and thus blocks of these nerves may be particularly useful. The posterior tibial nerve runs behind the medial malleolus just posterior to the easily palpated posterior tibial artery (**C**). The sural nerve courses with the short saphenous vein behind the fibula and lateral malleolus (**D**).

For a posterior nerve block, the patient should be positioned prone, with the foot extending beyond the end of the stretcher and held in slight dorsiflexion. After skin preparation, a 25- to 27-gauge needle is inserted perpendicular to the skin surface, at the level of the top of the malleolus just posterior to the arterial pulse (**C**). The tip of the needle is advanced to a position 1 mm from the underlying bone. If paresthesias are elicited, the needle is withdrawn 1 to 2 mm and, after aspiration to prevent intravascular injection, 3 to 4 mL of anesthetic is injected. If no paresthesia is elicited, 5 mL of anesthetic is injected as the needle is slowly withdrawn. For the sural nerve block, the skin is prepared and the patient positioned as for the posterior tibial nerve block. The needle is inserted just lateral to the Achilles tendon approximately 1 cm superior to the lateral malleolus (**D**). The needle is advanced subcutaneously toward the lateral malleolus. After aspiration, the block is created by injecting 3 to 5 mL of anesthetic in a subcutaneous band extending from the posterior aspect of the lateral malleolus to the anterior margin of the Achilles tendon. Both blocks become effective in 5 to 10 minutes and, if successful, may result in a foot skin temperature increase due to vasodilatation.

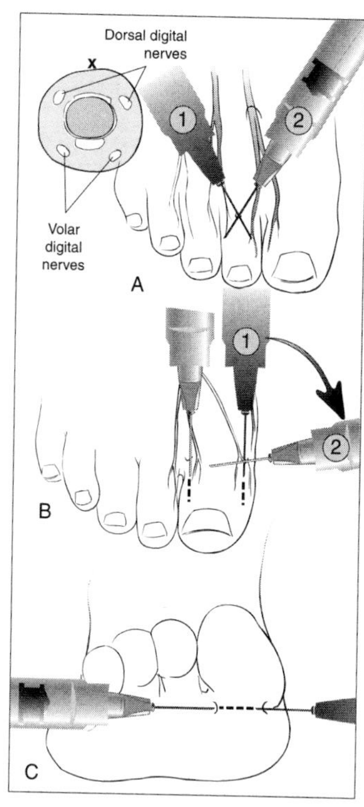

FIGURE 17.6 Digital toe blocks. As for finger digital nerves, each toe is supplied by four nerves positioned analogously to those described for the fingers (**A**). The digital nerve blocks are also accomplished in similar fashion, although because the proximal phalanx is relatively narrow for the small toes, both sides of these toes can be anesthetized from one insertion site (**A**). After skin preparation, the needle is inserted at the midline of the dorsal surface of the proximal portion of the phalanx and advanced to just under the volar skin surface, passing in close to the bone (**A**, *1*). After aspiration, 1 to 2 mL of anesthetic is injected as the needle is slowly withdrawn, thus blocking both volar and dorsal nerves. Then the needle is further withdrawn, without removing it from the skin, and redirected to the opposite side of the toe, where this process is repeated (**A**, *2*). The hallux toe has unique innervation and requires a circumferential ring of anesthetic for effective nerve block. After skin preparation, the needle is inserted in the dorsomedial aspect of the proximal portion of the toe and advanced toward the volar surface (**B**, *1*). After aspiration, 1 to 2 mL of anesthetic is injected as the needle is slowly withdrawn. Then, without removal, the needle is redirected across the dorsal surface of the toe laterally, and again 1 to 2 mL of anesthetic is injected as the needle is slowly withdrawn across the top of the toe (**B**, *2*). The needle may then be reinserted (through already anesthetized skin) at the dorsolateral surface of the toe, directed toward the volar surface, and the injection completed as was done for the medial side. Finally, the plantar surface of the toe is injected in the same way as the dorsal surface (**C**), completing the circumferential ring of anesthetic injection. Thus, only the initial needle puncture need occur through unanesthetized skin.

children older than 12 years, use 1 to 5 mL of 0.25% bupivacaine without epinephrine.

3. Insert needle 3 to 5 mm beneath skin, at the junction of the penile base and suprapubic skin at the 10 o'clock position. After a negative aspiration for blood, infiltrate half of the anesthetic dose.
4. Repeat step 3 at the 2 o'clock position and inject remaining anesthetic.
5. Wait 5 minutes and test for anesthetic effect before performing procedure.

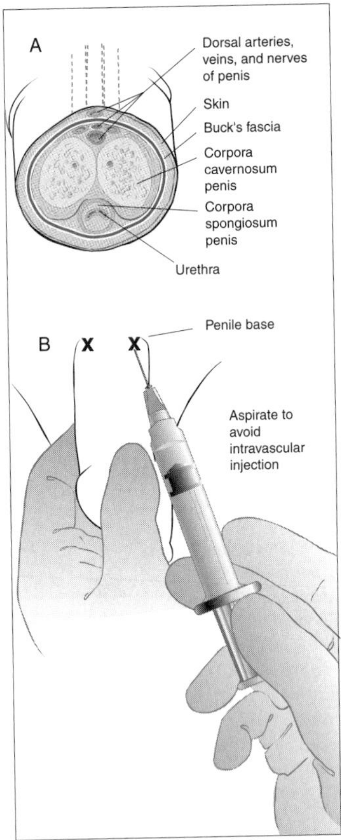

FIGURE 17.7 Penile nerve block. The dorsal nerves of the penis lie just lateral to the midline, adjacent to the dorsal arteries at the 2 and 10 o'clock positions beneath Buck's fascia (**A**). Penile nerve block is used to provide anesthesia for minor procedures of the penis, such as zipper entrapment of the foreskin or paraphimosis reduction. Using aseptic technique, the skin at the penile base is prepared with povidone–iodine. Lidocaine 1% without epinephrine is usually the anesthetic of choice, although 0.25% bupivacaine is longer lasting and might be preferred in adolescents. The volume of 1% lidocaine needed varies from 0.8 mL in neonates to 1 to 5 mL in older children. A 25-gauge needle is used and is inserted at the 2 or 10 o'clock position at the base of the penis [*x* in (**B**)]. At 3 to 5 mm penetration, a pop is felt as Buck's fascia is penetrated. Aspiration is done to avoid intravascular injection, after which half of the anesthetic is injected. The procedure is repeated on the other side. Alternatively, a subcutaneous ring of anesthetic can be injected circumferentially around the base of the penile shaft.

CHAPTER 18

Umbilical Vessel Catheterization

OVERVIEW

1. Place infant under radiant warmer in supine frog-leg position with cardiac monitor.

2. Prepare antiseptic field.

3. Determine distance to which catheter will be inserted.
   A. Arterial
      1) *Elective:* Use nomogram for umbilicus to lateral clavicle distance or, if less than 13 cm, insert catheter that distance plus 1 cm; if more than 13 cm, insert that distance plus 2 cm.
      2) *Emergent:* For subdiaphragmatic positioning, insert catheter until blood is obtained, then advance 1 cm.
   B. Venous
      1) *Elective:* Measure vertical distance from umbilicus to lateral clavicle and multiply by 0.6 for inferior vena cava positioning.
      2) *Emergent:* Pass the catheter 4 to 5 cm or until blood return is noted.

4. Loosely tie umbilical tape or pursestring suture at base of umbilical cord.

5. Cut cord transversely 0.5 to 2.0 cm from its base, and identify vessels.

6. Grasp and evert side(s) of umbilical stump with hemostat(s).

7. Dilate vessel lumen using curved iris forceps to accommodate 3.5- to 5-French catheter (artery) or 5- to 8-French catheter (vein).

8. Insert catheter tip into vessel lumen and pass catheter using gentle, constant pressure.

9. If there is resistance during arterial catheterization, use following techniques:
   A. Place tension cephalad on the cord.
   B. Apply twisting motion to catheter.
   C. Flush with 0.1 to 0.2 mL of 2% lidocaine.

10. Obtain radiograph of thorax and abdomen to confirm placement.

11. Secure catheter in place using pursestring suture and adhesive tape.

CLINICAL TIPS

1. In an emergent situation, subdiaphragmatic placement of an umbilical artery catheter is recommended and obviates the need for a radiograph before starting medications or fluids.
2. During emergent umbilical vein catheterization, the catheter is passed cephalad for 4 to 5 cm or until blood return is noted.
3. The umbilical artery can occasionally be accessed in neonates up to 7 days of age, the umbilical vein in neonates up to 14 days of age.
4. A twisting motion of the catheter often helps to overcome resistance when inserting an umbilical artery catheter.
5. Resistance as a result of vasospasm can sometimes be relieved by removing the catheter, filling its tip with 0.1 to 0.2 mL of 2% lidocaine, reinserting the catheter to the point of resistance, flushing the lidocaine into the vessel, and waiting 1 to 2 minutes before reattempting to advance the catheter.
6. Resistance at 5 to 10 cm in umbilical vein catheterization suggests the incorrect cannulation of a branch of the portal vein.
7. Vasospasm as a result of umbilical artery catheters often can be relieved with warm compresses applied to the contralateral extremity.

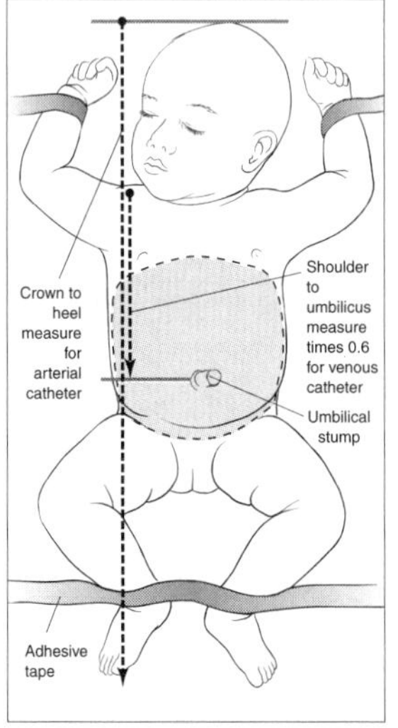

FIGURE 18.1 The infant is placed beneath a radiant warmer with extremities restrained as illustrated. Cardiac rate and adequate oxygenation should be monitored. The operator should wear surgical gown, gloves, mask, cap, and goggles. The shaded area is prepared with a bactericidal solution such as povidine–iodine, and then the umbilical area draped in sterile fashion. Note also shoulder-to-umbilicus and crown-to-heel measurements.

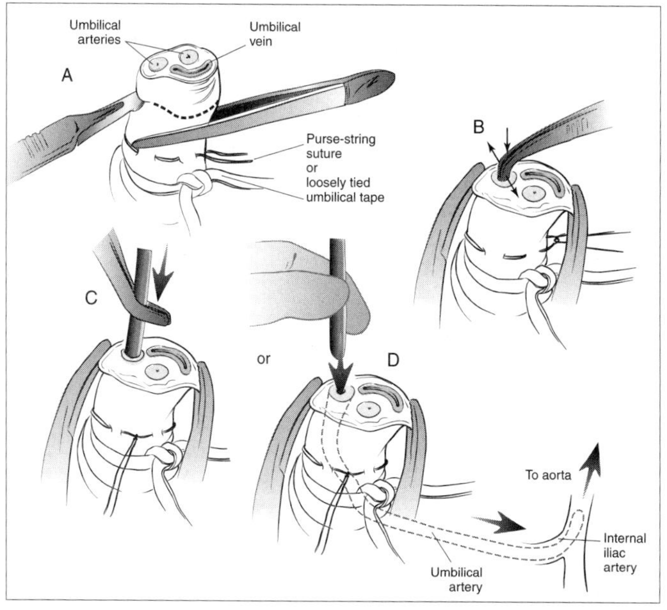

FIGURE 18.2 **A:** A pursestring suture or loosely tied umbilical tape is placed at the base of the umbilical cord. The cord is grasped full thickness with forceps between 0.5 and 2 cm from its base and cut by scalpel transversely at the top edge of the forceps. The vessels are then identified. **B:** Curved hemostats are used to grasp the cut edges of the cord as shown. The edges are everted and, using a curved iris forceps without teeth, approximately 1 cm of arterial lumen is gently dilated by repeated introduction and opening of the forceps. Alternatively, a pointed solid metal dilator can be used. **C,D:** Appropriate catheter sizes are 3.5 to 4 French for infants weighing less than 2 kg, and 5 French for those above 2 kg. The catheter, flushed with heparinized saline, is held 1 cm from its tip by thumb and index finger, or by small forceps, and is inserted into the artery. Gentle, steady pressure is used to advance catheter, with resistance commonly being felt at two points. At 1 to 2 cm, the artery curves toward the feet, and thus tension is placed in a cephalad direction on the cord, favoring catheter advancement toward the feet. At 5 to 6 cm, the artery joins the iliac artery, and some resistance may be overcome with a gentle twisting motion. Vasospasm may be relieved by the administration of lidocaine through the catheter. This requires removal of the catheter, filling its tip with 0.1 to 0.2 mL of 2% lidocaine without epinephrine, and then reinserting it to the point of resistance, flushing the lidocaine into the vessel, and attempting to advance the catheter after 1 to 2 minutes.

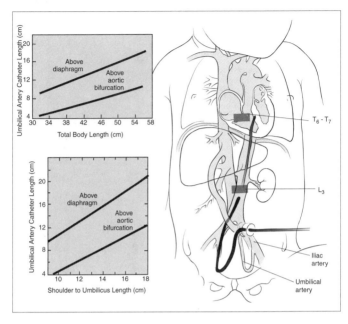

FIGURE 18.3 Nomograms for estimating umbilical artery catheter length. Two insertion depths are generally accepted. Optimal position above the diaphragm is at the level of the thoracic aorta between the ductus arteriosus and origin of the celiac axis (T6-9). Optimal position below the diaphragm is between the inferior mesenteric artery and the bifurcation of the aorta (L3-5). After placement, a radiograph is obtained to confirm placement. In an emergent situation, the instillation of medications or fluids without radiographic confirmation is less likely to be hazardous when a subdiaphragmatic placement is used. If a nomogram is not available, this can usually be achieved by advancing the catheter until blood is first obtained, and then 1 cm further. (Adapted from Dunn PM. Localization of the umbilical catheter by postmortem measurement. *Arch Dis Child* 1966;41:69.)

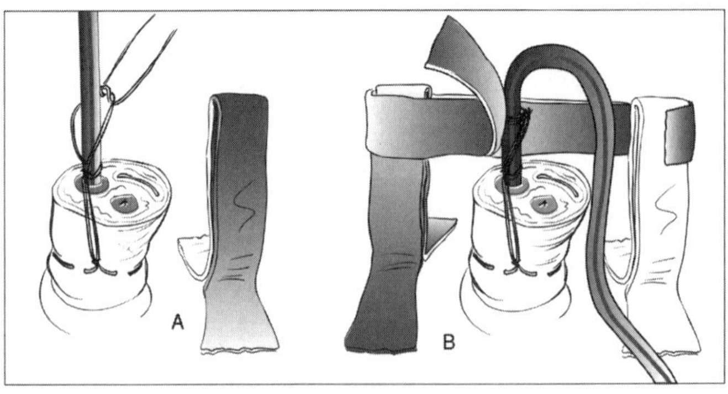

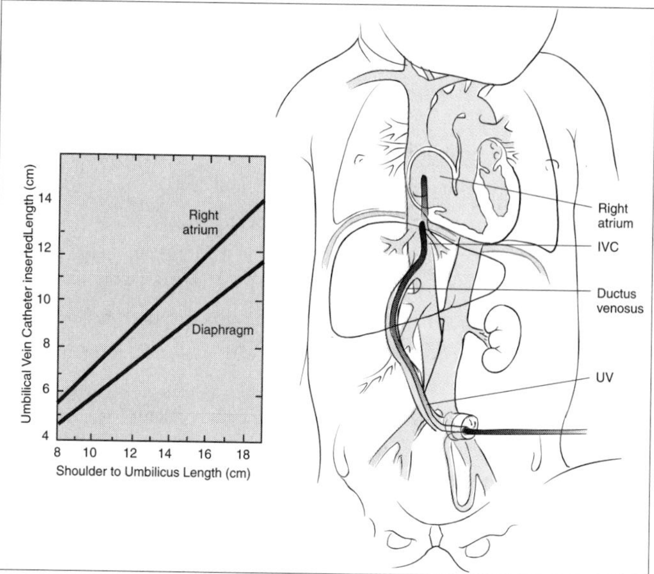

FIGURE 18.5 Nomogram for estimating umbilical venous catheter length. Umbilical venous catheterization is similar to that described for the artery, but the larger vein accommodates a larger catheter (5 or 8 French). The vein is entered, and emergent placement achieved when the catheter is gently passed 4 to 5 cm until blood return is noted. The nomogram-based length (or shoulder-to-umbilicus length × 0.6, usually 10 to 12 cm) approximates an above-the-diaphragm position at the junction of the inferior vena cava and right atrium, which is more suitable for long-term infusion of medications or hyperalimentation solutions, or for central venous pressure monitoring. However, an obstruction to passage at 5 to 10 cm suggests errant catheter passage into a portal vein branch within the liver. (Adapted from Dunn PM. Localization of the umbilical catheter by postmortem measurement. *Arch Dis Child* 1966;41:69.)

FIGURE 18.4 The catheter can be secured using the previously placed pursestring suture. The suture is tied in square knots around the catheter as shown, at the entrance into the vessel and 2 to 4 cm distal. An adhesive tape "bridge" is fashioned to secure further the suture and catheter, as illustrated.

CHAPTER 19

Lumbar Puncture

OVERVIEW

1. Determine patient ability to undergo lumbar puncture safely.
2. Explain procedure to parents and patient (if applicable).
3. Correctly position patient in lateral recumbent or sitting position.
4. With patient positioned, choose puncture site by lining up upper aspects of superior posterior iliac crests and finding L3-4 or L4-5 spinal interspace.
5. Cleanse area with iodine solution, drape, and relocate puncture site.
6. Anesthetize skin and subcutaneous tissue with 1% lidocaine infiltration (see Chapter 17).
7. For median approach (preferred if no ligamentous calcification), identify interspace with thumb of one hand and direct needle.
   A. Lateral recumbent position—parallel to bed and cephalad (toward umbilicus).
   B. Sitting—perpendicular to skin (slightly caudad).
8. For lateral approach, puncture skin just above transverse process of L3 or L4 and direct it medially and upward (cephalad).
9. Keeping stylet in place, advance spinal needle until a loss of resistance or a pop is felt; in infants, a pop may not be felt and the spinal needle should be advanced approximately 1 to 2 cm.
10. If performing manometry, attach manometer and stopcock to spinal needle; extend patient's neck and legs as much as possible and read the cerebrospinal fluid (CSF) pressure.
11. Remove stylet or manometer and collect fluid in sterile tubes.
12. Once fluid is obtained, remeasure CSF pressure (if indicated), replace stylet, and remove spinal needle.
13. Dress lumbar puncture site with adhesive bandage.

CLINICAL TIPS

1. Correct positioning of the patient with adequate flexion of the spine and good vertebral alignment is crucial to successful performance of a lumbar puncture.
2. Lidocaine anesthesia has not been shown to interfere with performance of a lumbar puncture.
3. If no fluid is flowing, the spinal needle should be rotated 90 degrees.

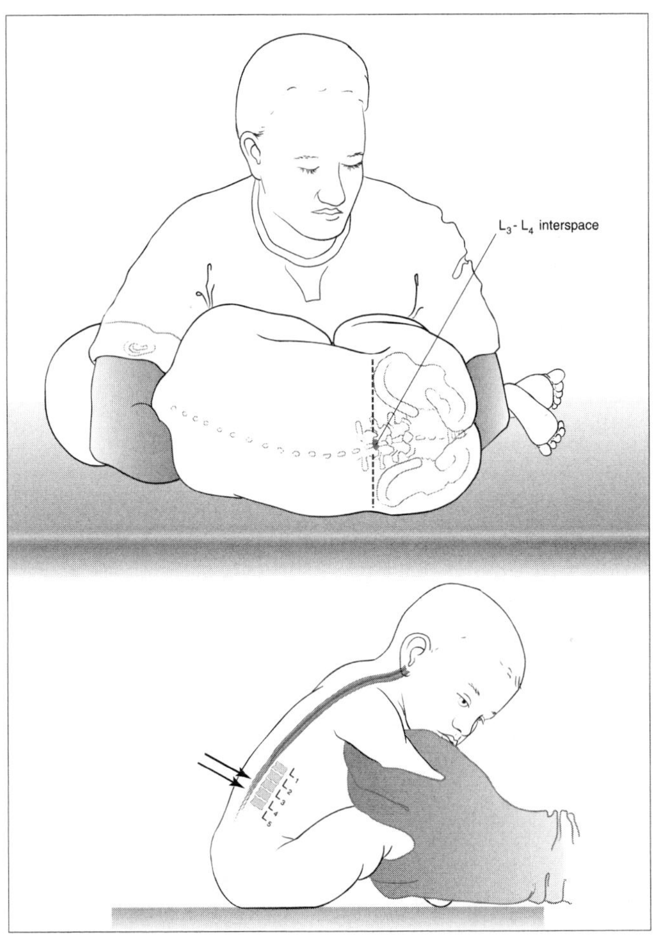

FIGURE 19.1 Achieving and maintaining correct patient position are the most crucial and challenging aspects of lumbar puncture in children. The goals of positioning are to stretch the ligamenta flava and to increase the interlaminar spaces. The two positions most widely used in the pediatric population are the lateral recumbent and the sitting positions. For the lateral recumbent position, the patient lays on his or her side near the edge of the examining table. An assistant places one arm under the patient's knees and the other arm around the posterior aspect of the patient's neck. By grasping his or her own wrists, the assistant can better control restraint of the patient. The sitting position can be used for older children who are cooperative and for very young infants who are unlikely to struggle. An older child may sit with feet over the side of the bed and with the neck and upper body flexed over a pillow. With an infant, the assistant holds the patient in a sitting position with an arm and a leg in each hand while supporting the patient's head to prevent excessive flexion of the neck.

4. If rotation of the spinal needle does not produce fluid, the needle is carefully inserted farther.
5. If CSF flow is slow in the lateral recumbent position, the patient may be moved to the sitting position.
6. If bony resistance is felt immediately below the skin, the puncture site is not over the spinal interspace.
7. If bony resistance is felt more deeply, the spinal needle should be withdrawn to the skin surface and redirected more cephalad while ensuring that the patient is properly flexed.
8. If bloody fluid that does not clear or that clots is obtained, the spinal needle should be withdrawn and the procedure attempted at a different lumber interspace.

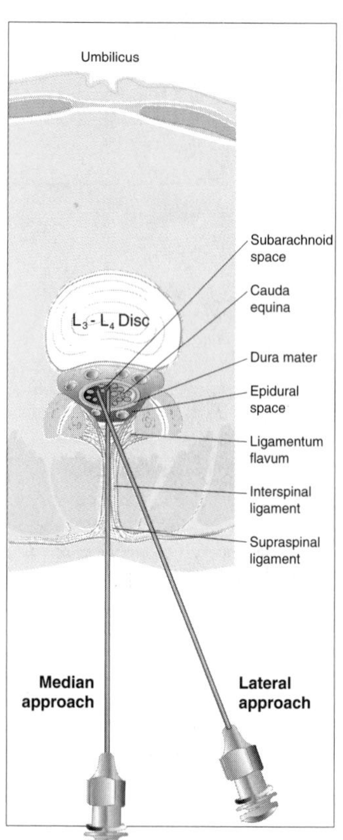

FIGURE 19.2 When placing the spinal needle, two possible approaches can be used. The median approach involves inserting the needle through the supraspinal ligament; with the lateral approach, the needle is inserted just lateral to the ligament. The median approach is used most commonly in children. In older patients, supraspinal and interspinal ligaments may be calcified, necessitating the lateral approach. However, this is rare in pediatric patients.

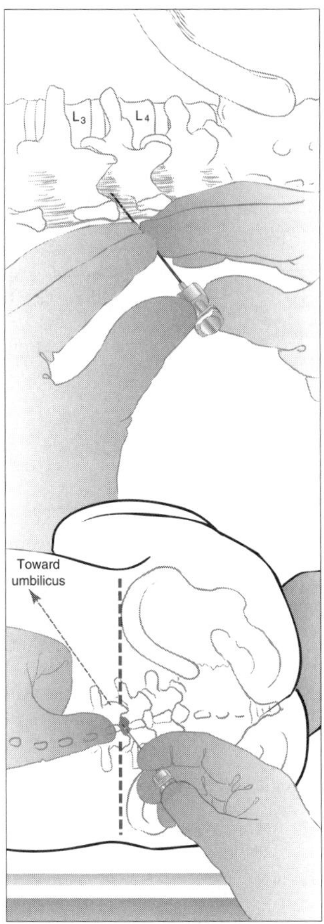

FIGURE 19.3 The spinal needle can be inserted using one or both hands. When using one hand, the clinician can ensure good alignment of the needle by placing the thumb of the other hand on the spinous process above the space being entered. When both hands are used to hold the needle, the thumbs are placed on either side of the needle hub, and the index fingers are used to support the needle.

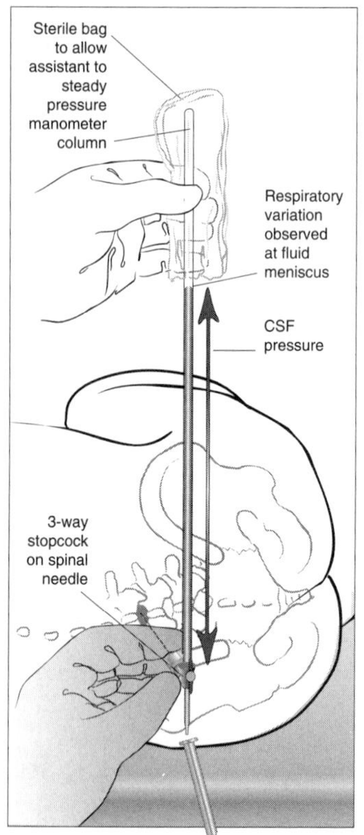

FIGURE 19.4 Measurement of the cerebrospinal fluid (CSF) opening pressure is recommended during a lumbar puncture in which it can be accurately performed. The struggling infant or child precludes the accurate measurement of opening pressure. The measurement is most reliable in a relaxed patient in the lateral recumbent position. When a free flow of CSF is obtained, the pressure manometer should be immediately attached to the needle hub by a three-way stopcock. CSF then fills the manometer column and is measured as the highest level achieved in the column. The measurement should not end until respiratory variation (rise and fall of the fluid meniscus with breathing) is determined. It is helpful to have an assistant hold the top of the manometer column so that the clinician performing the procedure can make the measurement and manipulate the stopcock for fluid collection.

TABLE 19.1 Spinal Needle Size by Age

Premature infant	22 gauge or smaller, 1.5 inch, plastic hub preferred
Neonate – 2 yr	22 gauge, 1.5 inch, plastic hub preferred
2–12 yr[a]	22 gauge, 2.5 inch
Over 12 yr	20 or 22 gauge, 3.5 inch

[a] May need larger needle depending on patient habitus.

CHAPTER 20

Ventricular Shunt and Burr Hole Puncture

OVERVIEW

Ventricular Shunt Puncture

1. Position child:
   A. Supine for frontal shunt.
   B. Lateral for posterior parietal shunts.
2. Clean shunt site and adjacent scalp with isopropyl alcohol.
3. Clip or shave a dime-sized area over reservoir.
4. Carefully clean site for several minutes with povidone–iodine and allow to dry.
5. For dome-shaped pumping reservoirs, insert needle tangentially approximately 2 to 5 mm; Rickham reservoirs should be punctured perpendicular to scalp.
6. Measure opening pressure by holding butterfly tubing perpendicular to floor and measuring from ear to top of cerebrospinal fluid (CSF) column in tubing.
7. Remove CSF until ventricular pressure is approximately 10 cm H_2O (10 to 20 mL). (Remember that slow flow may indicate a proximal obstruction and pressure measurement may be inaccurate in this setting.)
8. Transfer CSF into sterile test tubes for further studies.
9. Remove butterfly needle and apply sterile dressing.

Burr Hole Puncture

1. Locate burr hole.
2. Wash site with isopropyl alcohol.
3. Shave or clip hair in 3-cm circumference.
4. Wash site thoroughly with povidone–iodine.
5. Advance a 22-gauge, 3.5-inch spinal needle perpendicularly through burr hole; check every 0.5 cm for CSF flow up to 5 cm.
6. Withdraw fluid.
7. When pressure is relieved, replace stylet and slowly remove.

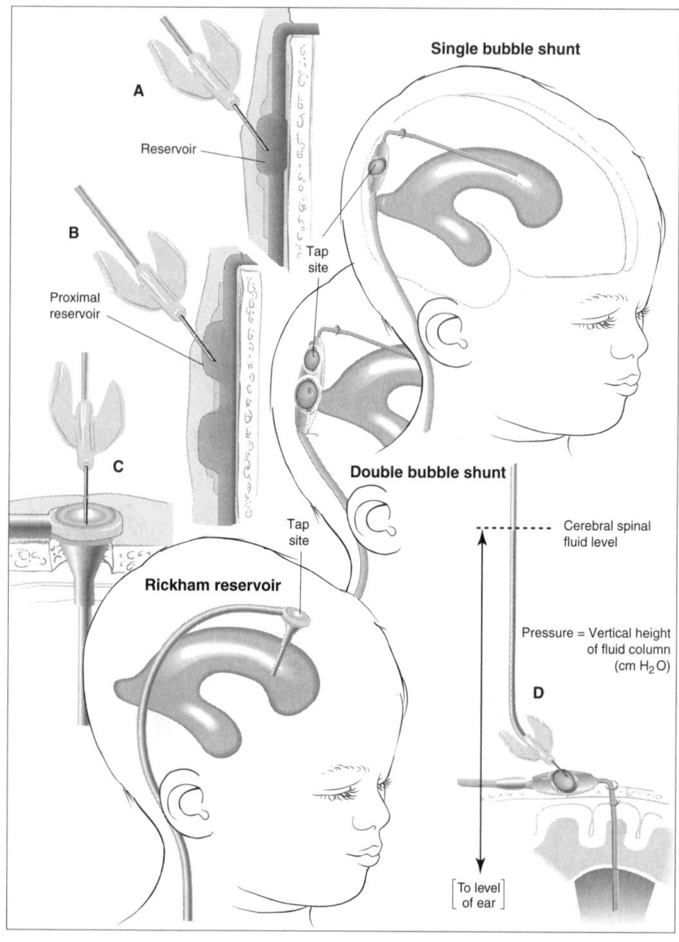

FIGURE 20.1 Puncture of a ventricular shunt reservoir allows collection of a sample of cerebrospinal fluid (CSF) as well as measurement of intracranial pressure. Slow flow of CSF into the butterfly tubing, with good respiratory variation and a normal pressure, is usually normal in the setting of small ventricles seen on brain imaging. Rapid flow of CSF under pressure suggests a shunt obstruction distal to the reservoir with a patent proximal shunt catheter. Slow or absent flow in the presence of enlarged ventricles (relative to the patient's baseline) indicates a proximal shunt obstruction, and pressure measurements are not accurate in this situation. A: Single reservoir shunt. B: Double reservoir shunt. C: Rickham reservoir. D: Measurement of CSF pressure during ventricular shunt tap.

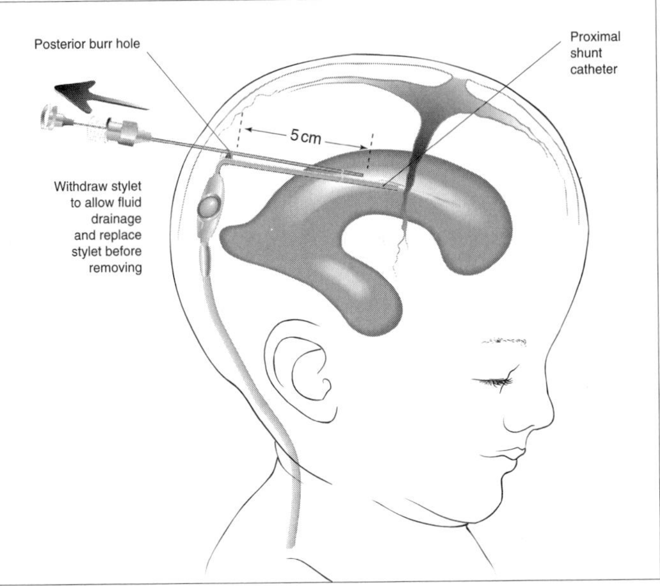

FIGURE 20.2 Ventricular puncture through a burr hole is indicated when signs of herniation are present and are not amenable to medical management (hyperventilation and diuretic therapy). The spinal needle is slowly inserted straight in, perpendicular to the skull, through either a frontal or occipital burr hole. In some shunts, the burr hole contains a reservoir, and this also is punctured by the spinal needle. The stylet is withdrawn after the ventricle is reached, and fluid is allowed to drain spontaneously until it begins to slow down, indicating relief of pressure. The stylet is then replaced and the needle is slowly withdrawn along its entry tract.

CLINICAL TIPS

Ventricular Shunt Puncture

1. No Flow
   A. The physician should ensure that the reservoir is being tapped.
   B. The angle or depth of the needle should be adjusted slightly to see if flow improves.
   C. In young infants, the physician can push on the fontanel.
   D. If the bubble collapses when suction is applied, the proximal catheter is likely to be blocked, and the procedure should be abandoned.
   E. In a child with signs of herniation, a ventricular tap through the shunt bur hole should be considered.

1. Slow Flow
   A. Partial proximal obstruction may be present.
   B. Low ventricular pressure may be present.

Burr Hole Puncture

1. The direction of the spinal needle should not be changed during the puncture to avoid shearing of brain parenchyma.
2. Burr hole puncture inevitably damages the shunt, necessitating operative intervention soon after alleviation of ventricular pressure.
3. Risk of intracranial injury after a ventricular puncture through the burr hole necessitates close observation and brain imaging after the procedure.

CHAPTER 21

Subdural and Ventricular Puncture

OVERVIEW

Subdural Puncture

1. Ensure that subdural puncture is appropriate; consider neurosurgical consultation, if time allows.
2. Immobilize patient in supine position and ensure appropriate monitoring, ancillary personnel, and resuscitation equipment.
3. Don a surgical mask and sterile gloves.
4. Prepare puncture site (lateral margin of the anterior fontanel) by shaving a small area of hair.
5. Vigorously clean the site with povidone–iodine solution applied in a circular fashion from puncture site outward.
6. Drape area with sterile surgical towels.
7. Inject local anesthetic intradermally; be sure to aspirate to ensure that inadvertent subdural injection does not occur.
8. Stretch skin overlying puncture site to aid in formation of Z-track.
9. Insert spinal needle and release skin.
10. Advance needle slowly to maximum depth of 1 cm at lateral margin of anterior fontanel at a 90-degree angle to the skull. If the fontanel is closed but the suture is fibrous (up to 18 months of age), insert needle in similar fashion 2 cm from the midline through the coronal suture.
11. Secure needle in place with hemostat applied at base of spinal needle.
12. Allow fluid to drain without using suction.
13. Apply gentle, sterile pressure dressing when procedure is completed.

Ventricular Puncture

1. Restrain patient to prevent inadvertent motion.
2. Position patient with head up at 30 degrees.
3. Prepare site (lateral border of anterior fontanel or coronal suture 2 cm from midline) using alcohol.
4. Shave or clip hair to provide 2-cm diameter site.

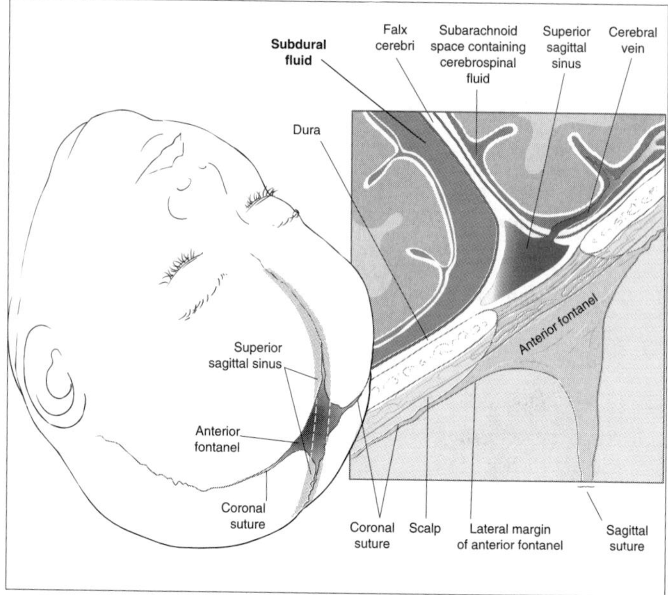

FIGURE 21.1 The subdural space lies beneath the skin, subcutaneous tissue, skull, and dura. In young infants, the major landmark for a subdural tap is the lateral margin of the anterior fontanel, which is formed by the coronal suture. Subdural fluid collections can be acute, subacute, or chronic. Disruption of the cerebral veins that traverse the dura is a major factor leading to subdural hematomas. Transudates and exudates can also occur and may be loculated. Identification of a subdural fluid collection as the etiology of increased intracranial pressure can allow rapid reversal of symptoms with the successful removal of fluid.

5. Cleanse puncture site vigorously with povidone–iodine.
6. Stretch skin over puncture site.
7. Puncture skin at lateral border of anterior fontanel or through coronal suture 2 cm from midline with 18-gauge, 2.5- or 3.5-inch spinal needle.
8. Release skin and direct and advance needle perpendicular to skull (straight in).
9. Advance needle slowly, checking for cerebrospinal fluid (CSF) return every centimeter *or* remove stylet and attach syringe and advance slowly with gentle suction.
10. Remove CSF until signs and symptoms of herniation subside.
11. Withdraw spinal needle slowly.

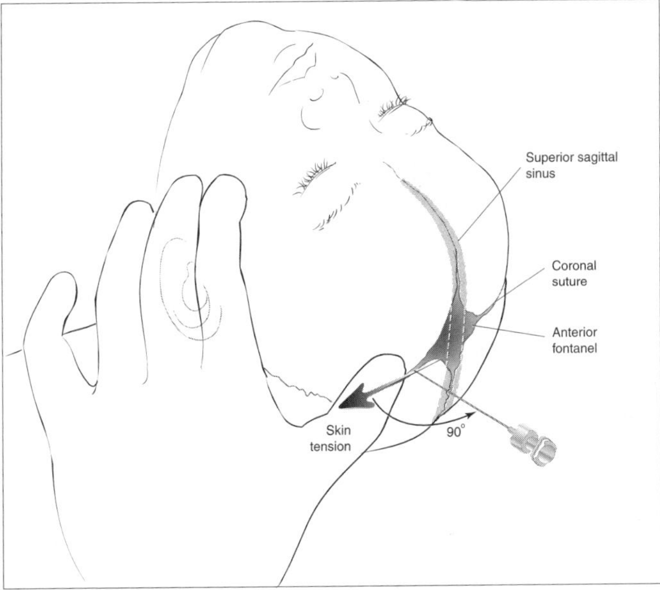

FIGURE 21.2 Subdural puncture. The patient should be secured supine in an immobilizer with additional head stabilization provided by an experienced assistant. A subdural needle (22-gauge, 1.5-inch spinal needle) is inserted at a 90-degree angle to the skull at the lateral margin of the anterior fontanel. The physician must not puncture too close to the sagittal midline where the venous sagittal sinus is located. The needle should be secured in the physician's hand with the heel of the hand against the infant's scalp to prevent a deep puncture with inadvertent head or table motion. The thumb of the other hand is used to provide skin tension during insertion. This effectively establishes a Z-track and helps minimize the possibility of postprocedural fluid leak.

CLINICAL TIPS

Subdural Puncture

1. If possible, a cerebral imaging study should be performed before subdural puncture, especially when intentional head trauma (child abuse) is suspected.
2. Bilateral or repeated subdural punctures are rarely needed.
3. Consultation with a pediatric neurosurgeon is indicated before a diagnostic or emergent subdural puncture, if time allows and if subdural fluid reaccumulates.

Ventricular Puncture

1. Once symptoms are relieved, the needle should be removed slowly until CSF flow ceases. The needle length is marked from skin edge to tip, thus estimating cortical width.
2. The direction of the spinal needle should not be changed nor should the needle be rotated in the skull. To change direction of puncture, the spinal needle must be removed to skin level.

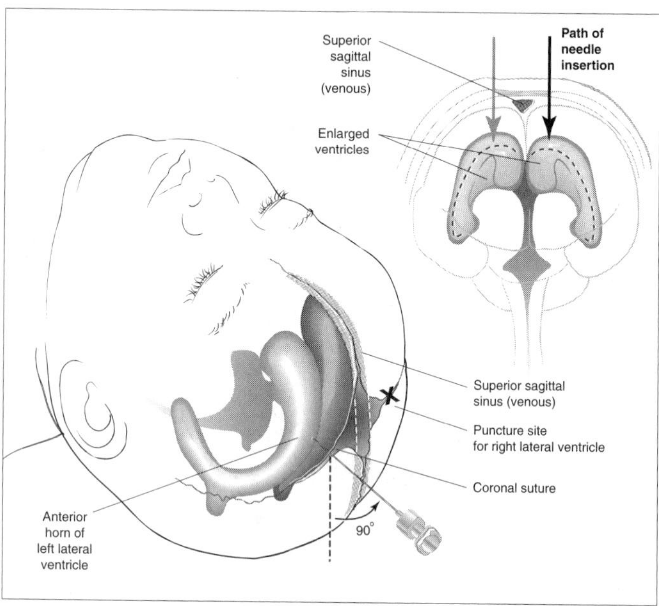

FIGURE 21.3 Ventricular puncture. For the child with severe hydrocephalus and cerebral herniation that is unresponsive to hyperventilation and diuretics, ventricular puncture and removal of cerebrospinal fluid can be life-saving. The patient should be secured supine in an immobilizer with additional head stabilization provided by an experienced assistant. Because performance of this procedure assumes ongoing herniation, the patient should be positioned head up at 30 degrees. The needle is inserted perpendicular to the skull at the lateral border of the anterior fontanel. If the anterior fontanel is closed, the needle may be inserted though the fibrinous coronal suture (up to 18 months of age) at least 2 cm from the sagittal midline. The physician must not puncture too close to the sagittal midline where the venous sagittal sinus is located. Skin tension is provided during needle insertion to establish a Z-track.

CHAPTER 22

Ophthalmologic Procedures

OVERVIEW

General Procedures

1. Opening the eye.
   A. Manually compress orbicularis muscle against bones and separate lids.
   B. Use cotton swabs with short sticks and roll skin toward lid margin to avoid eversion.
   C. Instill topical anesthetic before using lid specula or lid retractors.
2. Upper lid eversion.
   A. Recommended for lavage and identification of foreign body under lid.
   B. Have child look downward.
   C. Gently press cotton-tipped swab into body of upper lid and pull lashes to fold back upper lid.

CLINICAL TIPS

General Procedures

1. Opening the eye.
   A. Manual—no equipment, no pressure on globe.
   B. Cotton-tipped swabs—inexpensive, exerts pressure on globe.
   C. Lid specula—specialized equipment, no pressure on globe.
   D. Lid retractors—moderate expense, less discomfort than speculum; may fashion from paper clips.
2. Upper lid eversion.
   A. Keep reminding patient to look down during procedure.

OVERVIEW

Foreign Body Removal

1. Obtain a history. High-velocity injuries often result in penetration of the globe.
2. Assess for a ruptured globe. If at any point a penetrating injury is suspected, stop, shield the eye, and immediately call an ophthalmologist.

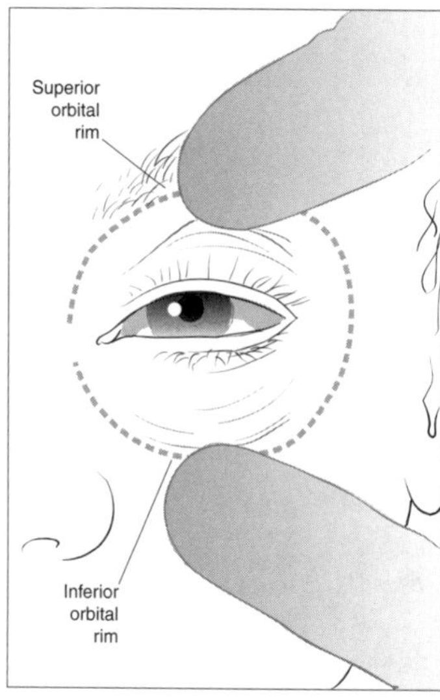

FIGURE 22.1 For rapid, although limited, eye exposure in a noncompliant child, manual lid opening is indicated. With the child's head gently restrained, the palm of one hand is placed on the forehead, and the fingers of the other hand are used to grasp the lower face, thus allowing stabilization of the head. The upper thumb is placed on the supraorbital rim (eyebrow) and the lower thumb on the infraorbital rim. Pressure is applied at these two locations, compressing the underlying muscle against the bone. As the pressure is applied, the two thumbs and underlying tissue are moved superiorly and inferiorly, exposing the eye. Care should be taken to avoid any pressure on the globe itself.

3. Anesthetize the eye.
4. Perform a thorough physical examination of the eye, including visual acuity testing and fluorescein examination.
5. Locate the foreign body. Evert the eyelids and inspect with magnification. Tiny foreign bodies adherent to the conjunctiva may be found by wiping a moist, cotton-tipped applicator across the superior fornix.
6. Remove superficial foreign bodies with irrigation.
7. Conjunctival foreign bodies may be removed with a moistened cotton-tipped applicator.
8. Embedded corneal foreign bodies in cooperative children may be removed with a 25-gauge needle on a syringe, or with a spud device.

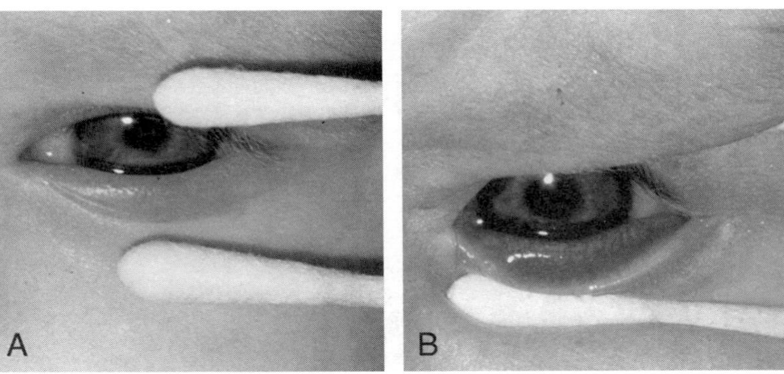

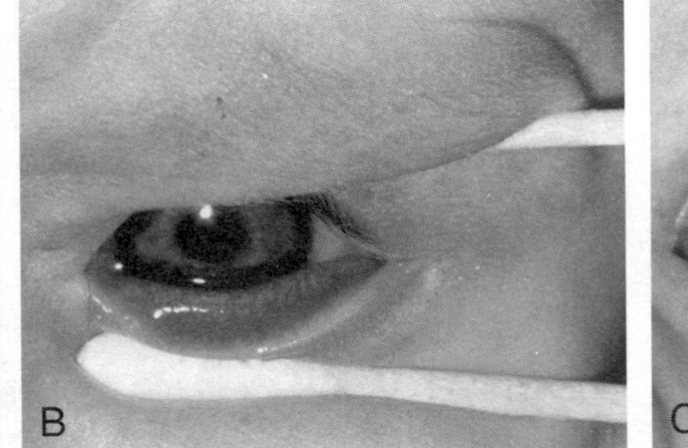

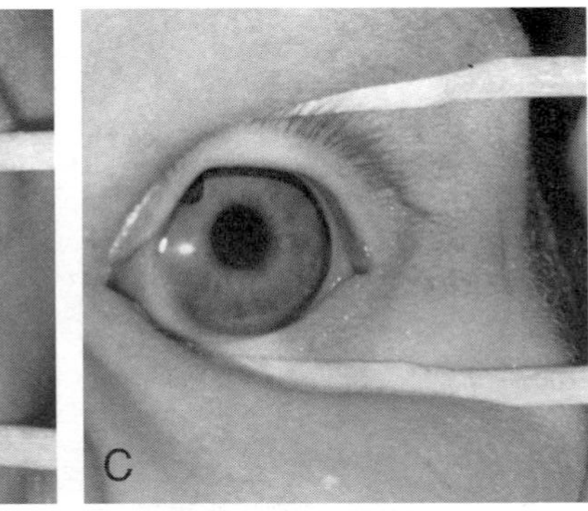

FIGURE 22.2 For wider lid separation, cotton-swab–assisted lid retraction is useful. However, this procedure, which places pressure on the globe, is contraindicated with a ruptured globe. The child is gently restrained in the supine position. One cotton swab tip is placed on the midbody of the upper lid, and the other similarly on the lower lid (**A**). With light pressure (enough to engage the skin), the tips are rotated one-quarter turn toward the lashes (**B**). This begins to separate the lid margins. Then the tips are depressed with gentle firmness posteriorly (direction of the globe), engaging the entire thickness of the lid, and the upper lid swab is moved superiorly and the lower swab inferiorly (**C**), effecting wide separation.

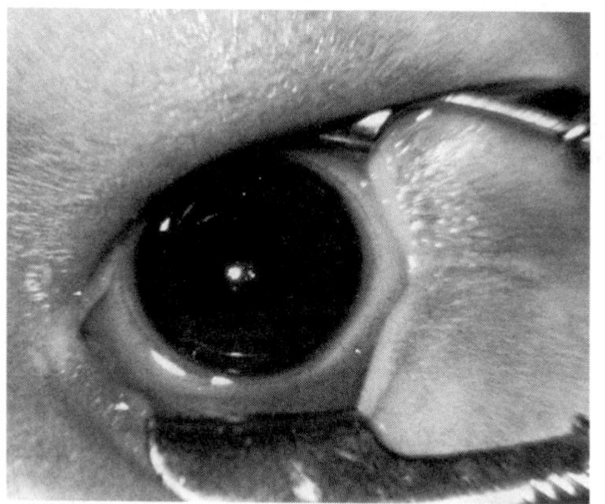

A

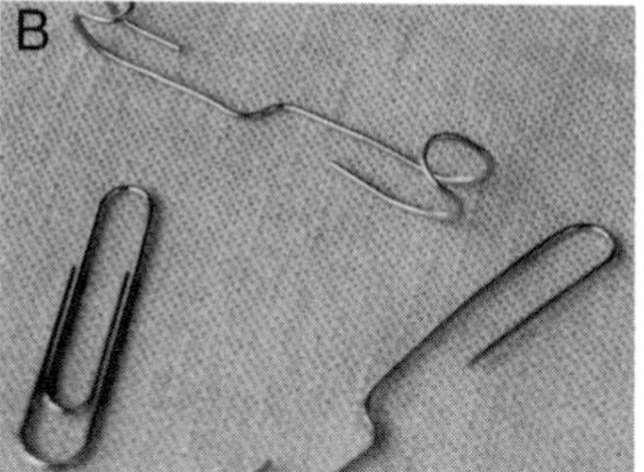

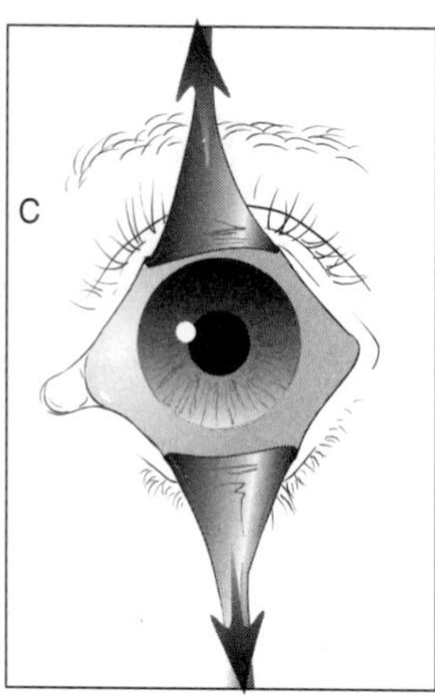

9. Perform a fluorescein examination after foreign body removal to detect a corneal abrasion.
10. Relieve pain of ciliary spasm or iritis with a drop of topical cycloplegic (homatropine 5%).
11. Prevent infection with instillation of antibiotic ointment or drops.
12. Consider patching the eye for corneal abrasions not caused by organic matter.
13. Arrange for reevaluation of the patient in 24 hours.

CLINICAL TIPS

Foreign Body Removal

1. Check the pupils carefully. A deformed pupil or an area of prolapsed iris may indicate a ruptured globe.
2. Beware of an intraocular foreign body if there is history of a high-velocity projectile. Plain radiographs or computed tomography can localize a foreign body. Magnetic resonance imaging is contraindicated with metallic foreign bodies.
3. If globe rupture is suspected, protect the eye with a shield and obtain immediate ophthalmologic consultation.

FIGURE 22.3 Lid retraction with specula and retractors. Specula and retractors do not put pressure on the globe and may be used in the patient with eye trauma. The child is typically restrained gently in the supine position. A drop of topical anesthetic (e.g., proparacaine, tetracaine) must be instilled. The speculum is grasped by thumb and forefinger. After approximately 30 seconds, one blade is inserted into either the upper or lower lid, and that lid gently retracted to allow the corresponding blade to be placed on the lid margin. The speculum is then compressed while pushing the engaged lid away, allowing engagement of the fellow lid. The speculum is then slowly and gently released to separate the lids (**A**). Retractors may cause slightly less stretching sensation to the patient. The retractors are used on one lid at a time, although two can be used simultaneously to retract both lids. If a commercial retractor is not available, a single-use, disposable retractor is easily constructed from paper clips (**B**). The paper clip type chosen should be smooth metal, not coated. Such a coating may fragment after bending and create particles that disperse onto the cornea; even after fashioning a smooth metal clip retractor, it is prudent to check for any sign of such particles and to prepare the bent clip with alcohol before use. Patient positioning and topical anesthetic use is the same as for speculum examination. The retractors are gripped by thumb and forefinger or as a pencil. The upper lid is approached at a 90-degree angle and the lid margin engaged by the retractor blade and then gently retracted away from the fellow lid, with care taken not to lift the lid too far off the eyeball surface (**C**).

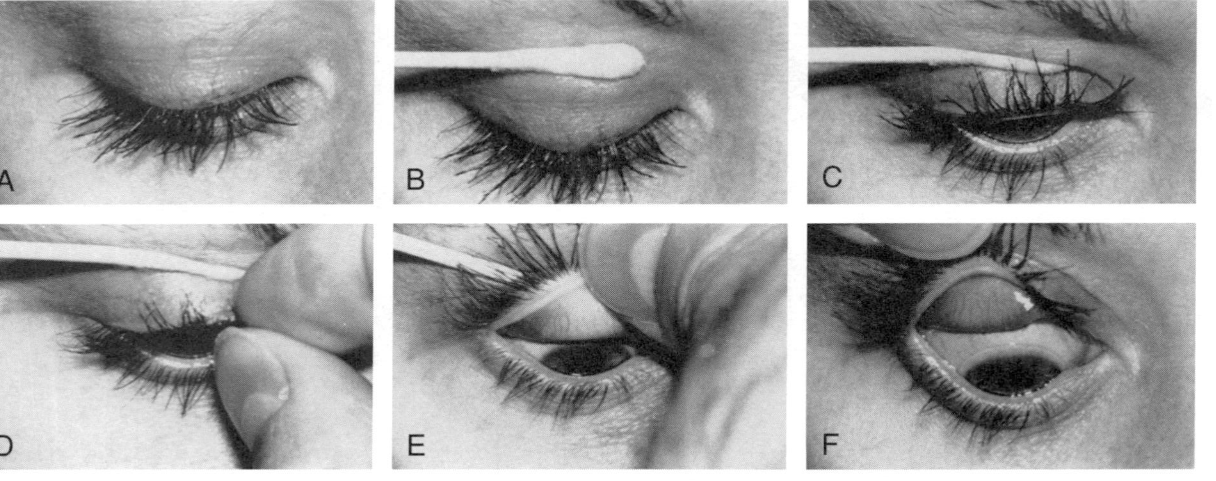

FIGURE 22.4 Upper eyelid eversion. This technique is very useful to search for foreign bodies, facilitate complete lavage after chemical exposure, and visualize the upper lid palpebral conjunctivae. **A:** The child is asked to look downward. **B:** A cotton-tipped applicator is placed on the midbody of the upper lid. **C:** The applicator is rotated toward the lid margin, causing the lid margin and lashes to rotate away from the eyeball. **D,E:** The lashes are grasped between the thumb and forefinger and pulled upward until the applicator tip is pushing into the body of the lid. **F:** The thumb pins the lashes against the superior orbital rim while the examination is conducted.

4. Cotton-tipped swabs may be useful for finding and removing conjunctival foreign bodies.
5. Consider ophthalmologic referral for the child with an embedded foreign body who cannot cooperate with examination.

OVERVIEW

Irrigation of Conjunctiva

1. Obtain brief history and examination as equipment is prepared.
2. If necessary, secure child and separate eyelids manually with gauze pads.

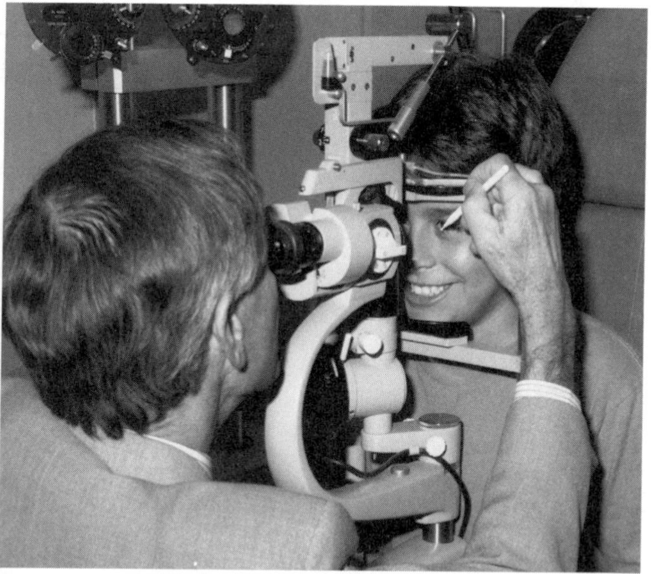

FIGURE 22.5 Ocular foreign body removal. Superficial foreign bodies are often easily removed by simple irrigation. Gentle dabbing with a premoistened cotton-tipped swab may also be effective for conjunctival foreign bodies, but can scratch the cornea. For embedded foreign bodies, ophthalmologic consultation is usually indicated, but in an older, cooperative child, a 25- or 27-gauge needle on small syringe or an eye spud device may be used in an attempt at removal. The child's head is secured against a slit lamp frame and the child instructed to focus on a distant object. The spud is held tangentially to the eye while the foreign body is gently scooped off the cornea. The physician's hand may be braced against the child's face during the procedure.

3. Check pH of conjunctivae.
4. Instill topical anesthetic.
5. Sweep away any particulate matter with moistened cotton-tipped swabs.
6. Irrigate with 1 to 2 L isotonic saline for approximately 20 minutes; direct saline over globe, into upper and lower fornices, and over canthi.
7. Measure pH of tears; if still alkaline or acidic, continue until pH normalizes to 7.4.
8. Recheck pH in 20 minutes.
9. Check for corneal abrasions with fluorescein.
10. Assess visual acuity.
11. Consult ophthalmologist as needed and arrange for follow-up.

CLINICAL TIPS

Irrigation of Conjunctiva

1. If in doubt—IRRIGATE.
2. Hold lids open with gauze pads.
3. Remove particulate matter from fornices.
4. Measure pH on completion and 20 minutes after irrigation.
5. Remember to assess for visual acuity and corneal abrasion.

OVERVIEW

Eye Patching and Guards

1. Eye patching
   A. Thoroughly examine eye before patching.
   B. Use at least two eye pads.
   C. Place over closed eyelid on angle with narrow end toward nose.
   D. Apply tape from forehead to zygoma, using benzoin if better adhesion is needed.

Eye Shielding

1. Place eye guard as soon as ruptured globe is suspected.
2. Ensure that eye guard does not contact eyelid or globe.
3. Apply tape from forehead to zygoma.

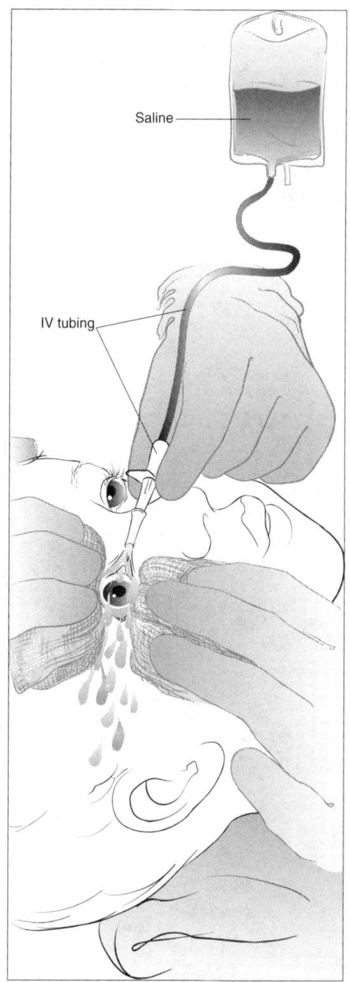

FIGURE 22.6 Irrigation of conjunctiva. The child is gently restrained in a supine position. An older child may lie with the head just off the end, facilitating drainage of irrigation fluid into a basin beneath the eye. Instillation of a topical anesthetic is advisable if not too time consuming. Saline is used with a standard intravenous setup to irrigate the eyes copiously. The end of the tubing is held just above the eyeball while the lids are held open. Gauze pads may enhance manual lid separation when the lids are wet. Saline should be directed over the entire globe, including both fornices and canthi, and, if cooperative, the child should look in all directions to facilitate such irrigation. Irrigation with 1 L of saline over 20 minutes usually is sufficient, although markedly acidic or alkaline chemicals may require more extensive irrigation, with postirrigation evaluation of the pH of the conjunctival fornices.

CLINICAL TIPS

Eye Patching and Guards

1. Do not place an eye patch on a child who may have a ruptured globe.
2. If the eye patch does not keep the eyelid completely closed, consider treatment without a patch.

3. Secure tape on eye patches and eye guards firmly. Supply parent with tape and patches in case the patch needs to be replaced.

4. If a patient with a simple corneal abrasion cannot or will not wear a patch, he or she should be managed without a patch.

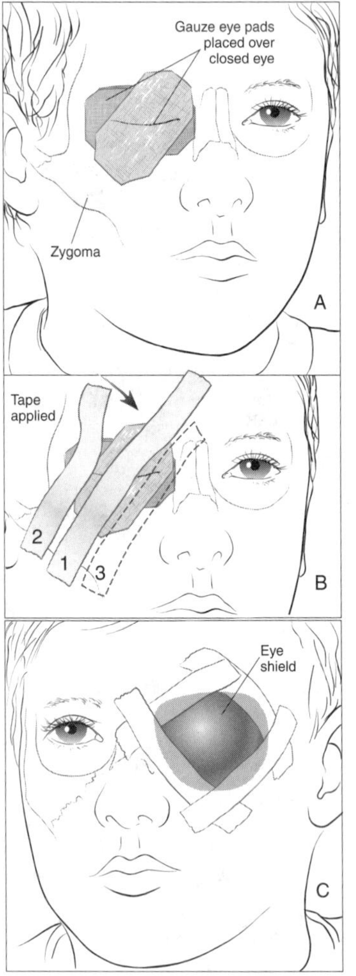

FIGURE 22.7 Eye patching and eye guards. Eye patches have traditionally been recommended for comfort in the treatment of minor, otherwise uncomplicated corneal abrasions (although usually not for those due to contact lens wear). Their value is currently somewhat controversial. If used, the eye is patched only after thorough ophthalmologic examination and instillation of warranted topical medications (e.g., cycloplegics, antibiotics). **A:** Eye pads can be fashioned from gauze if needed. At least two eye pads are placed on the closed eyelids. The pad is applied on a slant, with the narrow end toward the nose. **B:** Tape is applied from the center of the forehead to the zygomatic arch on the affected side and continued until the patch is securely taped. In contrast to patching, the purpose of the eye shield is to prevent the application of undue pressure to an injured eye. **C:** The shield is placed over the eye and tape is placed along the edges of the shield, securing it against the underlying bone. Pressure directly over the eye must be avoided. If an eye shield is unavailable, a plastic, paper, or Styrofoam cup may be used as a substitute.

OVERVIEW

Contact Lens Removal

1. All lenses/all patients.
   - A. Check patient's visual acuity and do complete eye examination.
   - B. Appropriately restrain patient, if necessary.
2. Hard contact lenses.
   - A. Cooperative patient.
     - 1) Pull eyelids from lateral palpebral margin to secure lids tightly against edges of contact lenses.
     - 2) Instruct patient to look toward nose, then downward.
     - 3) Grasp lens as it flips off eye.
     - 4) Alternatively, use suction device to remove lens.
   - B. Uncooperative patient.
     - 1) Place thumbs on upper and lower eyelids at lid margins.
     - 2) Open eyelids beyond margins of contact lens.
     - 3) Press both eyelids firmly on globe so lid margins touch contact lens edges.
     - 4) Press slightly more firmly on lower lid to work lower lid margin under lens edge.
     - 5) Move lids together so contact lens slides out and can be grasped.
     - 6) Alternatively, use suction device to remove lens.
3. Soft contact lenses.
   - A. Pull down lower eyelid.
   - B. Place tip of index finger on lower edge of contact lens.
   - C. Slide lens downward onto sclera and pinch between thumb and index finger or use pincer-type removal device.

CLINICAL TIPS

Contact Lens Removal

1. Assume that all unconscious adolescents are wearing contact lenses until an appropriate examination proves otherwise.
2. If the patient feels a foreign body in his or her eye, always determine the approximate location of the sensation before instilling topical anesthetic.
3. Do not hesitate to use fluorescein if a lens cannot be located. This stains a soft contact lens, but finding the displaced lens is more important.
4. Ensure that a proper eye examination is performed after the lens is removed. If the lens has been overworn, an underlying corneal infection is possible and should be diagnosed.

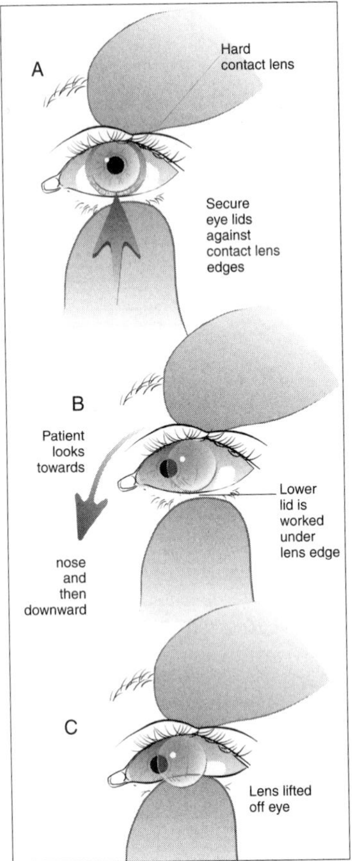

FIGURE 22.8 Contact lens removal. If possible, visual acuity is assessed before removal attempts. If globe perforation is suspected, an eye shield is placed (see Fig. 22.7C) and ophthalmologic consultation sought immediately. If not otherwise contraindicated, a topical anesthetic should be used before attempts to remove the lens. Hard contact lens removal in a cooperative child is illustrated here. The patient should hold his or her face over a table surface or clean cloth. The thumbs are placed on the upper and lower eyelids from the lateral palpebral margin and pulled to secure the lids tightly against the edges of the contact lens (**A**). The patient is instructed to look toward the nose and then downward (**B**). This maneuver allows the lower eyelid to work itself under the lower lens edge and lift the lens off the eye (**C**). If the patient is uncooperative, or must remain supine, the lens can be removed with a slight modification of this technique. The lens is located by shining a penlight across the eye surface. If the lens is properly positioned, the thumbs are placed on the upper and lower eyelid near the margins. The eyelids are opened so that the lid margins pull away beyond the lens edge. Both eyelids are then pressed gently but firmly on the globe so that the lid margins just touch the contact lens edges. Firmer pressure on the lower lid manually works the lid margin under the bottom lens edge. As the lower lens edge tips away from the surface of the eye, the lids are moved together and the contact lens slid out to where it may be grasped. Alternatively, lenses may be removed with specific suction cup devices or a cotton-tipped applicator. A lens may be floated into a position more amenable for removal by using drops of sterile saline or lubricating eye drops.

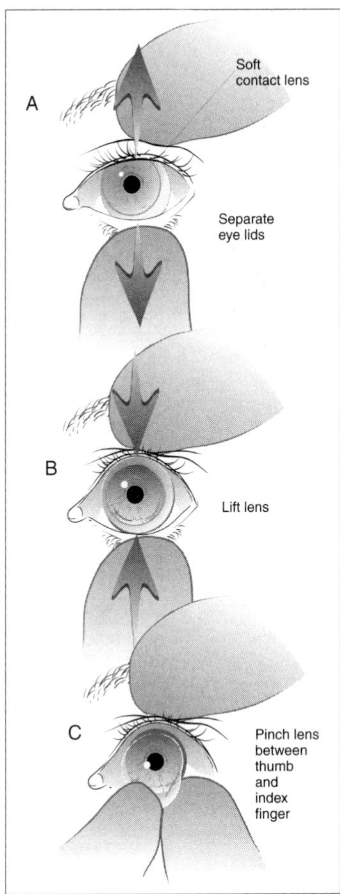

FIGURE 22.9 Soft contact lens removal. The same considerations before attempting removal apply as in hard lens removal (see Fig. 22.8). The lower eyelid is pulled down with the examiner's middle finger (**A**). Placing the tip of the index finger on the lower edge of the contact lens, the examiner then slides the lens downward onto the sclera (**B**). If the lens is dry and proves difficult to move, a drop of saline may help. Then, the lens is pinched between the thumb and index finger (**C**). The soft lens folds, allowing easy removal from the eye.

CHAPTER 23

Acute Upper Airway Foreign Body Removal: The Choking Child

OVERVIEW

First Aid for the Choking Infant Younger Than 1 Year of Age[a]

1. Hold infant head downward prone, resting on rescuer's forearm with head supported.
2. Deliver five back blows between infant's shoulder blades, using heel of hand.
3. Place free hand on infant's back and turn infant supine, with head dependent, across rescuer's thigh.
4. Perform five quick downward chest thrusts in same location as external chest compression (lower half of sternum, approximately one fingerbreadth below nipple line), but at a slower rate.
5. Attempt to provide rescue breathing. If airway remains obstructed and infant becomes unconscious, the rescuer should attempt to visualize foreign body and remove manually, then repeat sequence as necessary.

First Aid for the Choking Child Older Than 1 Year of Age[a]

Abdominal thrust with a conscious patient sitting or standing.

A. Stand behind child with arms directly under child's axillae and encircling chest
B. Place thumb side of one fist against patient's abdomen in midline, just above navel but below tip of xiphoid process
C. Grasp fist with other hand and exert five quick, upward thrusts
D. Continue thrusts until foreign body is expelled or five thrusts are completed. Attempts are made to provide rescue breathing. If airway remains obstructed, repeat sequence. If patient becomes unconscious, attempt to visualize foreign body and remove manually. If unsuccessful, modify approach as described in next section.

[a] Adapted from Committee on Pediatric Emergency Medicine. First aid for the choking child. *Pediatrics* 1993;92:477–479.

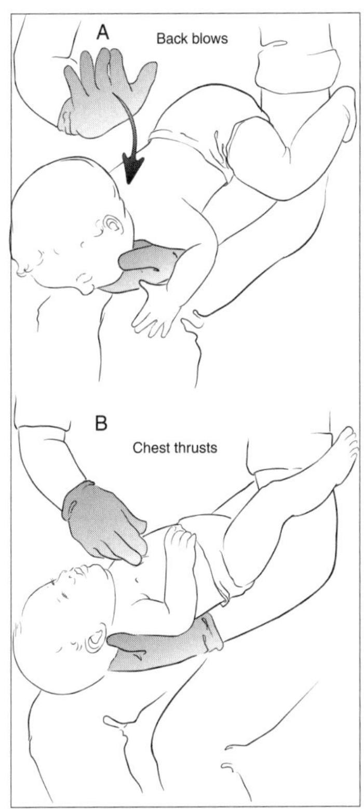

FIGURE 23.1 First aid for the choking infant (<1 year of age). **A:** The infant is initially held prone, resting on the rescuer's forearm. The infant's head is supported by firmly holding the jaw. Five back blows are delivered. The rescuer then places his or her free hand on the infant's back, holding the infant's head. The patient is thus held between the two hands of the rescuer—one supporting the neck, jaw, and chest, while the other supports the back. The infant is turned while the head and neck are carefully supported, and the infant is held in the supine position. **B:** Once the infant is supine, the head is turned to one side and held lower than the trunk. Five quick, downward chest thrusts are performed. The rescuer should use two or three fingers to compress the sternum approximately one-third to one-half the depth of the chest (0.5 to 1 inch).

Abdominal thrust with unconscious or conscious patient, lying down.

A. Place patient supine, with rescuer at patient's side or straddling patient's hips
B. Open patient's airway using chin lift or jaw thrust
C. Place heel of one hand on child's abdomen in midline just above navel and below costal margins and xiphoid. Place other hand on top of first hand
D. Press both hands into abdomen with quick, upward thrust in midline. If necessary, perform a series of five thrusts, with each thrust a separate and distinct movement
E. After delivery of five abdominal thrusts, attempt rescue breathing. If airway remains obstructed, the rescuer should attempt to visualize and remove foreign body manually. If unsuccessful, repeat sequence.

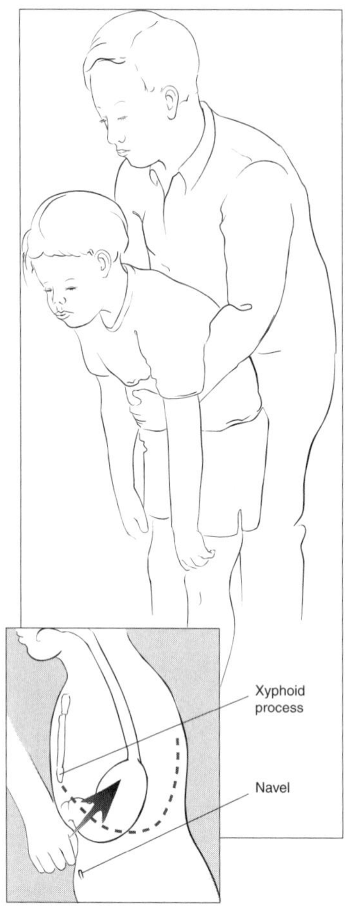

FIGURE 23.2 First aid for the conscious older child (>1 year of age) standing or sitting. The fist should not impact on the xiphoid process or the lower costal margins because force applied to these structures may damage internal organs. The rescuer should perform each thrust as a separate, distinct movement.

OVERVIEW

Laryngoscopic Foreign Body Removal

1. Assemble appropriate equipment for endotracheal intubation and surgical airway.
2. Carefully insert laryngoscope blade while visualizing oropharynx.
3. If foreign body is located, remove it with a Magill forceps (or Kelly clamp).
4. Intubate the trachea and perform positive-pressure ventilations.

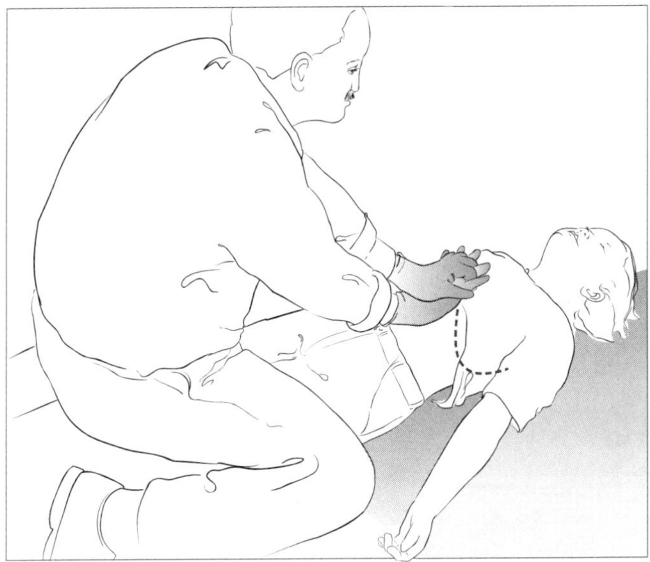

FIGURE 23.3 Abdominal thrusts with unconscious older child (>1 year of age) lying down. Thrusts are directed upward in the midline, and not to either side of the abdomen, to minimize the risk of damaging internal organs.

5. If the foreign body cannot be removed, intubate the trachea in an attempt to force the object more distally into one mainstem bronchus.
6. Attempt to ventilate one lung through the unobstructed mainstem bronchus.
7. If these efforts fail, immediately prepare to create a surgical airway.

CLINICAL TIPS

1. First aid airway maneuvering should not be performed in children with partial airway obstruction as evidenced by cough, presence of breath sounds, and maintenance of consciousness.
2. The abdominal thrust (Heimlich maneuver) is the mainstay for children older than 1 year of age.
3. Back blows and chest thrusts are the preferred maneuvers in children younger than 1 year of age.

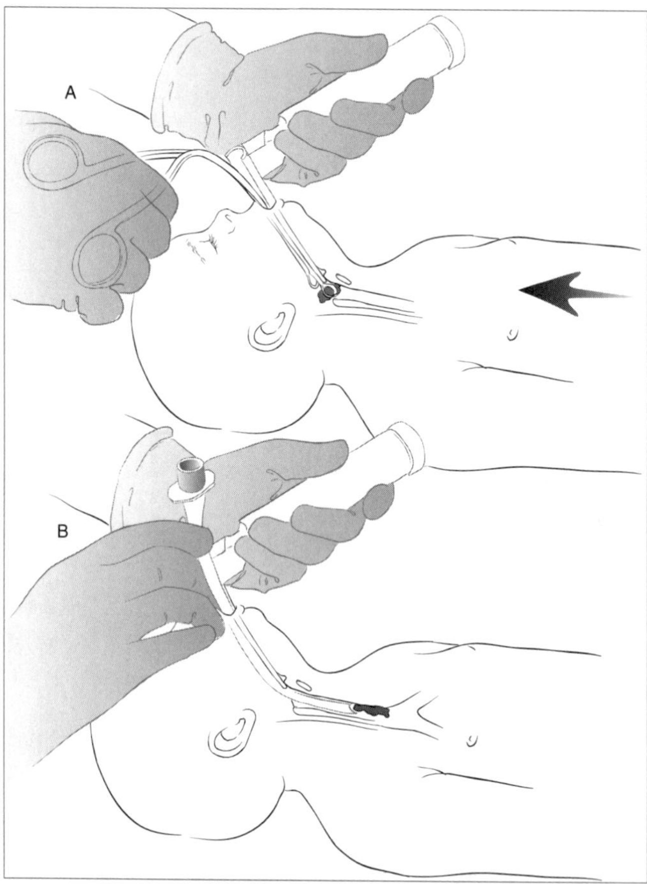

FIGURE 23.4 If back blows, abdominal thrusts, or chest thrusts are unsuccessful in expelling a foreign object from the airway, direct removal should be attempted. When appropriate equipment is available, this should be performed with a clamp or forceps under direct visualization by laryngoscopy. Laryngoscopy should be performed while carefully visualizing the oropharynx so the laryngoscope blade does not push a foreign body partly obstructing the airway further down and cause a complete obstruction. Most such foreign bodies are located at the base of the tongue or around the tonsillar pillars. **A:** If the foreign body is visualized, a Magill forceps (or Kelly clamp, if the Magill forceps is not available) is used in an attempt to grasp the foreign body and remove it. **B:** If direct removal is not possible, endotracheal intubation may force a subglottic foreign body distally enough to ventilate a child temporarily through one mainstem bronchus.

4. Each maneuver should be attempted five times in unconscious patients, and then ventilation reattempted. If possible, visualized foreign bodies may be removed by finger sweeping in the unconscious patient.
5. In the emergency department, prompt visualization of the airway by direct laryngoscopy and removal of the foreign body with Magill forceps should be attempted in the unconscious patient, while preparing for surgical airway interventions as necessary.
6. If the foreign body is not initially visualized during direct laryngoscopy, it is sometimes helpful to have an assistant perform abdominal or chest thrusts in an effort to move the object proximally, where it may be visualized and grasped.
7. If endotracheal intubation and ventilation through one mainstem bronchus is attempted, the pop-off valve of the bag-valve system should be occluded or disabled to deliver sufficient volume for effective oxygenation and ventilation.

CHAPTER 24

Removal of Cerumen/Foreign Body from the External Auditory Canal

OVERVIEW

Removal of a Cerumen Impaction

Syringing

1. Syringing solution may be saline or tap water at body temperature.

2. Necessary equipment includes 20-mL syringe attached to 16- or 18-gauge intravenous catheter or short section of butterfly needle tubing with attached hub.

3. Insert catheter 1.0 to 1.5 cm into auditory canal.

4. Direct stream posteriorly and superiorly.

Debridement

1. Initial attention to proper patient preparation and restraint ultimately results in a quicker, less traumatic, and much more likely successful procedure. Parents (and patients) should be warned that a certain minimal amount of unavoidable discomfort will occur, and bleeding postprocedure is common but usually not serious.

2. In blind debridement, brace hand holding curet against child's head, with child securely restrained and head held firmly against stretcher.

3. Gently lower curet into canal to estimate level of cerumen impaction, and then withdraw with scooping motion.

4. Frequently examine canal to ascertain if tympanic membrane is visible, even in absence of overt cerumen removal.

5. Debridement under direct visualization requires full patient cooperation and thus is rarely chosen for infants or toddlers. With visualization, cerumen may be removed by curet or alligator forceps.

Foreign Body Removal From the External Auditory Canal

Syringing

1. Irrigation is best used for nonvegetable foreign bodies.
2. Syringing solution may be saline or tap water at body temperature.
3. Necessary equipment includes 20-mL syringe attached to 16- or 18-gauge intravenous catheter or short section of butterfly needle tubing with attached hub.
4. Insert catheter 1.0 to 1.5 cm into auditory canal.
5. Direct stream posteriorly and superiorly.

Instrument Removal

1. Perform under direct visualization for foreign body removal.
2. Using curet, gently insert instrument into canal and attempt to pass hooked end beyond foreign body; after rotation, use hooked end to pull out object.
3. Alligator forceps are used optimally for irregular, graspable objects.
4. Suction and cyanoacrylate techniques are described for resistant cases.

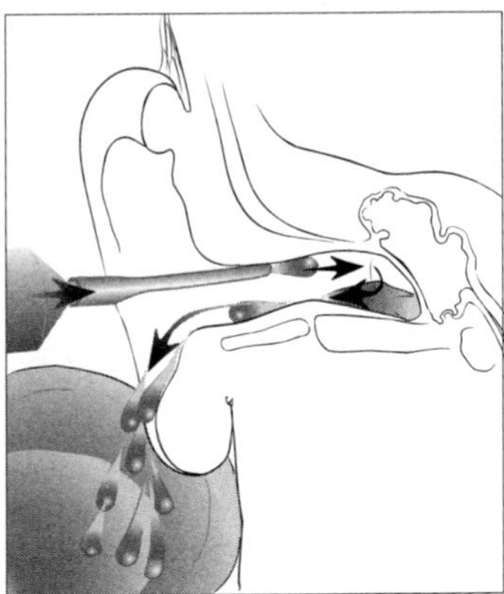

FIGURE 24.1 Syringing cerumen or a foreign body from the auditory canal with an intravenous catheter attached to a 20-mL syringe. The irrigating stream is directed at the posterior, superior wall of the canal.

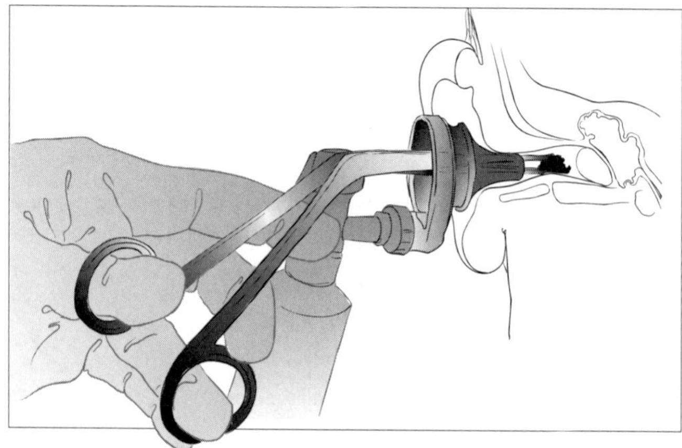

FIGURE 24.2 Cerumen or a foreign body is removed from the auditory canal under direct visualization with alligator forceps and an operating head otoscope.

Removal of a Cerumen Impaction

1. Instilling an emulsifying agent into the ear before debridement softens the cerumen, making it easier to remove.
2. Instilling Auralgan (antipyrine–benzocaine–oxyquinolone sulfate; Wyeth-Ayerst Laboratories, Philadelphia, PA) before debridement decreases pain.

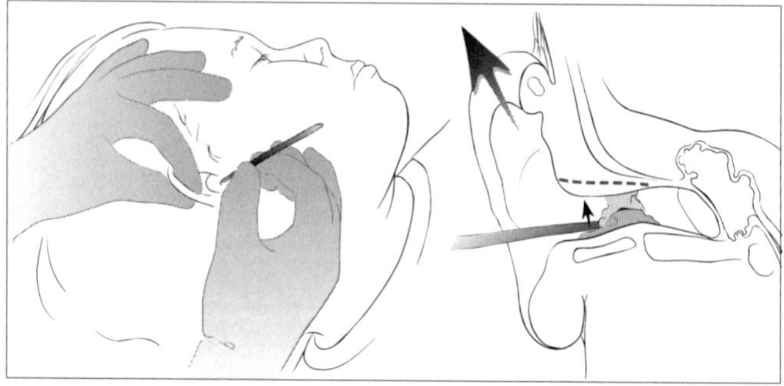

FIGURE 24.3 **A:** Blind removal of a foreign body or debridement of cerumen is accomplished with the child well restrained and the clinician's hand braced against the child's head. **B:** The cerumen spoon passes the foreign body or cerumen impaction and then is withdrawn slowly. The foreign body or cerumen is scooped out by applying gentle pressure toward the wall of the external canal as the cerumen spoon is withdrawn.

3. Ensuring proper positioning of the patient before debridement protects against sudden movements.
4. Straightening the auditory canal by applying traction to the auricle aids direct visualization or passing cerumen curet.
5. The irrigating syringe should be directed posteriorly while irrigating to prevent iatrogenic tympanic membrane injury.
6. Allowing gravity to guide the metal cerumen spoon in and down the auditory canal decreases complications.
7. If one tympanic membrane is visualized and the diagnosis of otitis media is made, it may not be necessary to débride the other side.
8. Allowing the child to see and touch the equipment such as the irrigating setup and the cerumen curet aids cooperation.

CLINICAL TIPS

Foreign Body Removal From the External Auditory Canal

1. Initial attention to proper patient preparation and restraint ultimately results in a quicker, less traumatic, and much more likely successful procedure.
2. Parents (and patients) should be warned that a certain minimal amount of unavoidable discomfort will occur, and bleeding postprocedure is common but usually not serious.
3. Reasonable limits must be set on time and number of attempts to retrieve a foreign body. Sedation or even general anesthesia should be considered after a failed attempt at instrument removal.
4. Live insects are optimally first killed with mineral oil, which quickly reduces patient discomfort and anxiety.
5. Button battery impaction is an emergency and requires immediate otolaryngologic consultation if emergency department removal is unsuccessful, as does any evidence of a middle ear pathologic process.

CHAPTER 25 •

External Ear Procedures

OVERVIEW

Regional Auricular Block

1. Restrain child appropriately and aseptically prepare the involved area.
2. For local anesthesia, infiltrate wound edges using 1% lidocaine so as to not distort wound edges.
3. For regional anesthesia of the ear, inject skin surrounding ear.
4. Wait several minutes for local anesthetic and 10 to 15 minutes for regional anesthetic to have maximum effect.

Auricular Hematoma Drainage

1. Properly restrain child.
2. Prepare area to be drained using aseptic technique and obtain sterile field.
3. If necessary, anesthetize area to be drained (frequently not required).
4. Drain hematoma completely using 18-gauge needle or no. 15 blade.
5. Apply manual pressure for 3 to 5 minutes and then place pressure dressing.
6. Follow-up within 24 hours to check for reaccumulation of fluid and/or blood.

Application of External Ear Pressure Dressing

1. Place two to four 4 × 4-inch gauze pads with the centers cut out around and under the external ear.
2. Place several saline-soaked cotton balls or petroleum gauze over the ear molded to fit all the contours of the external ear.
3. Place two to four intact sponges over the entire ear.
4. Wrap a 4-inch gauze bandage around the head and over the ear several times.

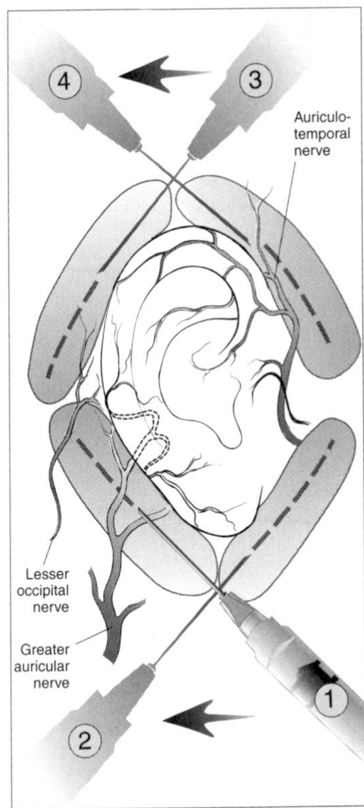

FIGURE 25.1 To perform a regional auricular block, the ear and surrounding skin are first prepared with antiseptic solution. A 10-mL syringe with a 1.5-inch, 27-gauge needle is filled with 1% lidocaine without epinephrine and is used to inject a track of lidocaine around the entire ear. This can be accomplished by initially entering a point just above the ear and fully inserting the entire length of the needle along the back of the ear. Lidocaine (2 to 5 mL) is injected as the needle is withdrawn. Without completely withdrawing the needle from the skin, a second track is made in front of the ear by fully inserting the needle and again injecting lidocaine as the needle is withdrawn. Similar tracks are made at the bottom of the ear by entering the skin just below the lobe in the sulcus. Injections are made both anteriorly and posteriorly to the ear, leaving a V-shaped track of anesthesia. Maximum anesthetic effect occurs in approximately 10 to 15 minutes.

CLINICAL TIPS

1. Because an auricular block is regional anesthesia, optimal anesthetic effect does not occur until 10 to 15 minutes after injection of lidocaine.

2. Always ensure that the amount of lidocaine used for an auricular block does not exceed the toxic dose for the patient.

3. Complete drainage of an auricular hematoma is mandatory for good outcome.

4. Follow-up after drainage of an auricular hematoma should occur within 24 hours to check for reaccumulation of fluid.

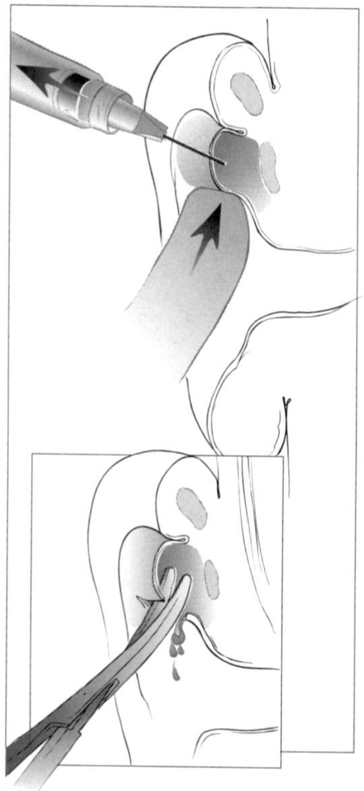

FIGURE 25.2 Evacuation of an auricular hematoma is performed by first preparing the overlying skin with antiseptic solution. An anesthetic may not be necessary if only a single-needle aspiration is to be performed. An 18-gauge needle attached to a 10-mL syringe is inserted into the area of the hematoma that is most fluctuant. The hematoma is then evacuated by applying negative pressure with the syringe and milking the hematoma using the thumb or index finger. If clot formation has occurred and complete evacuation is not possible by needle aspiration alone, a small incision should be made using a no. 15 blade, and a curved hemostat can then be used to break up and remove the clot. Complete evacuation is necessary to prevent potential cartilage necrosis. After the hematoma has been drained, a pressure dressing is applied to prevent reaccumulation of fluid. A repeat examination is required within 24 hours and, if fluid has reaccumulated, the ear must be drained again.

5. An external ear pressure dressing should apply even pressure over the entire ear (to provide structural support and prevent formation of a hematoma) without compromising blood flow.
6. All patients or parents should be educated about the signs and symptoms of perichondritis and chondritis: increasing pain over several hours, progressive swelling, redness, tenderness, and warmth.

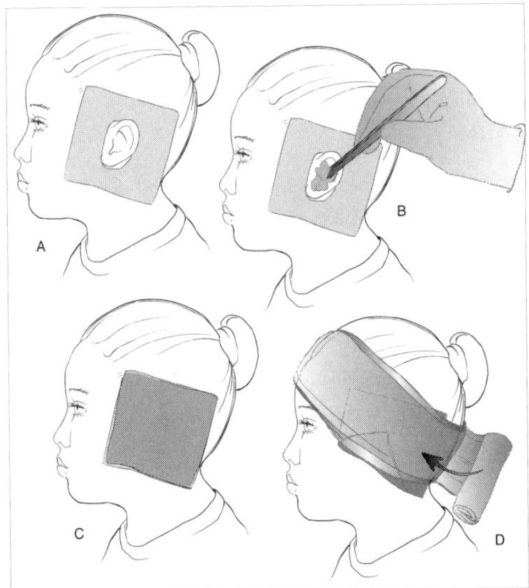

FIGURE 25.3 A pressure dressing is applied to the external ear to prevent fluid accumulation and to add structural support. This dressing should be used for any repair of a complicated ear injury or drainage of an auricular hematoma. **A:** Two to four 4 × 4-inch gauze pads with the centers cut out are first placed around (but not over) the entire external ear. This provides support behind the ear and prevents contortion of the ear or excessive pressure. **B:** Several saline-soaked cotton balls or petroleum gauze are then placed and molded to fit all contours of the external ear. **C:** Two to four intact sponges are placed over the entire ear. **D:** A 4-inch gauze bandage is wrapped around the head and over the ear several times. The desired effect is to apply even pressure without compromising blood flow. Close follow-up must be ensured to assess wound healing and prevent possible perichondritis or chondritis.

CHAPTER 26

Tympanocentesis

OVERVIEW

1. Obtain 22-gauge, 3.5-inch spinal needle bent 30 degrees 3 to 4 cm from distal end attached to 1-mL syringe.
2. Restrain patient well and use sedation if needed.
3. Prepare external canal by removing cerumen and then cleanse canal with 70% alcohol.
4. Visualize tympanic membrane using otoscope with operator head.
5. Insert needle with direct visualization of landmarks along inferior aspect of ear canal.
6. Pierce membrane in anterior-inferior quadrant and apply negative pressure.
7. Send aspirate for Gram stain and culture using nonbacteriostatic saline as needed to obtain small amount from spinal needle.

CLINICAL TIPS

1. Control of the child to avoid an unexpected movement is critical during tympanocentesis. Appropriate restraint is essential, and conscious sedation should be considered if necessary.
2. The superior quadrants of the tympanic membrane must be carefully avoided to prevent injury to important middle ear structures.
3. If continued drainage of the ear is desirable, consultation with an otolaryngologist should be sought for possible myringotomy.

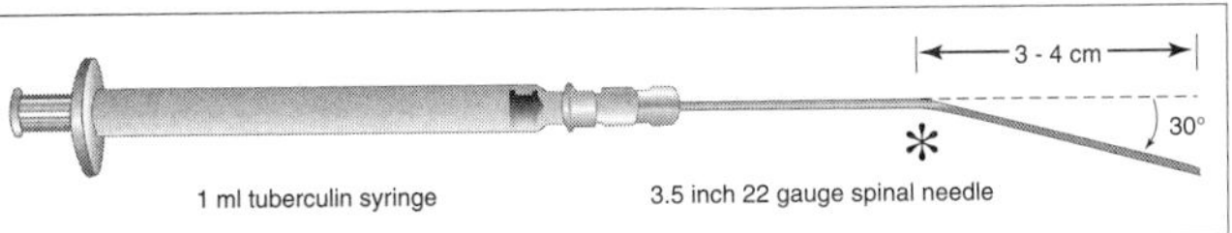

FIGURE 26.1 Tympanocentesis can be performed using a tuberculin syringe and a 3.5-inch, 22-gauge spinal needle with the stylet removed. The needle is bent to a 30-degree angle approximately 3 to 4 cm proximal to the tip. Bending the needle in this way allows a better view of the tympanic membrane during the procedure.

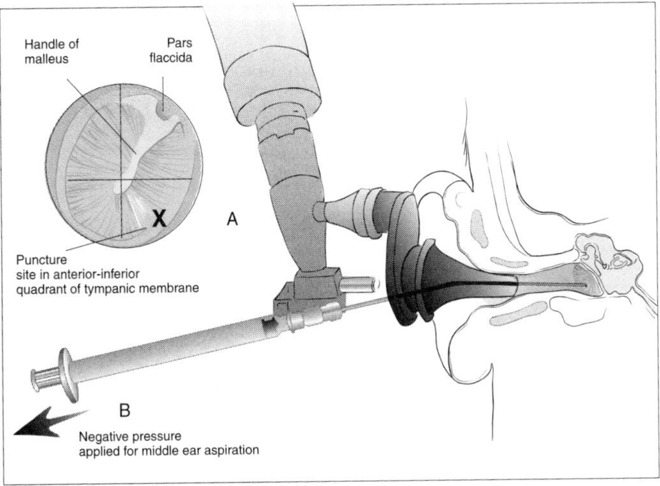

FIGURE 26.2 Before performing a tympanocentesis, the child should be securely restrained (usually with a papoose) and conscious sedation should be administered as necessary. Cerumen in the canal should be removed and the external canal should be cleansed with 70% alcohol. Any remaining fluid should then be suctioned from the canal. **A:** The puncture site for tympanocentesis is in the anterior-inferior quadrant of the tympanic membrane. This can be located by imagining horizontal and vertical lines drawn through the tip (umbo) of the malleus. Insertion of the needle anterior and inferior to this important landmark minimizes the possibility of damaging underlying structures of the middle ear. **B:** Using an operating otoscope, the entire tympanic membrane is visualized by the operator using both eyes, so that depth perception is maintained. The spinal needle is advanced down the inferior aspect of the canal to the anteroinferior quadrant of the tympanic membrane. The tympanic membrane is then punctured and negative pressure is applied to the syringe to obtain a fluid specimen. After the procedure is completed, the ear should be rechecked for bleeding or signs of significant tympanic membrane trauma.

CHAPTER 27

Management of Epistaxis

OVERVIEW

Anterior Nasal Packing

1. Position patient sitting upright facing clinician whenever possible. Younger patients who are unable to cooperate may be positioned supine with appropriate restraint. A sedative may be administered as needed.
2. Apply topical vasoconstrictor and topical anesthetic to nasal mucosa.
3. Locate site of bleeding and cauterize as well as possible.
4. Coat petroleum gauze (0.25- or 0.5-inch) with antibiotic ointment.
5. Insert nasal speculum into nostril and open vertically to expose septum.
6. Grasp gauze with bayonet forceps 5 to 7 cm from end and insert it straight back on floor of nose. Approximately 2 to 3 cm of gauze should protrude from nose.
7. After first layer is placed, remove speculum and replace it on top of gauze to pack it down gently as next layer is placed in accordion fashion.
8. Continue applying layers of gauze until nasal cavity is filled.
9. Place a piece of tape on gauze protruding from nose to stabilize pack.

OVERVIEW

Posterior Nasal Packing[a]

1. Position patient sitting upright facing clinician whenever possible. Younger patients who are unable to cooperate may be positioned supine with appropriate restraint. A sedative may be administered as needed.
2. Apply topical anesthetic to nasal mucosa.
3. Tie two silk sutures or umbilical tapes around cylindrically rolled 2 × 2-inch gauze pads or an open gauze pad wrapped around cotton filling, leaving a long (8 to 12 inches) length of tie on each end.
4. Insert small (8 to 10 French) red rubber catheter through anesthetized

[a] A simplified method of placing a posterior nasal pack using a Foley catheter is shown in Fig. 27.3.

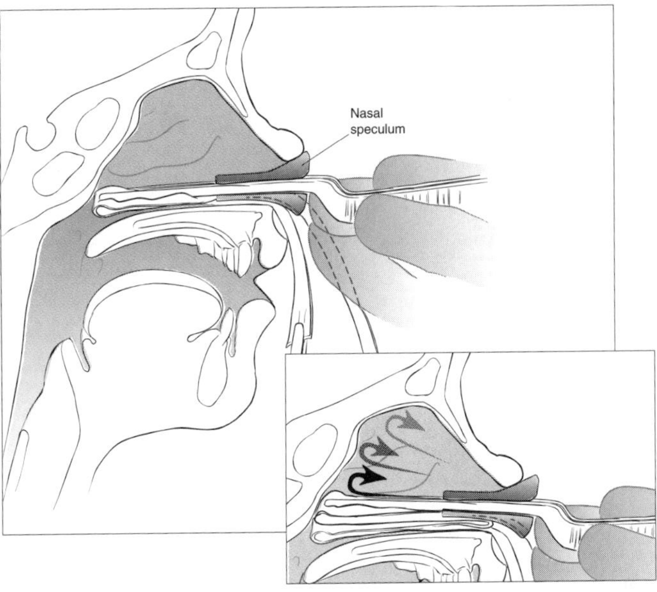

FIGURE 27.1 Traditional method of placing an anterior nasal pack using petroleum gauze. A bayonet forceps is used to insert the gauze straight back along the floor of the nasal cavity. The speculum is removed after each layer is applied and then reinserted to pack the gauze down gently. The gauze is layered in accordion fashion until the nasal cavity is filled.

bleeding nostril until it can be retrieved from posterior pharynx through mouth.

5. Fasten one end of a tie to catheter and withdraw catheter so tie protrudes from nostril.
6. Repeat same procedure on opposite side using one end of other tie.
7. When one end of each tie protrudes through each nostril, draw pack into posterior pharynx and quickly position it manually against vomer.
8. Tape opposite end of ties (protruding from mouth) to cheek so that they can be used later in removing pack.
9. Pack anterior nose.

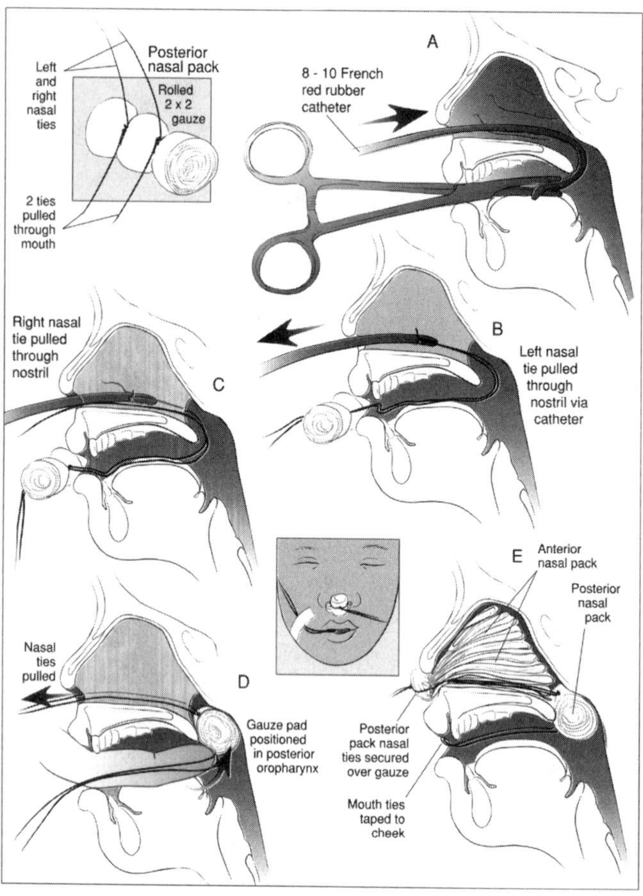

FIGURE 27.2 Traditional method of placing a posterior nasal pack using gauze pads. **A:** A small catheter is inserted into one nostril, advanced to the posterior pharynx, and withdrawn through the mouth. **B:** One end of a tie is then fastened to the end of the catheter and the catheter is removed to pull the tie out through the nose. **C:** This is repeated on the opposite side using one end of the other tie. **D:** The pack is drawn into the posterior pharynx by pulling both ties and positioned manually against the vomer. An anterior nasal pack is then applied. **E:** The ends of the ties protruding from the mouth are taped to the cheek. The ends protruding through the nostrils are tied around a gauze pad under the septum of the nose.

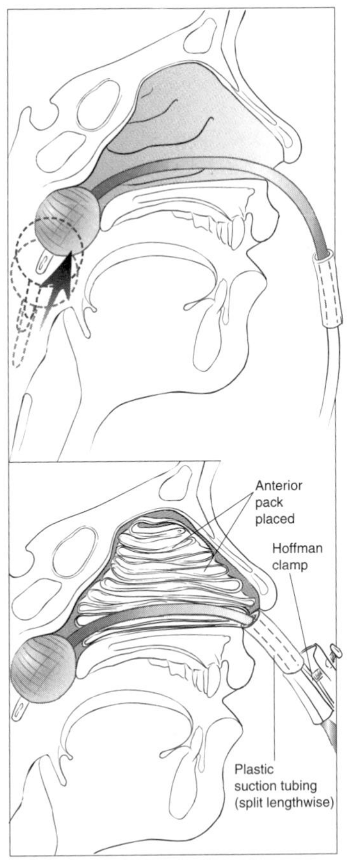

FIGURE 27.3 An alternative to the traditional rolled gauze method involves using a Foley catheter as a posterior nasal pack. This method is usually less time consuming and technically easier to perform. A catheter should be selected that approximates the diameter of the external nares (10 to 16 French). Before using the catheter, the balloon should be inflated to ensure that no air leak is present, and the end of the catheter distal to the balloon should be cut off to prevent irritation of the posterior pharynx. The catheter is lubricated with antibiotic ointment and inserted into the anesthetized bleeding nostril until the balloon is visible in the posterior pharynx. The balloon is then inflated with 10 to 15 mL water or saline, and the proximal end of the catheter is withdrawn until the balloon is snug against the vomer. If the pressure exerted by the balloon causes any significant pain, the balloon should be deflated slightly. The catheter may be secured by placing a length of plastic suction tubing, split lengthwise, around the catheter just under the nostril. A Hoffman clamp, umbilical clamp, or hemostat fastened under the plastic cuff is used to hold the catheter in place. An anterior pack should then be placed around the Foley catheter.

10. Secure nasal ties of posterior pack over a rolled gauze pad placed under nostrils.

CLINICAL TIPS

1. When the patient has a known history of an intranasal lesion (e.g., a polyp or hemangioma) or a known bleeding disorder, otorhinolaryngologic consultation should be sought before attempting to cauterize or pack the affected area.
2. When using a speculum to examine the nose, the blades should be opened

vertically rather than horizontally so that the septum is better visualized without being directly instrumented.

3. When using silver nitrate to perform chemical cautery, it should be applied to the affected area in concentric circles, starting at the outer limits of the area and working inward. Cautery of both sides of the septum can lead to necrosis. Circumferential cautery around the entire margin of one nostril can lead to scarring and stenosis.
4. Patients with packs in place for more than a few hours should be placed on oral antibiotics to prevent sinus infection and toxic shock syndrome.
5. Posterior nasal packs are known to cause hypoxia and hypoventilation and may cause significant pain, dysphagia, and infection. In addition, accidental dislodgment of the pack into the hypopharynx can cause airway compromise. Patients with a posterior pack should therefore be monitored in the hospital.
6. The risk of rebleeding after treatment may be minimized by having the parents humidify the child's home environment, by lubricating the anterior septum with petroleum or water-based jelly, and by preventing the child from picking his or her nose.
7. With younger patients who are unable to cooperate, it may be necessary to administer conscious sedation to perform the procedures used for managing epistaxis.
8. Although complete systemic absorption of cocaine and lidocaine does not occur after topical administration, the maximum allowable dose of these agents (3 mg/kg for cocaine and 5 mg/kg for lidocaine) should not be exceeded.

CHAPTER 28

Nasal Foreign Body Removal

OVERVIEW

1. Ascertain nature of foreign body, if possible.
2. Explain procedure to parent and child.
3. Assemble necessary equipment.
4. Restrain child appropriately; assign one assistant to stabilize child's head.
5. Perform conscious sedation as necessary.
6. Insert nasal speculum and visualize object to determine size, location, and orientation.
7. Apply topical anesthesia (4% cocaine or 4% lidocaine) as needed.
8. Apply topical vasoconstrictor [0.25% phenylephrine (Neo-Synephrine; Sanofi Winthrop Pharmaceuticals, New York, NY)] as needed.
9. Remove foreign body.
   A. For hard, smooth foreign bodies, insert removal instrument parallel to nasal turbinates (straight in) until tip is behind object and pull outward.
   B. Grasp soft objects with forceps and remove.
10. Reinspect nasal cavity after removal to ensure the object(s) are completely removed and mucosa has not been injured.

CLINICAL TIPS

1. A nasal foreign body should never be intentionally pushed back into the hypopharynx in an attempt to remove it because this may result in aspiration of the object into the proximal airway.
2. If it is apparent that a foreign body is only being pushed further into the nasal cavity during attempted removal, the procedure should not be continued. In such cases, removal by an otolaryngologist in the operating room may be necessary.
3. Visualization of the object usually can be improved by (a) applying a topical vasoconstrictor to the nasal mucosa, (b) using a high-intensity light source (a head lamp is ideal), and (c) using suction to remove any blood or secretions.

4. The child must be very still during this procedure to prevent injury to the nasal cavity, and the clinician should take appropriate measures to accomplish the goal (restraint, and if necessary, sedation). If the clinician is not confident that the child will remain motionless, the procedure should likely be performed in the operating room.
5. With a verbal child, explaining each step of the procedure in a friendly, calming voice is often the most effective means of avoiding any sudden movements by the patient.
6. A firm, smooth foreign body that cannot be readily removed using a curet or right-angle curet can often be retrieved by applying histacryl blue ("super glue") to the tip of a wooden stick, pressing the tip against the object for 15 to 30 seconds to form a secure bond, then slowly withdrawing the stick.
7. Although total systemic absorption of cocaine and lidocaine does not occur after topical administration, the maximum allowable doses of these agents (3 mg/kg for cocaine and 5 mg/kg for lidocaine) should not be exceeded.

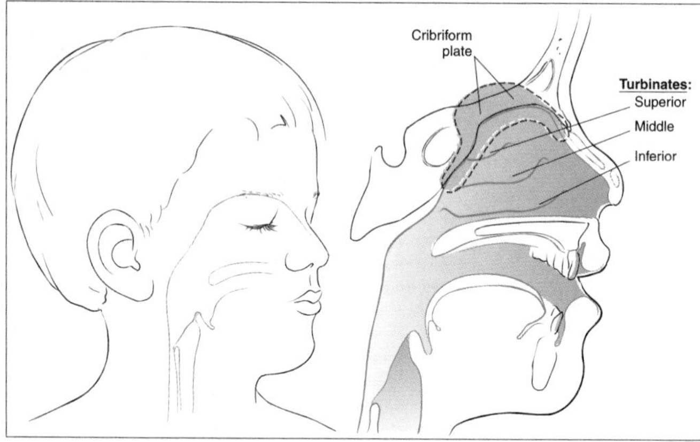

FIGURE 28.1 A good view of the nasal cavity should always be obtained before any instrumentation. Blind passage of removal devices is rarely successful and increases the risk of injury. The three nasal turbinates are essentially perpendicular to the face. Instruments inserted into the nose to remove a foreign body should therefore be oriented in an anteroposterior direction (i.e., straight in). The area superior and medial to the middle turbinate is immediately adjacent to the cribriform plate and as such represents a danger zone. Overzealous instrumentation with a metal probe can result in puncture of this thin segment of bone. For this reason, a foreign body lodged in this position should be removed only by an otolaryngologist.

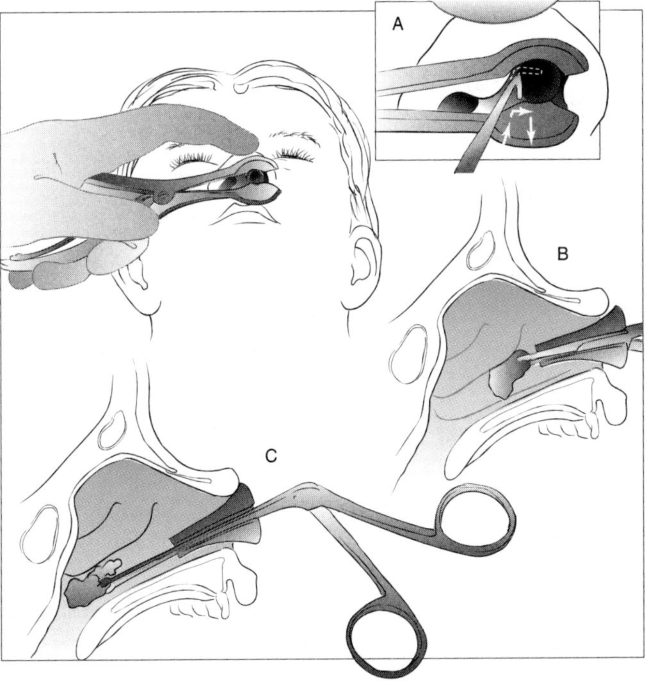

FIGURE 28.2 For removal of an intranasal foreign body, the patient should be positioned supine with appropriate restraint. **A:** A right-angle curet can be used to remove firm or rounded objects. **B,C:** Forceps (bayonet or alligator) can be used to remove softer materials (e.g., rubber or paper).

CHAPTER 29 •

Incision and Drainage of a Peritonsillar Abscess

OVERVIEW

1. Assemble required equipment (including airway equipment) at bedside.
2. Have patient positioned with head firmly against the stretcher.
3. Use appropriate restraint methods (e.g., assistant holding patient's head, papoose board) as necessary.
4. Use needle guard or tape scalpel blade to control depth of incision.
5. To perform three-point needle aspiration, insert needle first at superior pole of tonsil and aspirate. If pus is not obtained, insert needle 0.5 to 1 cm inferior to first site and aspirate. If again unsuccessful, insert needle 0.5 to 1 cm inferior to second site and aspirate (inferior pole).
6. If aspiration is successful, evacuate as much pus as possible and send to laboratory for cultures. If pus cannot be adequately drained using needle aspiration, perform incision and drainage.
7. To perform incision and drainage, first make a 1- to 2-cm vertical incision through the mucosa overlying point of greatest fluctuance. Then insert a curved hemostat through incision and gently spread to break loculations. Suction with rigid suction as necessary.
8. Send samples of purulent material to laboratory for aerobic and anaerobic culture.

CLINICAL TIPS

1. Signs and symptoms characteristic of a peritonsillar abscess include trismus, dysphagia, odynophagia, drooling, fever, "hot potato" voice, deviation of the uvula away from the abscess, and bulging of the posterolateral soft palate.
2. A needle guard can be made by trimming the terminal portion of the plastic needle cover so that 0.5 to 1 cm of the needle protrudes. This is then taped in place so that it will not be dislodged. A blade guard is made by simply wrapping adhesive tape around the blade several times so that 0.5 to 1 cm of the blade tip is exposed.
3. If pus is not obtained after three-point aspiration, the swelling and erythema most likely represent a cellulitis rather than an abscess. In such

cases, patients usually should be admitted to the hospital, started on parenteral antibiotics, and reassessed in 24 hours for possible abscess formation.

4. Up to 90% of peritonsillar abscesses are localized in the superior pole; this is the optimum site for aspiration or incision.
5. Take care during these procedures to avoid laterally directed aspiration or incision. Branches of the facial artery are just lateral to the constrictor muscles and the carotid vessels are located no more than 2 cm lateral to the tonsillar fossae.
6. Be prepared to manage a compromised airway and have all equipment at hand. Have suction readily accessible.

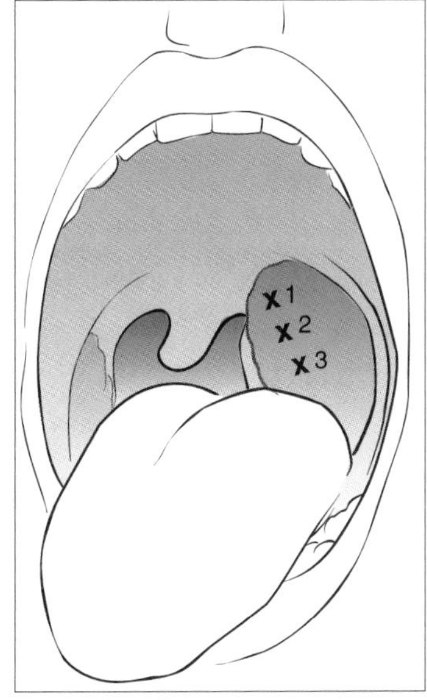

FIGURE 29.1 Aspiration of a peritonsillar abscess is performed using a 3.5-inch, 20- or 22-gauge needle (a spinal needle will suffice) attached to a Luer-Lok 3- or 5-mL syringe. A needle guard should always be used to prevent arterial puncture (see Fig. 29.2). The first attempt in the typical three-point needle aspiration of a possible peritonsillar abscess is made at the supratonsillar area of the greatest pharyngotonsillar bulge. This is superior and medial to the tonsil, at the junction of the anterior tonsillar pillar and the soft palate. The second aspiration is made 0.5 to 1 cm below the first if pus is not obtained; a third attempt may be performed 0.5 to 1 cm lower, near the inferior pole. As much pus as possible should be drained, and the aspirated fluid should be sent to the laboratory for aerobic and anaerobic cultures. If the purulent material cannot be adequately drained by needle aspiration, incision and drainage should usually be performed.

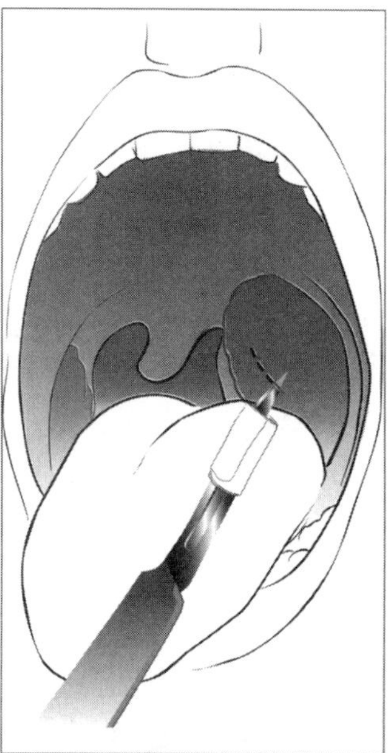

A

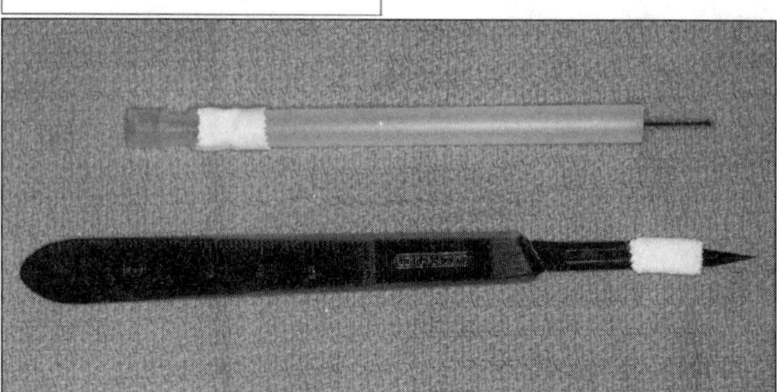

B

FIGURE 29.2 As with any other type of abscess, the optimal site for incision and drainage of a peritonsillar abscess is at the point of maximal fluctuance. **A:** A no. 11 or 12 surgical scalpel blade with an adhesive tape blade guard is used to incise 1 to 2 cm of mucosa overlying the area of greatest pharyngotonsillar bulge. A curved hemostat is then placed though the incision and gently spread to extend the incision and break loculated abscess pockets. The abscess cavity should be swabbed for cultures. Large amounts of drainage should be suctioned using a rigid Yankauer suction device. **B:** Needle guard and blade guard.

CHAPTER 30 •

Diagnostic Laryngoscopic Procedures

OVERVIEW

Diagnostic Laryngoscopy Using a Flexible Fiberoptic Laryngoscope

1. Apply topical vasoconstrictor and anesthetic to one or both nares using cotton pledgets or a spray device—1% ephedrine sulfate and 2% tetracaine hydrochloride is a good combination. Allow 5 to 10 minutes to achieve full effects of these agents.
2. Before inserting fiberoptic laryngoscope, view an object through eyepiece to ensure that tip is clean and focal length is correct.
3. Deflect tip back and forth using control lever on head of laryngoscope to determine force necessary to move tip a given amount.
4. While viewing through eyepiece, insert fiberoptic laryngoscope along floor of nasal cavity parallel to septum and medial to inferior turbinate. Examine entire nasal cavity, noting adenoid size, patency of eustachian tube orifice, nasal polyps, etc.
5. At posterior nasal cavity, deflect tip of fiberoptic laryngoscope inferiorly and advance tip around posterior aspect of soft palate. Landmarks at this point are base of tongue and medial aspect of each tonsil.
6. Advance laryngoscope into supraglottic region and carefully examine all important structures. Deflect tip and rotate laryngoscope in a systematic fashion to obtain a complete view of area. Note any abnormal lesions, injuries, presence of a foreign body, etc.
7. Assess vocal cord function. With infants and younger children, observe movement of cords with phonation or crying. With older children and adolescents, have the patient say "EEEEE" and whistle (or hum) a tune.

CLINICAL TIPS

1. Because indirect laryngoscopy with an angled mirror requires significant cooperation from the patient, this procedure is not appropriate for infants and younger children. These patients usually can be examined successfully using a flexible fiberoptic laryngoscope.
2. Diagnostic laryngoscopy should not be performed in the outpatient setting when the patient is in significant respiratory distress due to airway ob-

struction. In such cases, the patient should be transferred to the operating room, where rigid bronchoscopy and emergent tracheostomy can be performed if necessary.

3. Significant adenoid hypertrophy, particularly when the orifice of the eustachian tube is occluded, warrants referral to an otolaryngologist.

4. Foreign bodies of the supraglottic region not identifiable on plain radiographs (e.g., a wooden splinter, fish bone) are commonly found using diagnostic laryngoscopy.

5. Inadvertently introducing a fiberoptic laryngoscope at or below the level of the vocal cords can in rare cases precipitate laryngospasm. Consequently, this procedure is contraindicated in situations when advanced airway management techniques would not be possible.

6. If a laryngeal mirror warmer is not available, the angled mirror can be placed under warm running water and dried before use to prevent fogging.

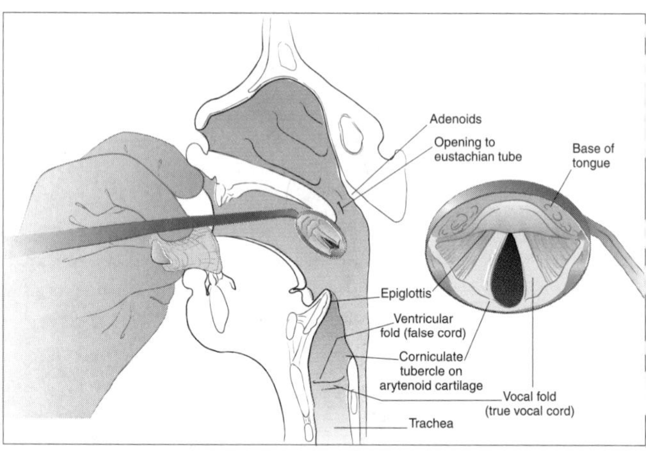

FIGURE 30.1 Indirect laryngoscopy with an angled mirror should be performed with the patient seated and leaning forward in the "sniffing position" [i.e., the head slightly extended (rotated) and the neck flexed]. Spraying Cetacaine (Cetylite Industries, Pennsauken, NJ) or another topical anesthetic may be helpful in controlling the patient's gag reflex. The airway is illuminated with a strong light source (usually an electric head light) focused on the mirror. The tongue is grasped with gauze and gently pulled forward. The mirror is then inserted into the patient's mouth and positioned over the back of the tongue. The larynx and surrounding structures can be visualized by tilting the mirror back and forth as necessary.

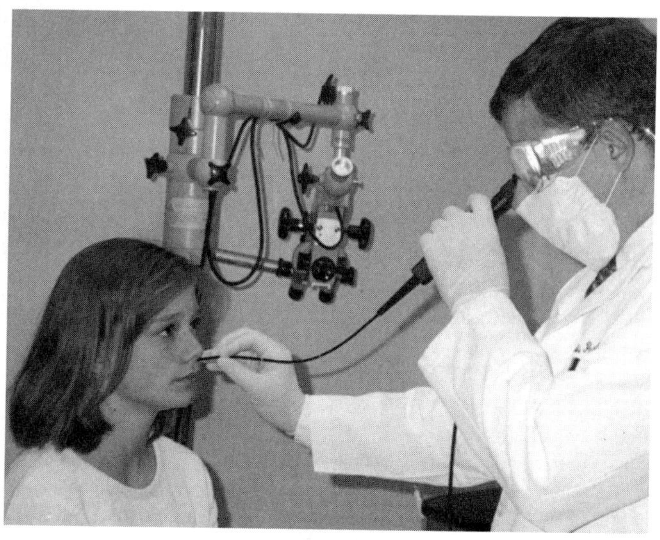

FIGURE 30.2 Positioning for flexible fiberoptic laryngoscopy.

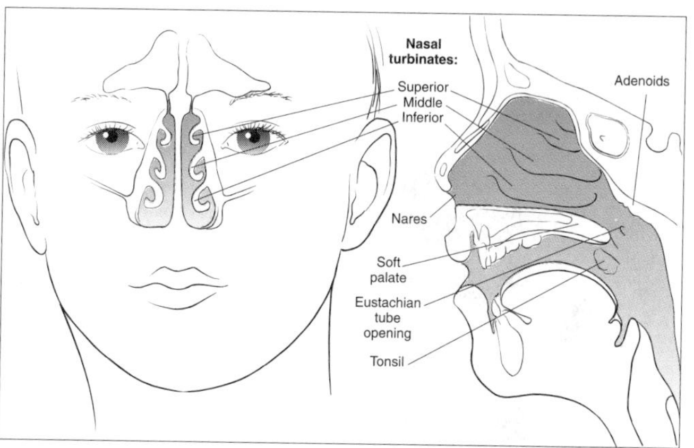

FIGURE 30.3 Anatomy of the nasopharyngeal cavity.

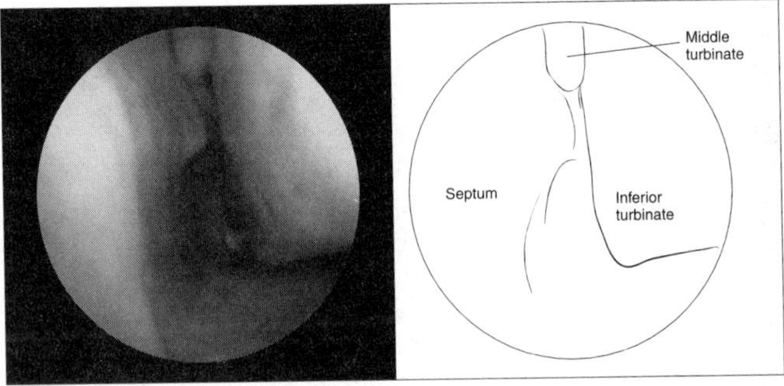

FIGURE 30.4 View of the nasal cavity with fiberoptic laryngoscopy.

7. Special care must be taken when cleansing the insertion tube of a fiberoptic laryngoscope. Grasping it with a gauze and pulling vigorously causes the material covering the fiberoptic bundles to bunch at the tip, making subsequent passage difficult. In addition, bending the insertion tube excessively can break the glass bundles.

8. Having the patient hum or whistle a tune causes adduction and abduction of the vocal cords throughout the full range of motion.

9. The fiberoptic laryngoscope should never be advanced blindly because this increases the likelihood of injury to the nasal or pharyngeal mucosa.

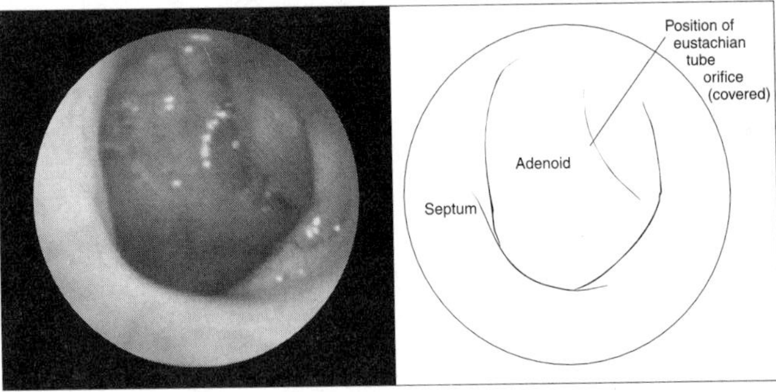

FIGURE 30.5 Adenoid hypertrophy.

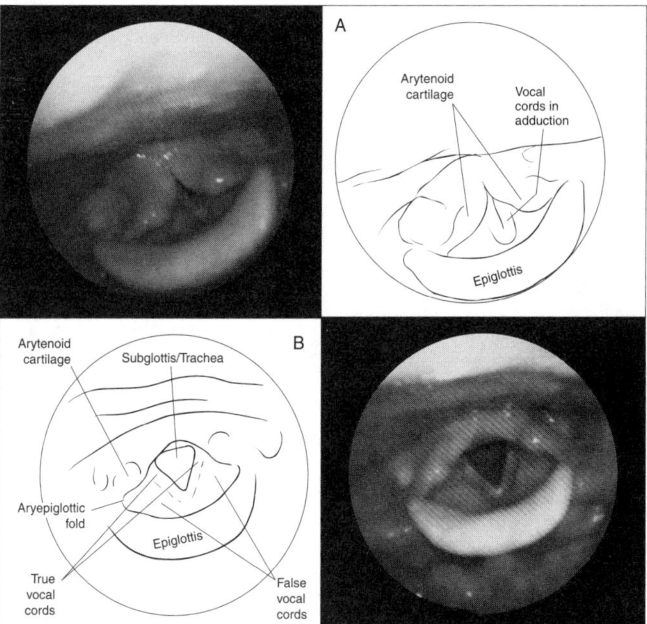

FIGURE 30.6 View of the larynx with fiberoptic laryngoscopy. **A:** Adduction of vocal cords. **B:** Abduction of vocal cords.

CHAPTER 31

Orofacial Anesthesia

OVERVIEW

Infraorbital Nerve Block

1. Locate site of infraorbital foramen by palpation and mark spot with thumb or middle finger.
2. Apply topical anesthesia to mucous membrane.
3. Insert needle at mucolabial fold just anterior to first premolar. Needle axis should follow axis of tooth pointing toward finger marking infraorbital foramen. Do not insert needle more than 2 cm because this increases risk of entering orbit.
4. When needle tip has contacted bone at foramen, aspirate, then slowly inject 1 to 2 mL of anesthetic.
5. Withdraw needle, wait 5 minutes, then test for anesthesia.

Inferior Alveolar Nerve Block

1. Grasp mandibular ramus between thumb and index finger. Determine approximate location of mandibular sulcus on interior surface of ramus midway between thumb and index finger and just above or below level of occlusal plane of teeth, depending on child's age.
2. Apply topical anesthesia to mucous membrane.
3. Hold barrel of syringe over contralateral molars of patients, with needle tip just over mucosa that overlies mandibular sulcus.
4. Advance needle through mucosa until bone is contacted (approximately 15 mm); withdraw needle approximately 1 mm, aspirate, and then inject 1 to 1.8 mL of anesthetic over approximately 1 minute.
5. To guarantee anesthesia of lingual nerve, withdraw needle to half insertion depth and instill additional anesthetic.
6. Withdraw needle, wait approximately 5 minutes, then test for anesthesia by absence of sensation on ipsilateral lower lip.

Infiltration Dental Anesthesia

1. Apply topical anesthesia to mucous membrane.
2. Grasp lip with piece of gauze, and retract it to expose mucobuccal fold.

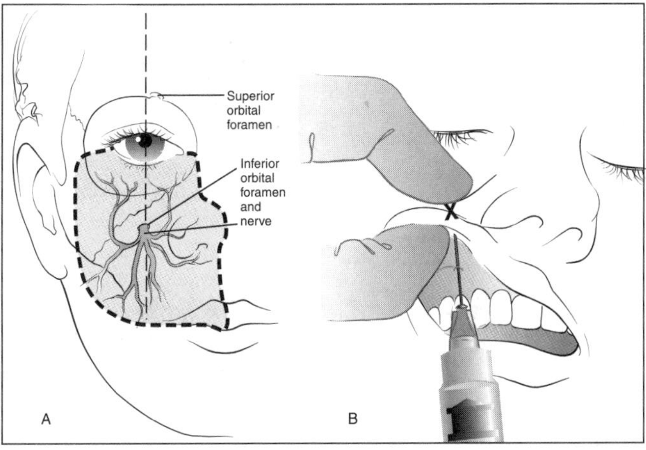

FIGURE 31.1 Infraorbital nerve block. **A:** The primary landmark for an infraorbital nerve block is the inferior orbital foramen. Following an imaginary line drawn perpendicular to the face that intersects the pupil, a shallow depression can be palpated approximately 0.5 cm down from the inferior rim of the orbit. The inferior orbital foramen lies within this depression. **B:** One finger is used to mark the site of the foramen while the other fingers retract the lip. The needle is inserted in the mucolabial fold (where the mucosal aspect of the upper lip meets the maxillary bone) just anterior to the apex of the first premolar tooth. The needle tip should be advanced along the axis of the tooth toward the infraorbital foramen. After aspirating to exclude intravascular needle placement, approximately 1 to 2 mL of anesthetic is slowly deposited. The needle should never be advanced more than 1 to 2 cm from the insertion point to avoid entry into the orbital cavity.

3. Insert needle through mucobuccal fold with bevel oriented toward bone.
4. Advance needle to level of apex of tooth (2 mm for primary anterior maxillary teeth, 1.5 cm for permanent teeth).
5. Aspirate, then inject 1 to 2 mL of anesthetic over 1 minute.
6. Withdraw needle, then wait 5 to 10 minutes for anesthesia to take effect; confirm anesthesia by the absence of pain with manipulation.

CLINICAL TIPS

1. Younger or uncooperative patients may require sedation using nitrous oxide or intravenous conscious sedation.
2. It may be helpful to suggest that the child close his or her eyes just before

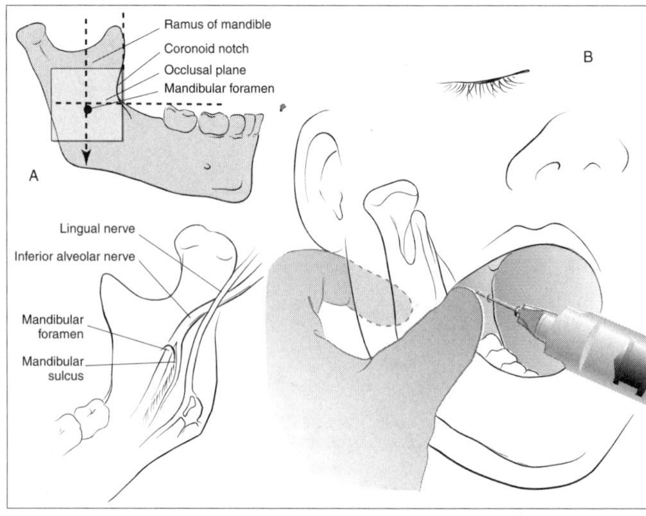

FIGURE 31.2 Inferior alveolar nerve block. **A:** The goal of this block is to place the anesthetic in the mandibular sulcus, the notch that funnels into the mandibular foramen. This site can be found by drawing an imaginary line perpendicular to the face originating at the deepest portion of the anterior aspect of the ramus (coronoid notch). The mandibular sulcus lies at the point along this line halfway between the anterior and posterior aspects of the ramus of the mandible. **B:** With the barrel of the syringe positioned over the contralateral mandibular canine tooth (or primary molar in younger children), the needle is inserted at the coronoid notch and advanced until it contacts the bony surface of the inner aspect of the mandible. The needle is then withdrawn approximately 1 mm. Intravascular needle placement is excluded by aspiration, and up to 1.8 mL of anesthetic (or maximum dose based on patient's weight) is injected over 30 to 60 seconds.

the injection. The child should be warned of the pinch or pain that is about to occur. The needle should be concealed as long as possible to reduce anxiety.

3. Distraction techniques can be very effective. Singing or talking to the child by the physician or parent may make the patient more comfortable. Another technique involves pressing the lip firmly at some site away from the injection site. While inserting the needle and injecting the anesthetic, the lip is gently shaken.
4. Having an uncooperative patient keep the mouth open may difficult. This can be facilitated using a mouth prop. This device is commonly used by dentists and is available in various sizes. Alternatively, several tongue

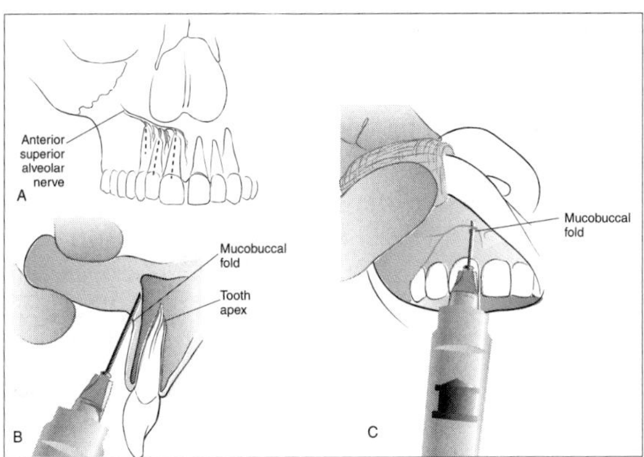

FIGURE 31.3 Supraperiosteal infiltration. **A:** Nerve supply of maxillary teeth. **B:** Needle insertion at the mucobuccal fold allows deposition of anesthesia close to the tooth apex. **C:** Minimal depth of needle insertion (approximately 2 mm) is required for the anterior primary maxillary teeth.

blades covered with layers of gauze and held together by tape may serve the same purpose.

5. Younger and uncooperative children should be restrained appropriately to avoid unexpected movements. Both the injecting and supporting hands should be anchored against the patient's face or teeth when anesthetic is injected.

TABLE 31.1 Characteristics of Common Dental Anesthetics

Anesthetic Agent	*Relative Toxicity*[a]	*Maximum Dose (mg/kg)*	*Maximum Total Dose (mg)*	*Class*
Lidocaine 2%	2	4.0	300	Amide
Lidocaine 2% with epinephrine	2	4.0	500	Amide
Mepivacaine 3%	1.5	6.6	400	Amide
Mepivacaine 2% with epinephrine	1.5	6.6	400	Amide
Bupivacaine 0.5%	3+	2	175	Amide
Bupivacaine 0.5% with epinephrine	3+	2	225	Amide
Procaine[b] 4%	1	20	1000	Ester[c]

[a] Refers to cardiac and neurologic toxicities.

[b] Novocain (Sanofi Winthrop, New York, NY).

[c] The esters have a much greater allergic potential than the amides.

Adapted from Bennett CR. *Monheim's local anesthesia and pain control in dental practice*, 7th ed. St. Louis: CV Mosby, 1984.

6. Treatment should begin immediately after the onset of anesthesia. Delay from the time of anesthesia to the start of treatment is a common cause of anesthesia failure. This is especially true in children because both diffusion and absorption of anesthetic may be more rapid.
7. When performing a nerve block, injecting anesthetic directly into the neural foramen should be avoided because this can damage the nerve. If the patient complains of paresthesias at any time, the needle has likely entered the nerve and should be withdrawn (until no paresthesias are felt) before injection of anesthetic.

CHAPTER 32

Incision and Drainage of a Dental Abscess

OVERVIEW

1. Provide sedation when necessary.
2. Apply topical anesthesia followed by local infiltrative anesthesia or regional nerve block.
3. Make horizontal incision through area of fluctuance; have suction or gauze sponge ready to catch any pus and extend incision to bone for periapical abscess.
4. Widen incision with hemostat; dissect through bone for periapical abscess when possible.
5. Irrigate wound with saline through a 20-gauge angiocatheter.
6. Place drain or packing (if desired); suture drain into place.
7. Begin 5-day course of oral antibiotics.
8. Encourage warm-water rinses for first 24 hours.
9. Refer for dental follow-up at 24 to 48 hours.

CLINICAL TIPS

1. Acute drainage in the emergency department is indicated only in stable patients for whom dental referral will be delayed, or when pain relief is necessary and a dentist is unavailable.
2. Carious teeth suggest a periapical rather than a periodontal abscess.
3. Good anesthesia is crucial. Treatment is rarely successful if a child feels any significant pain.
4. All patients require dental follow-up for more definitive treatment.

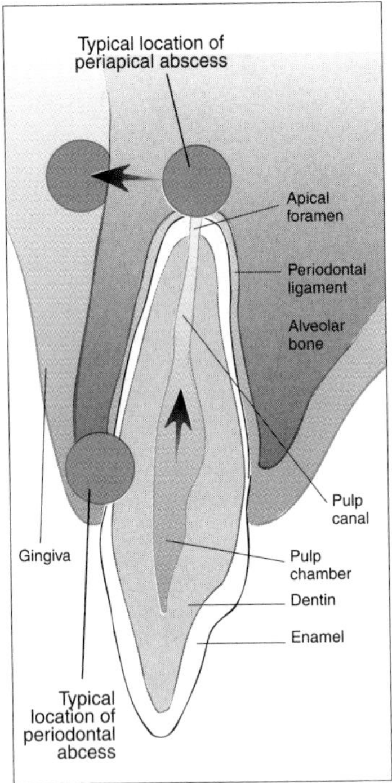

FIGURE 32.1 Periodontal abscesses are commonly located along the margin of the gingiva where the tooth emerges. Unlike in adults, periodontal abscesses in children are not associated with periodontal disease. Often a cause cannot be elucidated, but frequently they are due to impaction of a foreign body in the periodontal tissue. Periapical abscesses, as the name implies, occur at the apex of the tooth. A periapical abscess can be seen externally when pus tracks through the alveolar bone and forms a collection within the gingival tissue. In contrast to a periodontal abscess, a periapical abscess is almost always associated with a nonvital tooth.

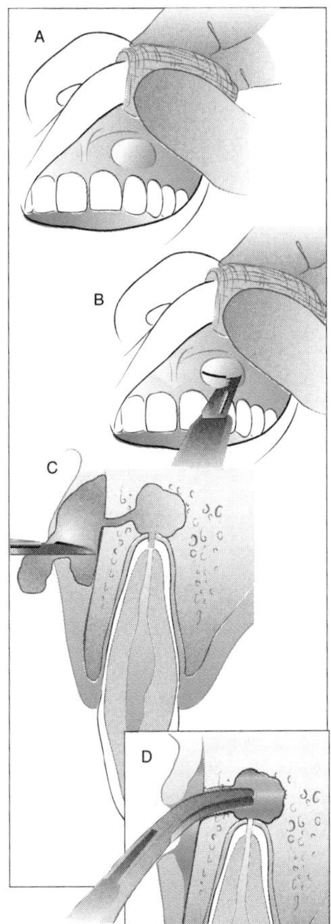

FIGURE 32.2 Before incision and drainage of a dental abscess, local or regional anesthesia should be administered for the affected area. Children should be appropriately immobilized as needed. A bite block (a rubber block that is placed between the molars) or a mouth prop (an adjustable metal prop) may also be required. **A:** Incision and drainage should be performed at the point of maximal fluctuance or swelling. **B:** With the scalpel blade perpendicular to the bone, a horizontal incision is made through the gingiva. **C:** For periodontal abscesses, entry into the abscess cavity is sufficient. For a periapical abscess (as illustrated), the incision should extend down to the alveolar bone and should be long enough to allow proper drainage without premature closure. **D:** The incision should be widely opened by dissection using a hemostat along the abscess tract. For periapical abscesses, the dissection should proceed through the bone to the periapical area to allow adequate drainage of the source of infection.

CHAPTER 33 •

Management of Dental Fractures

OVERVIEW

1. Account for any missing tooth fragments.
2. Use restraint, conscious sedation, and bite block as needed.
3. Inject regional or local anesthesia.
4. Irrigate fractured tooth and surrounding area with normal saline.
5. Dry fractured tooth and surrounding area with suction and gauze pads.
6. Apply calcium hydroxide or glass ionomer product to fracture with applicator stick or wooden end of a cotton-tipped swab

CLINICAL TIPS

1. Follow-up care with a dentist is essential for optimal outcome.
2. Extreme sensitivity is common after a tooth fracture involving dentin or pulp.
3. Prognosis for teeth with pulpal exposure or deeper dentin involvement is time dependent.
4. Calcium hydroxide or glass ionomer application is not indicated if delay in treatment is greater than several hours, or if the tooth is grossly contaminated, because more extensive pulp treatment will be required.
5. Visualization of a central pink area or bleeding from the tooth is diagnostic for pulp involvement.

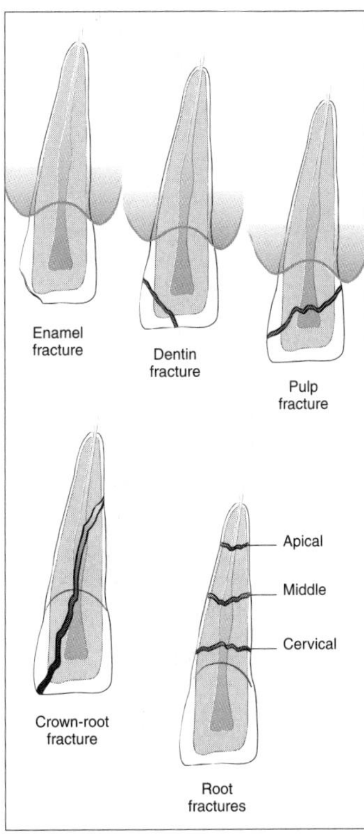

FIGURE 33.1 Dental fractures are classified as complicated or uncomplicated depending on whether the pulp is exposed. The simplest fractures are those involving only the enamel. Fractures that involve the dentin can be identified by the presence of a yellow area within the fracture site and an associated sensitivity of the tooth. Fractures resulting in pulp exposure are identified by the presence of a pink area or an actual bleeding spot located in the center of the tooth. Crown-root fractures are visible above the gingiva but extend into the root of the tooth. They involve the enamel, dentin, and frequently the pulp. Root fractures are classified according to their location along the length of the root. The cervical third of the root is adjacent to the clinical crown, and the apical third is located at the root apex.

TABLE 33.1 Differentiating Characteristics of Primary and Secondary Teeth

Characteristics	*Primary Teeth*	*Secondary Teeth*
Age	<6 yr	>6 yr
Color	Milky white, opalescent	White to yellowish-gray
Size	Smaller	Larger
Clinical crown length	Shorter	Wider
Shape	Smooth	Ridged
Radiographic appearance	Developing permanent tooth visible	No apical structures visible

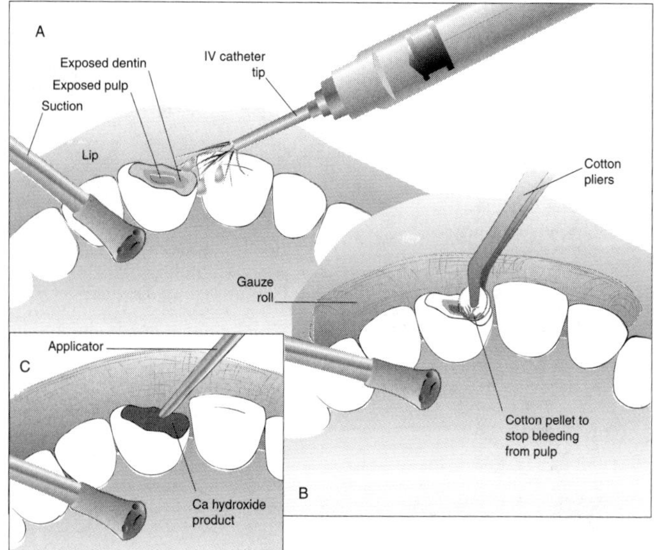

FIGURE 33.2 Dental fractures of secondary teeth that expose dentin or pulp sometimes require application of a temporary protective coating. Measures that facilitate this procedure include appropriate restraint (as needed), a mouth prop, and liberal anesthesia of the affected area. This is only a temporizing procedure, and follow-up with a dentist should occur within 24 hours. **A:** The fractured tooth and surrounding area are irrigated with normal saline though a syringe and intravenous catheter while oral suction is used simultaneously to remove any loose material or blood. **B:** Once the area has been cleaned, it is dried but not desiccated using a combination of a suction catheter and gauze pads. Gauze rolls are placed between the lip and tooth and generous oral suction is used to prevent contamination of the tooth by oral secretions. Any bleeding from the pulp can usually be controlled with pressure from cotton pellets on the end of cotton pliers. **C:** Calcium hydroxide base and catalyst or glass ionomer product is mixed on a mixing pad and a thin layer is applied directly to the pulp and surrounding 2 mm of dentin using the applicator or the wooden end of a cotton-tipped swab. The material should be allowed to dry for a few minutes before the mouth prop is removed.

TABLE 33.2 Eruption Schedule for Secondary Dentition

	Age (yr)	
	Lower	*Upper*
Central incisors	6–7	7–8
Lateral incisors	7–8	8–9
Cuspids	9–10	11–12
First bicuspids	10–12	10–11
Second bicuspids	11–12	10–12
First molars	6–7	6–7
Second molars	11–13	12–13
Third molars	17–21	17–21

TABLE 33.3 Emergency Department Management of Dental Fractures

Injury Type	*Clinical Findings*	*Treatment Options*
Primary teeth	See Table 33.1	• Extraction • Dental referral
Secondary teeth		
Enamel	• Chip of top layer	• Dental referral
Dentin	• Exposed yellow area below enamel • Tooth sensitivity	• Dental referral • Temporary $Ca(OH)_2$ or glass ionomer coating
Pulp	• Exposed pink area • Frank bleeding dot • Tooth sensitivity	• Temporary $Ca(OH)_2$ or glass ionomer coating
Crown-root fracture	• Fracture line visible above gingiva and extends into root	• Dental referral
Root fracture	• Tooth mobility • Bleeding at gingiva • Fracture on radiograph	• Splinting for cervical and middle third root fractures

CHAPTER 34

Reimplanting an Avulsed Permanent Tooth

OVERVIEW

1. Always handle tooth by its crown.
2. Inspect tooth for fractures.
3. Cleanse tooth by gently swirling it in normal saline solution or a commercial medium.
4. Locate empty socket; for better visualization, lightly suction or swab surrounding area.
5. Position tooth at socket opening.
6. Reinsert tooth smoothly, applying firm but gentle pressure.
7. Hold tooth in place manually or have child bite on gauze pad until dentist arrives.

CLINICAL TIPS

1. Reimplantation is indicated only for an avulsed permanent tooth, not for a deciduous (primary) tooth.
2. The tooth must be reimplanted immediately. Delay reduces the chance of success.
3. If the physician cannot reimplant the tooth, it should be stored in milk.
4. The tooth must always be handled by its crown. The root should never be touched.
5. The dentist should be consulted as soon as the physician is notified about the case.

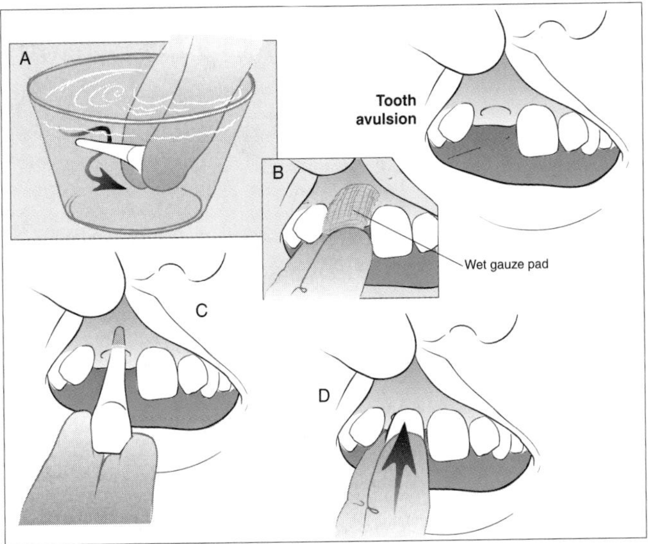

FIGURE 34.1 A permanent tooth should be reimplanted in the socket as soon as possible after avulsion. After identifying it as a permanent tooth, it should be inspected for fractures. Reimplantation is contraindicated if a root fracture or a vertical fracture more than half its length is identified. **A:** The best way to cleanse debris off the tooth is to hold it by the crown and gently swirl it in Hanks' balanced salt solution, normal saline, or milk. The tooth must never be scrubbed because this injures the periodontal ligament fibers. **B:** Before reimplanting the tooth, the area surrounding the socket can be gently swabbed with a wet gauze or cleared with low suction. Usually, the socket itself does not require suctioning, even when a clot has formed, because newly formed clots tend to be soft and displace easily during reimplantation. A hematoma or ecchymosis of the mucosa apical to the socket suggests the possibility of an alveolar bone fracture. **C:** To reimplant the tooth, it is first positioned and aligned correctly at the socket opening. Administering a sedative or local anesthetic before reinsertion usually is not indicated. **D:** With firm but gentle pressure, the tooth is reinserted into the depth of the socket. If the child resists reinsertion, the alveolus should be inspected for fractures. Often the reimplanted tooth protrudes a little more than its nonavulsed equal. The tooth must be stabilized until a splint can be applied by the dentist; the child can bite on a gauze pad, or a responsible adult can hold the tooth in place with finger pressure.

CHAPTER 35

Repair of Lip Lacerations

OVERVIEW

1. Assess and stabilize life-threatening injuries.
2. Examine injuries for presence of underlying fractures or foreign bodies.
3. Document sensory and motor examination of cranial nerves.
4. Administer conscious sedation as needed.
5. Physically restrain patient with papoose board if necessary.
6. Place bite block or stent mouth open with taped tongue depressor.
7. Administer regional nerve block or local infiltrative anesthetic as indicated.
8. Carry out any necessary debridement or excision.
9. Irrigate wound with saline.
10. Identify and mark vermilion border before initiating anesthesia or débridement.
11. Prepare wound borders with povidone–iodine solution.
12. Reapproximate vermilion border.
13. Reapproximate inner fibrofatty junction with resorbable 3-0 or 4-0 suture using interrupted stitches with inverted knots.
14. Close outer fibrofatty junction in same manner.
15. Unite fibrofatty junction at free edge.
16. Close dermal-fat junction with inverted interrupted resorbable 4-0 sutures.
17. Ensure vermilion border is reapproximated exactly.
18. Close epidermal-dermal layer sewing "away from" vermilion border using 5-0 nonresorbable sutures.
19. Close remaining vermilion with 5-0 nonresorbable suture if laceration is limited to dry vermilion, or 4-0 resorbable suture if it extends to wet vermilion.

Tongue Lacerations

1. Optimize visualization using bite block or 3-0 silk suture placed through tip of tongue and used for retraction.
2. Close small lacerations with interrupted 3-0 or 4-0 sutures placed through mucosa and muscle and tied with inverted knots.
3. Close larger lacerations in two layers with 3-0 or 4-0 resorbable sutures in inverted interrupted stitches.

Buccal Mucosa Lacerations

1. Close only external skin surface when possible.
2. When necessary, close internal mucosa first using 3-0 or 4-0 resorbable sutures in interrupted or continuous fashion.
3. Repeat irrigation of wound with saline through external surface.
4. Close muscle layer using 3-0 or 4-0 resorbable sutures in inverted interrupted stitch.
5. Reapproximate external skin surface using 5-0 or 6-0 nonresorbable sutures.

Postclosure Care

1. Consider using prophylactic antibiotics.
2. Recommend liquids until anesthetic effect has resolved, and then soft diet for 1 or 2 days.
3. Administer tetanus booster as necessary.

CLINICAL TIPS

1. The vermilion border should be marked or approximated before infiltration anesthesia or débridement.
2. Using epinephrine in infiltration anesthesia obscures the vermilion border.
3. Using a regional anesthetic block avoids distortion of soft tissue landmarks.
4. Inverted sutures and multiple knots are useful to avoid untying.
5. The orbicularis oris must be approximated or it will result in a depressed scar when in motion.

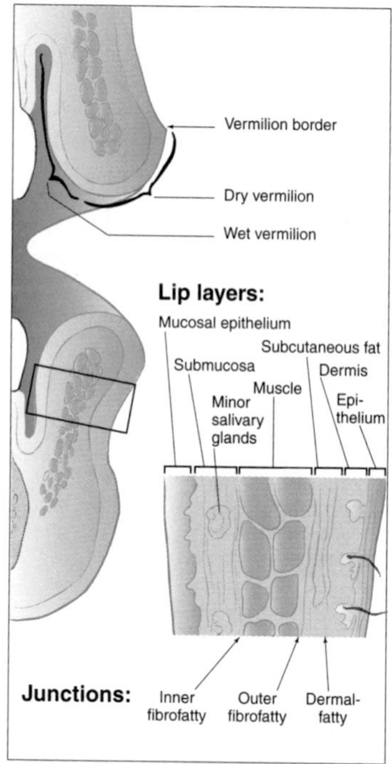

FIGURE 35.1 The structure of the lip is multilayered, with the skin comprising the external layer and the mucosa the internal layer. The middle layer is composed of muscle (the orbicularis oris), which encircles the mouth. A fibrofatty junction borders both the inside and the outside surfaces of the muscle. Between the inner fibrofatty junction and the mucosa, a layer of submucosal or minor salivary glands is present. The vermilion border is the mucocutaneous junction of the lips where the mucosa meets the skin. The most common lip injury treated in the emergency department is a through-and-through laceration. These lacerations often involve the vermilion border, which is a fixed and obvious landmark.

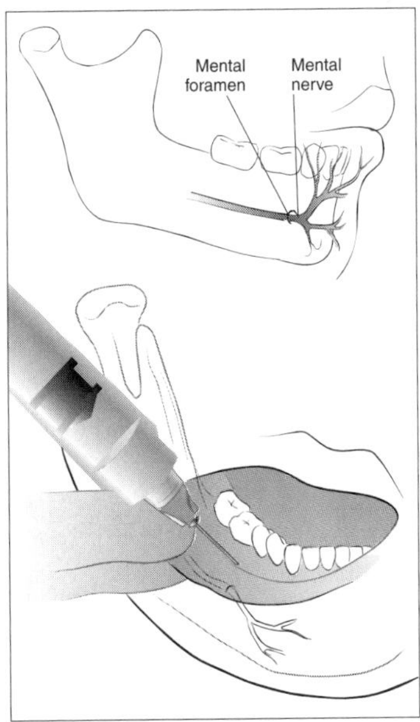

FIGURE 35.2 A mental nerve block may be used for lacerations of the lower lip. It produces less distortion of soft tissue landmarks and requires less total anesthetic injection than direct infiltration. A mental nerve block results in anesthesia of the buccal gingiva anterior to the mental foramen, as well as the mucosa and skin of the lower lip from the midline to the labial commissure on the side of the injection. The mental foramen can be palpated near the apex of the second primary molar of a young child or near the apex of the second premolar of an adolescent. The lip and buccal tissues are tautly retracted using the fingers of the nondominant hand. A 25-gauge or smaller needle is inserted at the reflection of the buccal and gingival mucosa, angled slightly anterior to the mental foramen. The needle is advanced approximately 5 mm and, if no blood is aspirated, 0.5 to 1 mL of 1% lidocaine is injected. If paresthesias are described by the patient indicating entry of the needle into the nerve or foramen, the needle should be withdrawn slightly before injection of lidocaine.

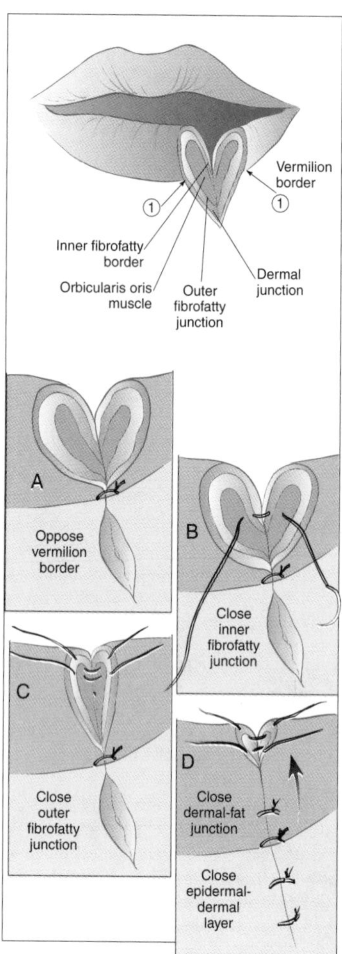

FIGURE 35.3 Closure of a through-and-through lip laceration should occur in three layers. **A:** A stitch that aligns the vermilion border may be placed at the beginning of the closure. **B:** The inner fibrofatty junction at the wound apex is then reapproximated using a resorbable 3-0 or 4-0 suture. Interrupted sutures with inverted knots provide adequate reapproximation without protrusion of the knots through the wound. **C:** The outer fibrofatty junction is approximated next, and the two fibrofatty junctions are united at the free edge. **D:** The dermal-fat junction is then closed with an inverted interrupted stitch using resorbable 4-0 suture. Alignment of the vermilion border must remain perfect before and after this layer is sutured. Finally, the epidermal-dermal layer is approximated by suturing "away from" the vermilion-cutaneous junction toward the wound apex in the skin using a 5-0 nonresorbable material such as nylon.

CHAPTER 36

Reduction of Temporomandibular Joint Dislocation

OVERVIEW

1. Administer conscious sedation as needed.
2. Position patient upright in chair and straddle patient's lap.
3. Protect thumbs by generously wrapping them in gauze.
4. Place thumbs against lower posterior molars and wrap fingers around angle and body of mandible.
5. Apply slow, steady pressure, first downward and then posteriorly.

CLINICAL TIPS

1. Use of sedation is highly recommended to alleviate anxiety and decrease the degree of muscle spasm.
2. Stimulation of the gag reflex has been described in adults as a successful alternative to manual reduction.
3. Gentle rocking of the mandible or digital massage may fatigue muscles that are in spasm and ease reduction.
4. With a bilateral dislocation, reduction of one condyle at a time may be useful when spasm is severe.
5. Dislocations associated with fractures should be referred to an oral surgeon for reduction.

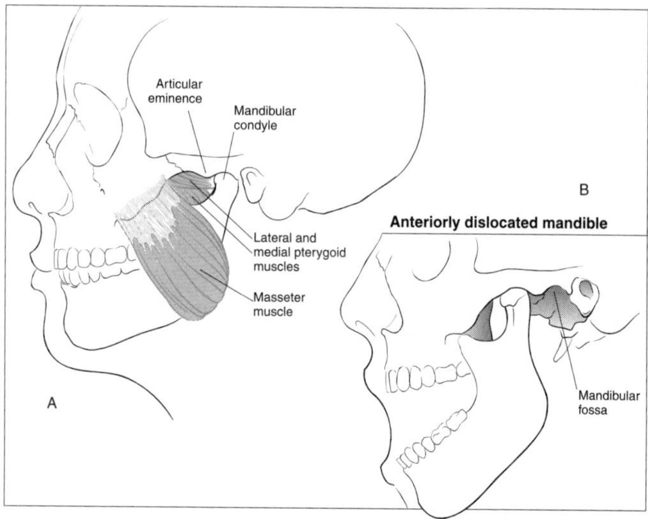

FIGURE 36.1 **A:** Anatomy of the temporomandibular joint. **B:** Anterior dislocation of the temporomandibular joint.

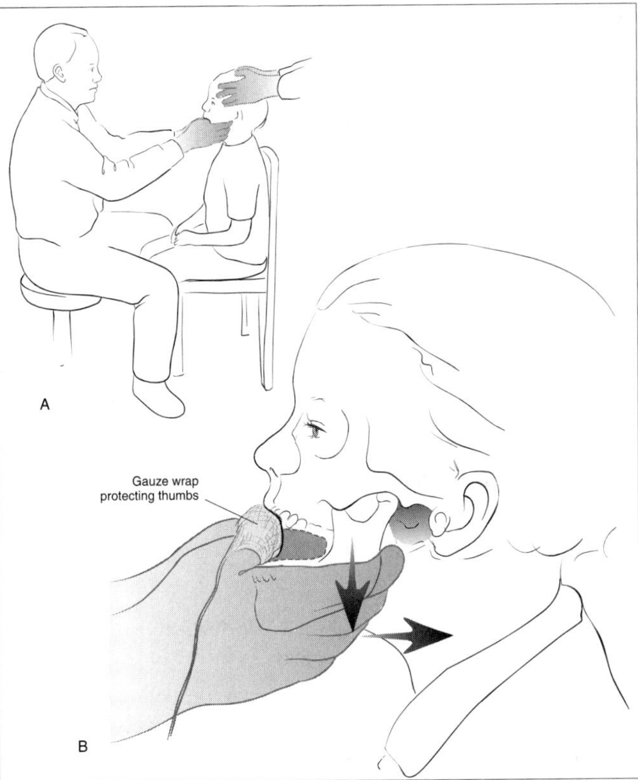

FIGURE 36.2 Technique for reduction of temporomandibular joint dislocation. **A:** The patient is positioned in a chair facing the clinician. The head is held firmly by an assistant or stabilized posteriorly against a wall or head rest. Further control is gained by straddling the patient's lap. **B:** Both thumbs are swathed in gauze to avoid injury when the mandible snaps back into place. The thumbs are placed against the surface of the lower molars as far posteriorly as possible. The fingers of each hand are wrapped under the angle and body of the mandible. Pressure is applied first in a downward motion to release the condyle from the articular eminence, and then posteriorly to move the condyle back into the fossa.

CHAPTER 37

Converting Stable Supraventricular Tachycardia Using Vagal Maneuvers

OVERVIEW

1. The child is assessed for appropriateness of vagal maneuvers in the particular clinical context (see Clinical Tips 1 through 3 and Fig. 37.1).
2. An intravenous access line is placed.
3. Monitoring and resuscitation equipment and medications are made available at the bedside.
4. The ice bag (Fig. 37.2, infants and younger children) or carotid massage (Fig. 37.3, older children) procedure is performed.

CLINICAL TIPS

1. Vagal maneuvers are indicated only in stable children who do not exhibit signs of severe hemodynamic compromise.
2. Patients with congestive heart failure or shock require immediate cardioversion.
3. In stable supraventricular tachycardia (SVT), vagal maneuvers are attempted first, but if unsuccessful are followed by adenosine.
4. All children with SVT deserve cardiology consultation even after successful return to sinus rhythm. Many patients warrant a detailed diagnostic workup, including electrophysiologic studies.
5. Vagal maneuvers may be only temporarily effective, and long-term medical therapy is often indicated.
6. Vagal maneuvers often are not effective in young infants.
7. Proper monitoring, intravenous access, and resuscitation equipment and medications must be available for the uncommon, but serious, complication of prolonged asystole.

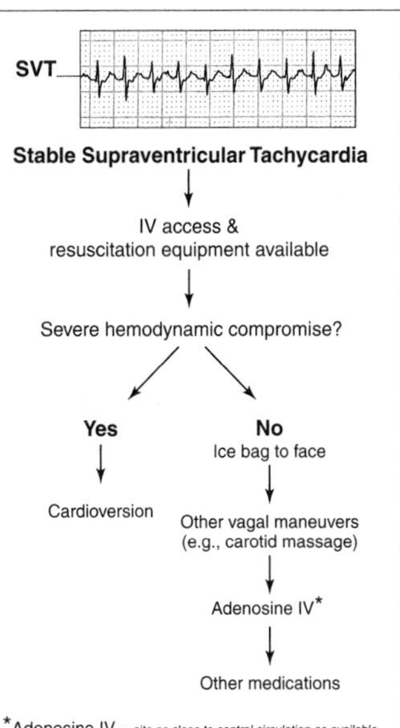

FIGURE 37.1 The child with stable supraventricular tachycardia is approached as illustrated in this algorithm. If hemodynamic status becomes compromised at any point, immediate cardioversion is indicated. If the child remains stable, sequential use of ice bag technique, followed by other vagal maneuvers, intravenous adenosine, and other medications may be used.

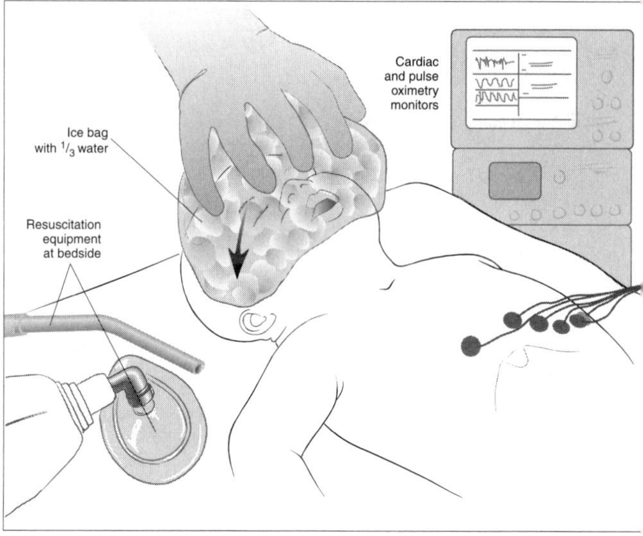

FIGURE 37.2 Ice bag technique. The infant or child should have intravenous access, continuous electrocardiographic monitoring, and pulse oximetry in place. Resuscitation equipment and medications should be available at the bedside. A plastic bag is filled one third with water and an equal volume of ice. The bag should be large enough to completely cover the child's face and overlap the preauricular area. Older children are asked to hold their breath in end-inspiration. Younger children are immobilized. The bag is applied so that it covers the mouth and nose and prevents breathing for a maximum of 15 seconds. If conversion to sinus rhythm occurs sooner, the bag is immediately removed.

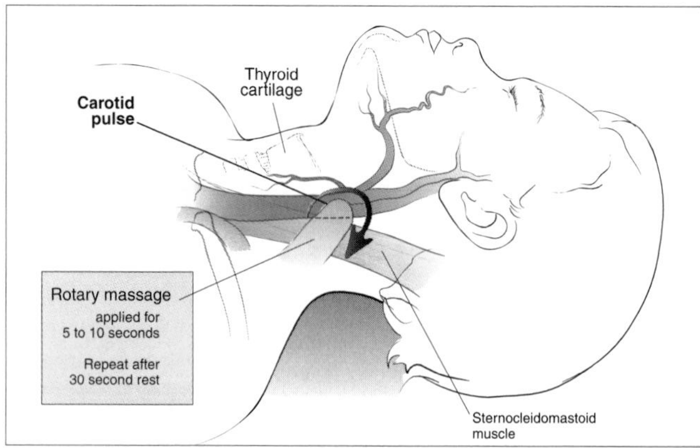

TABLE 37.1 Vagal Maneuvers: Complications

Vagal Maneuver	*Advantage*	*Possible Disadvantage*
All	**Noninvasive**	• **Transient effect** • **Asystole** • **Dysrhythmias**
Ice bag to face	Most successful	• Apnea • Unpleasant
Immersion of face in iced saline with breath holding	Older children can perform themselves	• Unpleasant • Aspiration
Carotid massage	Easy to perform on older children	• Transient ischemic attack/cerebrovascular accident • Not with digoxin toxicity
Rectal stimulation	Can be used in noncooperative or young child	• Tissue trauma • Unpleasant
Valsalva	Older, cooperative child	• Subconjunctival hemorrhages • Rupture of tympanic membrane • Syncope
Antishock trousers	Easy to use	• Limited to toddler size and older
Coughing	Older, cooperative child	• Aspiration • Subconjunctival hemorrhage • Ruptured tympanic membrane • Syncope
Gag reflex	Easy to perform on all ages	• Tissue trauma • Emesis/aspiration • Unpleasant

FIGURE 37.3 Carotid massage technique. The same initial preparations and monitoring are made available as for the ice bag conversion. Carotid massage may be effective in older children with long, narrow necks, but is considered contraindicated in patients with digitalis toxicity. The child's head is turned to the left and tilted backward slightly. The carotid pulse is located, and firm but gentle rotary motion or massage is applied with the fingertip for 5 to 10 seconds without complete occlusion of the pulse. If unsuccessful, the procedure may be repeated after 30 seconds of rest. Simultaneous, bilateral carotid massage should never be done. Additional vagal maneuvers are summarized in Table 37.1.

Emergent Pericardiocentesis

OVERVIEW

1. Assess patient: airway, breathing, circulation.
2. Recognize presence of cardiac tamponade.
   A. Beck's triad—distant heart sounds, increased jugular venous distention, hypotension.
   B. Suspect in appropriate clinical setting in absence of Beck's triad.
3. Position patient in reverse Trendelenburg position to maximize succes rate.
4. Select appropriate sizes of equipment for age; consider using catheter over-wire system if there is chronic effusion to allow continued drainage.
5. Attach needle to grounded electrocardiograph (ECG) lead (if time allows using chest lead.
6. Insert needle at 45-degree angle 1 cm to left of xiphoid process; conside parasternal approach in adolescents.
7. Advance needle (with constant traction on plunger) until fluid is obtaine and withdraw needle a short distance if ECG changes occur; redirect whe ECG changes are ascertained.
8. Assess patient response.
   A. Pulses, blood pressure.

FIGURE 38.1 Pericardiocentesis from substernal approach. Emergent pericardiocentesi is indicated for relief of life-threatening cardiac tamponade (pericardiocentesis is per formed also for less critical indications, typically by subspecialists in the cardiac catheter ization laboratory or operating room after ultrasound imaging). The patient is place supine, or preferably in slight reverse Trendelenburg position if this position can be tol erated. An adequate airway is ensured, and the patient is monitored continuously wit electrocardiography (ECG) and pulse oximetry. Parenteral sedation is required in all bu the most critically ill patients. The operator should don sterile gloves, mask, and gown. I time allows, the needle hub (18- to 20-gauge, 2.5-inch spinal needle, or comparabl Seldinger kit needle) should be attached by alligator clip to a grounded precordial ECC lead. The needle should be equipped with a suitably large syringe (20 to 50 mL). The ski is prepared and, if time permits, anesthetized along with the subcutaneous muscle layer The needle entry site in children is just inferior and 1 cm to the left of the xiphoid pro cess. The needle is directed cephalad toward the tip of the patient's left scapula, at a 30 to 45-degree angle to the skin surface. The plunger of the syringe should be withdraw

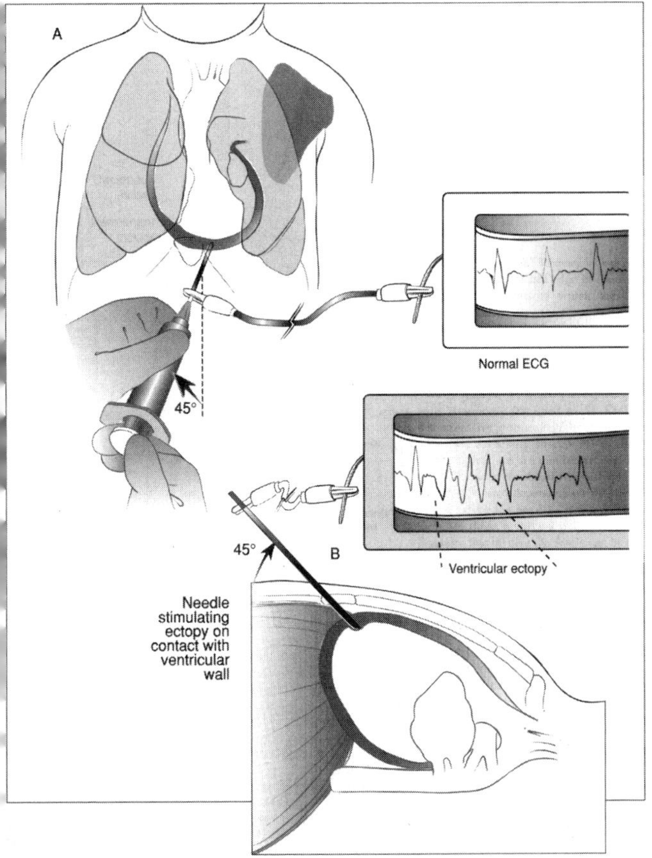

slightly and continuously as the needle advances. The needle is advanced until pericardial fluid is obtained or ECG changes are noted. If fluid is obtained, as much is drained as possible. Optionally, a wire-guided catheter may be placed using the Seldinger technique, attached to a stopcock, and left in place for repeated aspirations as needed. If acute ECG changes are noted, the needle is withdrawn a small distance until baseline ECG pattern returns, then slightly redirected. If clinical circumstances preclude attachment of the precordial ECG lead to the pericardiocentesis needle, at a minimum an assistant should continuously observe the cardiac monitor to visualize immediately any pattern change.

B. Heart sounds.
C. Jugular venous distention.

9. After procedure, follow up with appropriate monitoring in critical care setting or operative intervention.

CLINICAL TIPS

1. Know how to recognize cardiac tamponade—the only indication for emergent pericardiocentesis (distant heart sounds, increased jugular venous distension, and hypotension).
2. Ensure airway control before initiating the procedure.
3. Place the patient in reverse Trendelenburg position to maximize success rate.
4. Two-dimensional echocardiography during the procedure can be valuable to enhance success and to minimize complications.
5. Aim the needle 45 degrees from perpendicular 1 cm left of the xiphoid process. Advance toward left scapula.
6. Observe the ECG for premature ventricular beats, ST-T segment changes, or QRS widening while advancing the needle. Withdraw a short distance when ECG change occurs, then redirect and try again.

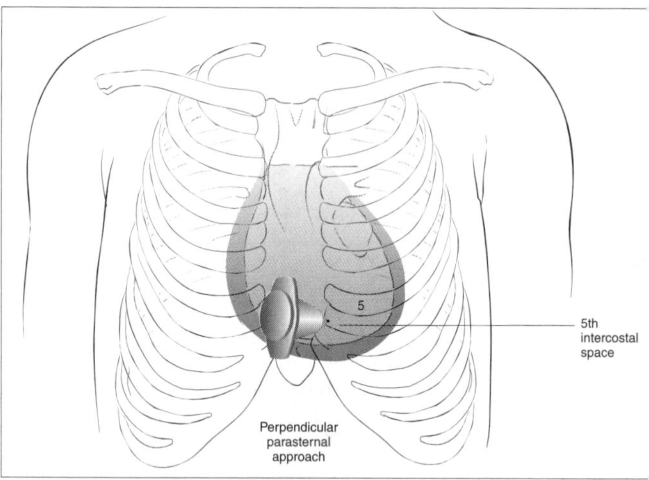

FIGURE 38.2 Pericardiocentesis from parasternal approach. Recent studies using echocardiographic guidance on adult patients have advocated the parasternal approach. This may be more appropriate in older children and adolescents. The same general positioning, preparations, and monitoring considerations apply as for the substernal approach. The needle is inserted perpendicular to the skin surface into the left fifth intercostal space just lateral to the sternum, and advanced slowly with continuous aspiration on the syringe plunger.

CHAPTER 39

Arterial Puncture and Catheterization

OVERVIEW

1. Assess indications and contraindications for arterial puncture or catheterization.
2. Identify optimal site for arterial access.
3. Maintain sterile preparation and technique throughout procedure.
4. Use finger of nondominant hand to locate most superficial (easily palpable) course of artery.
5. Approach skin at 30- to 45-degree angle from horizontal; when attempting catheterization, lower angle slightly once flashback is observed and advance catheter into lumen of artery.
6. Advance catheter over needle; do not withdraw needle until hub of catheter is at skin.
7. Secure catheter to skin with nylon or silk suture material (4-0 or 5-0) and sterile transparent dressing.
8. Connect catheter to appropriate extension or pressure tubing.
9. Use heparinized (2 U/mL) saline to prevent clotting of catheter.

CLINICAL TIPS

Arterial Puncture

1. Site selection is important; know the anatomy. The most commonly used sites in the child include the radial, femoral, and posterior tibial arteries.
2. Failure to detect a pulse may be due to low blood pressure, occlusion of an artery by firm pressure by the assistant, or ill-timed inflation of a blood pressure cuff.
3. Perform and document an Allen test for ulnar collateral flow if the radial artery is to be used for puncture or catheterization.
4. Local infiltration of lidocaine may optimize success of arterial puncture or catheterization.
5. After puncture, apply direct pressure over any arterial site after catheter withdrawal for a full 5 minutes.

Arterial Catheterization

1. Once a flash of blood appears in the transparent chamber, lower the angle of the catheter to the skin and advance 1 to 2 mm to ensure that the catheter is in the lumen of the artery.
2. Do not withdraw the needle; stabilize the needle while advancing the catheter over the needle into the artery.

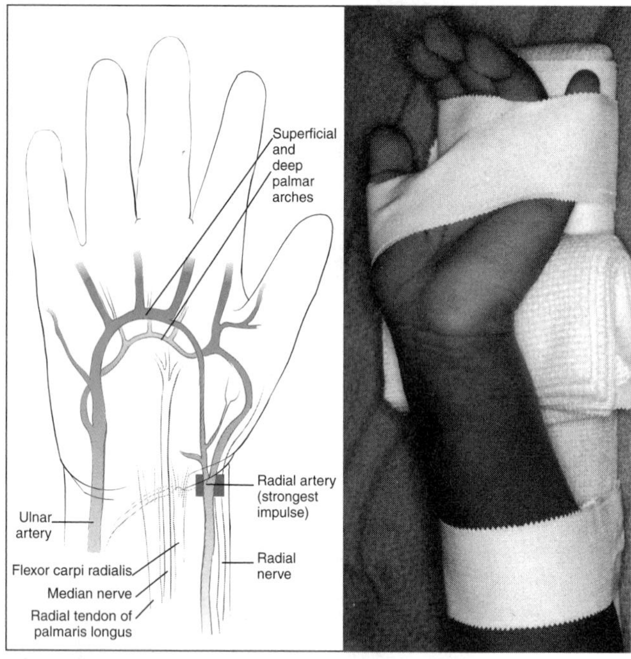

FIGURE 39.1 Radial artery anatomy and positioning for access. The radial artery lies just lateral to the flexor carpi radialis tendon at the second skin crease proximal to the hand. In children, it is often helpful to stabilize the hand and wrist on an armboard, placing the wrist in 30 to 45 degrees of extension over several gauze pads, as illustrated.

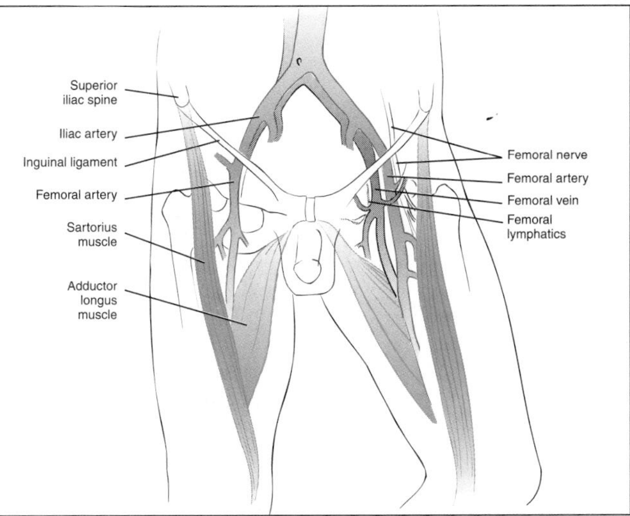

FIGURE 39.2 Femoral artery anatomy. The femoral artery courses through the femoral triangle, and is usually easily palpated there just below the inguinal ligament, at the midpoint between the anterior superior iliac spine and the symphysis pubis.

3. Failure to observe pulsatile blood flow from the catheter may indicate that the back wall of the artery has been punctured. Slowly withdraw the catheter and advance again when pulsatile blood appears in the hub.
4. Secure the catheter with a transparent dressing such that a "window" is available to observe blanching of the skin around the site of the catheter.

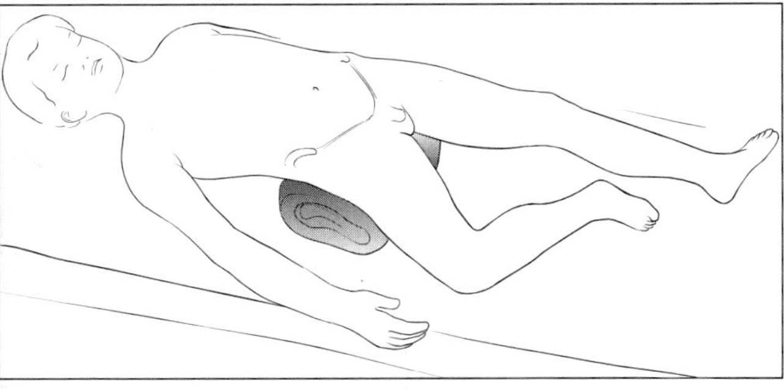

FIGURE 39.3 Positioning of the patient for femoral artery access. The optimal position in children is achieved by externally rotating the leg at the hip and comfortably flexing the leg at the knee.

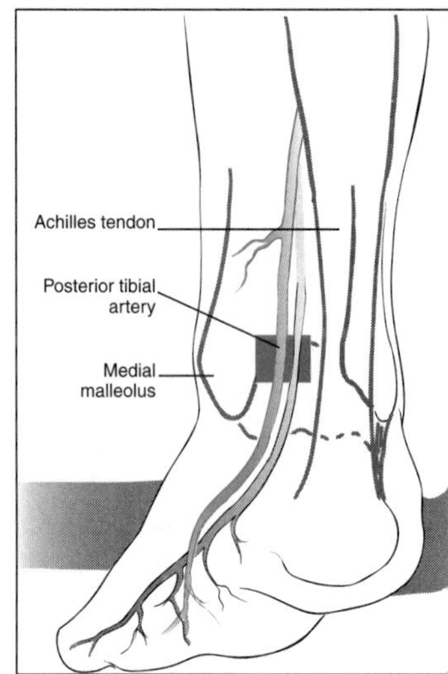

FIGURE 39.4 Posterior tibial artery anatomy. The most accessible site is a point between the medial malleolus and the calcaneus tendon. Cannulation may be facilitated by holding the foot in comfortable dorsiflexion.

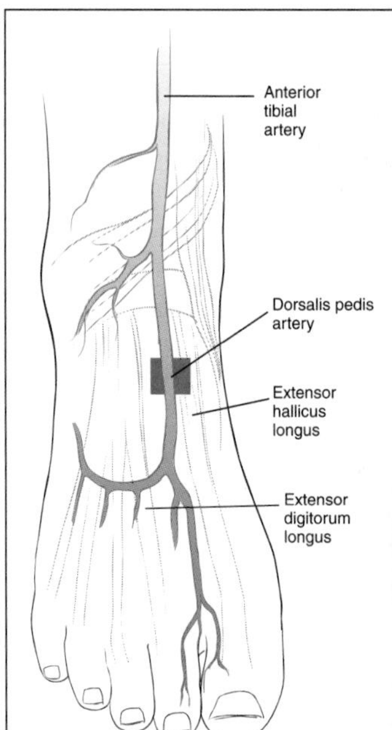

FIGURE 39.5 Dorsalis pedis artery anatomy. Cannulation of the dorsalis pedis is best done at the dorsal midfoot, where the artery courses parallel to the extensor hallucis longus, between it and the extensor digitorum longus. Access is facilitated by holding the foot in mild plantar flexion.

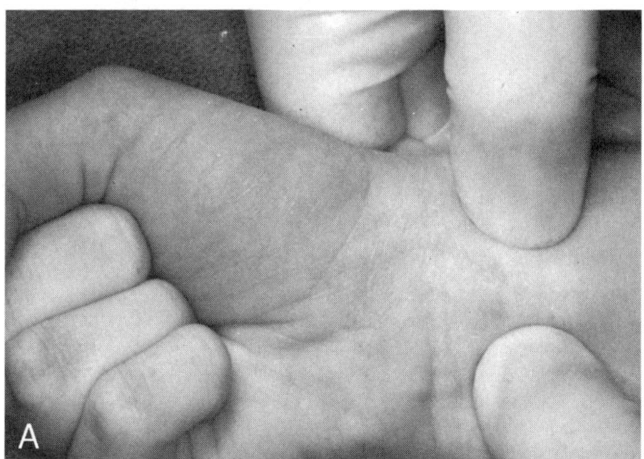

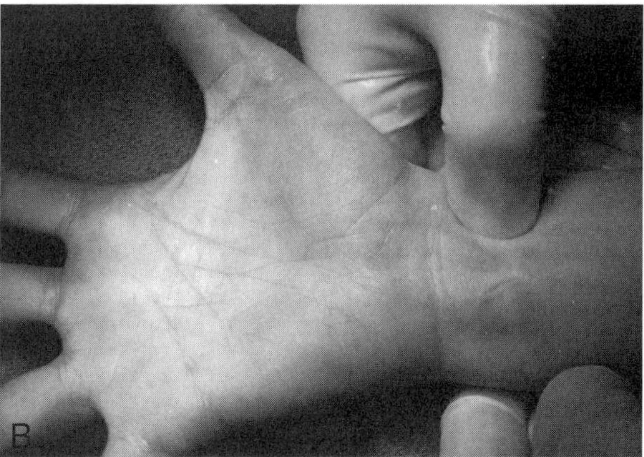

FIGURE 39.6 Allen test for ulnar collateral flow. The test begins by having the patient clench the fist to exsanguinate the hand. In a young, uncooperative, or unconscious patient, exsanguination is effected by manually "milking" the clenched hand or using an elastic bandage wrapped around the hand. Firm digital pressure is then used to occlude the radial and ulnar arteries at the pulse over the wrist (**A**). The hand is opened without hyperextending the fingers and the occlusion of the ulnar artery is released (**B**). The open hand is examined for return of perfusion (rubor). The Allen test is normal if pallor resolves and rubor returns within 5 seconds, indicating adequate collateral flow. The radial artery flow should then be checked to be sure that radial artery pulsation is not due solely to ulnar flow.

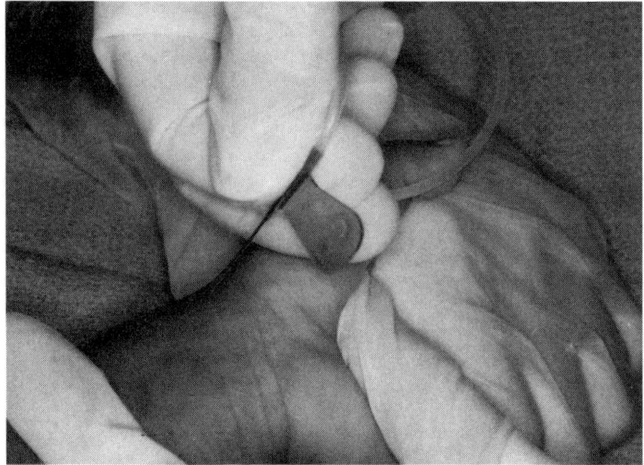

FIGURE 39.7 Arterial puncture. The arterial pulse is located (radial artery illustrated here), and the skin prepared with povidone-iodine. A small amount of 1% lidocaine without epinephrine may be used to anesthetize the skin puncture site. With an uncapped butterfly needle or prepackaged needle and syringe, the skin is approached at a 30- to 45-degree angle to the skin, aiming the needle toward the pulse identified by the proximal finger. The needle is advanced slowly toward the pulse until arterial blood flows into the tubing. At this time, a heparinized syringe is attached to the tubing hub and blood is aspirated. With the prepackaged needle and syringe, the blood passively flows into the syringe once the artery has been entered. After the needle is withdrawn, manual pressure should be applied to the puncture site for 5 minutes.

FIGURE 39.8 Peripheral arterial catheterization. The arterial pulse is located (radial artery illustrated here), and the skin is prepared and may be anesthetized as for arterial puncture. The approach is at a 30- to 45-degree angle to the skin, entering the artery with an over-the-needle catheter as described for puncture (see Table 39.1 for appropriate catheter sizes). Bright red blood should appear in the catheter flash chamber. At this point, it is helpful to lower slightly the angle of the catheter and advance it slightly to ensure that the catheter itself is within the arterial lumen. The catheter is then advanced over the stabilized needle. Pulsatile blood should appear at the catheter hub when the needle is withdrawn. If blood does not appear, puncture through the posterior wall of the artery may have occurred. In this case, the catheter should be slowly withdrawn and pulsatile flow may reappear, at which time the catheter is advanced slowly into the lumen. This latter technique is actually an accepted alternative method of arterial catheterization preferred by some operators. The catheter is secured using nylon or silk suture material. Sutures are placed in the skin, tied, then looped around the suture ring of the catheter hub or through the fenestrations in the catheter wing clips. Antibiotic ointment may be applied to the catheter entry site, followed by application of a transparent sterile dressing. The catheter hub and extension tubing are then further secured with tape.

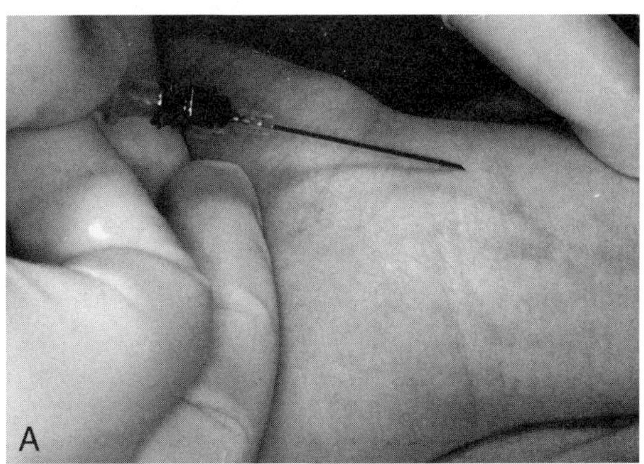
A

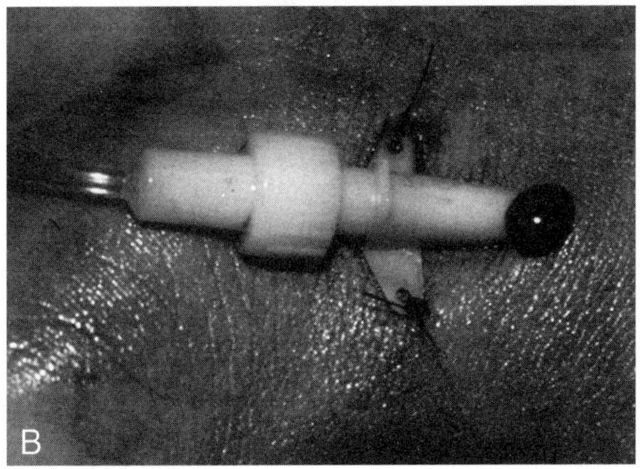
B

TABLE 39.1. Arterial Catheter Sizes by Site and Body Weight

	INFANTS <10 KG		*10–40 KG*		*>40 KG*	
Site	*Catheter Size*	*French Size*[a]	*Catheter Size*	*French Size*	*Catheter Size*	*French Size*
RA, PTA, DPA, TA	Angiocath 24/22 gauge		Angiocath 22 guage		Angiocath 22/20 gauge	
Femoral artery, axillary artery	Angiocath 20/18 gauge	3.0/4.0	18/16 gauge	4.0/5.0	18/16/14 gauge	5.0/5.5 6.0
Umbilical artery		Umbilical catheter 3.5/5.0				

RA, radial artery; PTA, posterior tibial artery; DPA, dorsalis pedis artery; TA, temporal artery.

[a] Single-humen central catheters are manufactured in standard French size and lengths: 3.0 French (5 or 8 cm); 4.0 French (12 cm); 5.0 French (15, 20, or 25 cm); 5.5 French (5 cm with introducer); 6.0 French (15, 20, or 25 cm). The diameter of wires used for over-the-wire catheter technique correspond to the inner diameter of the catheter used; 3.0 French: 0.018 inch; 4.0 French: 0.021 inch; 5.0 French: 0.035 inch; 6.0 French: 0.035 inch.

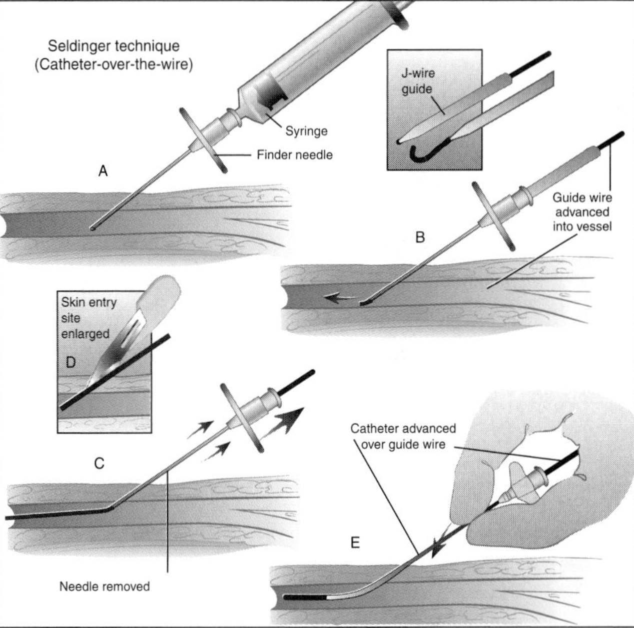

FIGURE 39.9 Seldinger over-the-wire catheter technique. An alternative method of arterial catheterization uses the Seldinger technique of introducing a catheter over a guide wire. This procedure is detailed in Chapter 7 (see Fig. 7.1 and text). Briefly, an introducer needle attached to a non–Luer Lok syringe is placed in the lumen of the selected artery, stabilized on aspiration of arterial blood into the syringe, and the syringe disconnected. A guide wire is then directed through the introducer needle into the lumen of the artery. The needle is withdrawn over the guide wire, taking care to control both the proximal and distal ends of the wire. A catheter is threaded over the guide wire into the artery, keeping the distal end of the wire beyond the catheter hub. The guide wire then is removed and the catheter connected to the appropriate tubing.

CHAPTER 40 •

Venipuncture and Peripheral Venous Access

OVERVIEW

1. Prepare patient and equipment at bedside. Ensure good lighting and appropriate assistance to maximize immobilization.
2. Look for best vein before starting.
3. Always follow universal precautions—don gloves.
4. Immobilize and then apply tourniquet/rubber band to visualize vein.
5. Clean area with povidone-iodine and allow to dry, then cleanse with alcohol; make skin taut.
6. Insert needle 0.5 to 1 cm distal to actual point of entry, bevel up. When vein is collapsed or small, a bevel-down entry is recommended.
7. Puncture vein and, after flashback, insert device into vein 1 to 2 mm further to ensure that both needle tip and catheter end are in vein.
8. Thread catheter in vein by feeding catheter over needle by thumbnail of nondominant hand while stabilizing needle.
9. Attach hub to T-connector and syringe after flushing with saline. Flush catheter to make sure catheter is still in vein.
10. If blood needs to be drawn, T-connector is not purged beforehand and it is attached to a syringe and blood is drawn into syringe by slow negative suction. Alternatively, blood samples can be collected from blood dripping from catheter hub.
11. Secure intravenous site, either with adhesive tape alone or tape and a clear dressing. Tape T-connector tubing away from intravenous site.
12. Tape extremity to intravenous board when necessary.
13. Consider protecting site with plastic cover, especially on scalp.
14. Attach to intravenous fluids or convert intravenous catheter to heparin lock.

CLINICAL TIPS

1. Prepare the parents and patient; this helps the procedure go smoother.
2. Prepare all necessary equipment beforehand. Ensure good lighting.
3. Immobilize the patient well.

4. Clinician should be comfortable.

5. Choose the best vein available, using peripheral veins first. Try not to use the hand of thumb suckers, a toddler's feet, or a vein that crosses joints.

6. To increase visualization of the vein:
   A. Use tourniquet on extremities or a rubber band on the scalp.
   B. Tap vein gently to enhance filling.
   C. Keep extremity in dependent position.
   D. Apply warm compresses to enhance vasodilation.
   E. In a darkened room, place flashlight under extremity to light blood in vein.
   F. Place dab of 4% nitroglycerin cream to cause vasodilation.

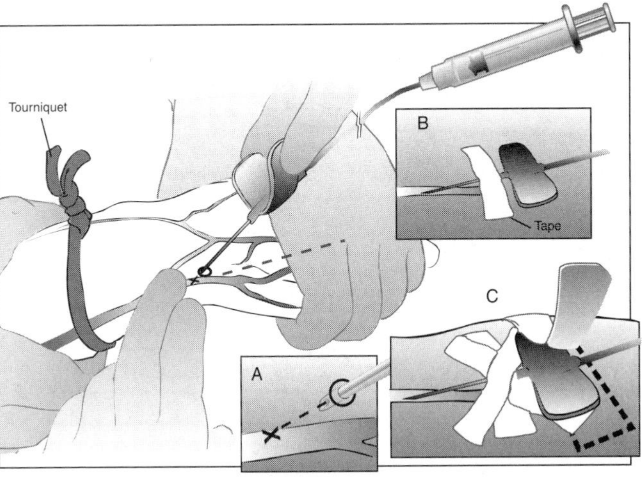

FIGURE 40.1 Venipuncture and peripheral venous access with butterfly needle. A tourniquet is applied proximal to the selected vein. The skin is prepared with alcohol for general venipuncture, and povidone-iodine, possibly followed by alcohol, for blood cultures or venous catheterization. The butterfly needle, typically 23 or 25 gauge, is often preferred for venipuncture to obtain blood samples in young children. The butterfly tubing is attached to a syringe of appropriate size. Tension is applied to the skin and vein distal to the puncture site, and the needle tip is inserted into the skin at a 30- to 45-degree angle, 0.5 to 1.0 cm distal to the intended vein entry site (**A**). The skin is firmly pierced, the needle slightly redirected to be more parallel with the skin surface, and the vein is slowly entered. For venous blood sampling only, the needle is advanced only if necessary for adequate blood flow (**B**). A small piece of clear tape may help to stabilize the needle and facilitate completion of an adequate blood draw. For indwelling intravenous placement, the butterfly is lifted slightly by its wings and advanced carefully, then taped in place (**C**).

7. If veins are not visualized at all, veins with relatively fixed locations can be used for attempts (i.e., long saphenous, median cubital, or cephalic vein proximal to the thumb).
8. After flashback of blood is seen, enter 1 to 2 mm further into the vein to ensure that the intracatheter also has entered the vein, and not only the needle tip.
9. When the clinician has difficulty feeding the catheter over the needle, rotating the catheter or flushing with saline helps make feeding the catheter into the vein easier.
10. Secure with tape and a transparent dressing (i.e., Tegaderm).

FIGURE 40.2 Over-the-needle intravenous catheter placement. The over-the-needle catheter is preferred for intravenous infusions in most instances. Many sizes are available, ranging from 24 gauge intended for neonates to 14 to 16 gauge for large-volume infusions in older children and adolescents. Skin preparation, tourniquet placement, and needle insertion approach are as described for venipuncture (**A**). The needle bevel is kept up for skin puncture, but some experts believe a bevel-down entry into the vein itself helps to avoid tearing the opposite vein wall, especially when the vein is very small (e.g., smaller than the catheter caliber). After skin puncture, the needle angle is lowered slightly to be more parallel with the skin surface, and advanced slowly to puncture the vein (**B**). A flash of blood in the clear hub signals vein entry. The needle is then advanced carefully an additional 1 to 2 mm to ensure catheter entry into the vein lumen. The catheter is then fed over the needle while the needle is held steady (**C**). Slight resistance to full threading of the needle may be overcome in some cases by removing the needle and tourniquet and flushing the catheter with saline as further advance is attempted. When the catheter is fully advanced, a T-connector is attached, the tourniquet removed, and an attempt to flush the line with saline is made to verify intraluminal placement. The catheter hub and tubing are then further secured with tape alone, or tape and a clear dressing (Fig 40.1C).

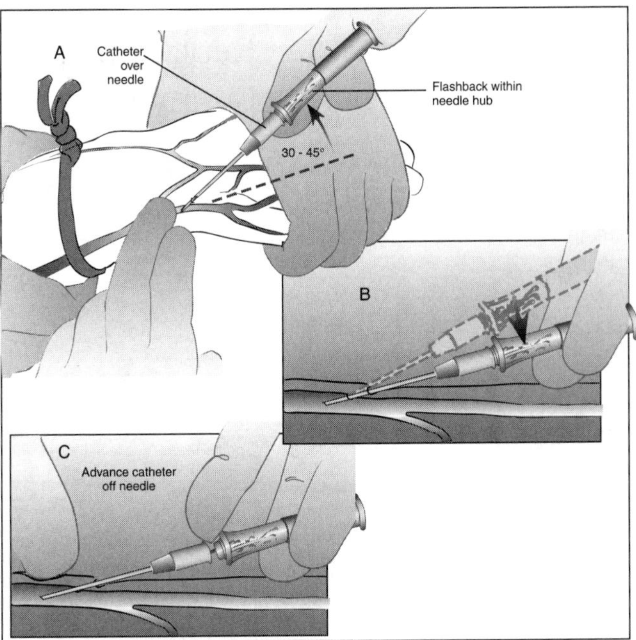
A
Catheter over needle
Flashback within needle hub
30 - 45°
B
C
Advance catheter off needle

Replacement of Tracheostomy Cannula

OVERVIEW

1. Assess patient—airway, breathing, circulation.
2. Position patient with head and neck hyperextended (place roll under shoulder).
3. Oxygenate with 100% O_2 by nose, mouth, or stoma.
4. Determine if tracheostomy cannula is dislodged or obstructed.
   A. Attempt to pass suction catheter.
   B. Try to ventilate using cannula.
   C. Remove inner cannula and repeat steps A and B.
5. Remove complete tracheostomy tube if dislodged or unable to clear obstruction.
6. Recannulate:
   A. Select tracheostomy tube, preferably same size and model as original tube (parents often carry a spare one; Table 41.1).
   B. Remove inner cannula of new tube, if present, and place obturator within outer cannula before insertion.
   C. Lubricate tip of cannula.
   D. Insert gently in a posterior then caudal direction in one sweeping motion.
   E. Remove obturator and replace inner cannula (if needed).

   Note: DO NOT FORCE cannula into place.
7. If difficult insertion:
   A. Use smaller tracheostomy tube or endotracheal tube.
   B. Consider passing catheter (ideally connected to oxygen source) and use as a stylet. Insert it and oxygenate; cut it longer than cannula length outside of stoma entry and pass tube or cannula over it into airway.
   C. If unsuccessful, bag and mask from above while stoma is covered, until further airway management is undertaken.
8. Secure tracheostomy cannula.
   A. Cut cloth tape at a length long enough to wrap around neck twice, allowing an additional 6 to 8 inches to tie (cut ends on diagonal).
   B. Thread one end through an eyelet and pull ends even (hemostats can assist threading).
   C. Slide both ends under head and around neck, then thread one end of tie through second eyelet.

TABLE 41.1 Approximate Size of Tracheostomy Cannulas, Endotracheal Tubes, Suction Catheters

	Shiley	*Holinger*	*Portex*[a]	*Bivona*[a]	*Berdeen*[a]	*Endotracheal Tube*[a]	*Suction Catheter*
Premature	00[b]	00	3.0	2.5–3.0[b]	—	2.5–3.0	6 Fr
Newborn	0	0	3.0	3.0–3.5	3.5	3.0–3.5	6 Fr
0–6 mo	0–1	1–2	3.5	3.5–4.0	3.5–4.0	3.5–4.0	6–8 Fr
6–12 mo	1–2	2–3	4.0	4.0–4.5	4.0–4.5	4.0–4.5	8 Fr
12 mo–2 yr	3	3	4.5	4.5–5.0	5.0	4.5–5.0	8 Fr
3–6 yr	4	4	5.0	5.0	5.0	5.0	8–10 Fr
7–10 yr	4	5	5.0	5.0–6.0	6.0	6.0	10 Fr
10–12 yr	6	6	6.0	6.0–7.0	6.0	7.0	10 Fr
12–14 yr	6	6	7.0	7.0	7.0	7.5	10 Fr

Note: Tracheostomy tubes in infants and young children are usually uncuffed because the airway lumen is small with cricoid ring as the narrowest portion.

[a] based on internal diameter in millimeters.

[b] Have neonatal series with shorter lengths.

D. Pull ends snugly with neck in *flexed* position (leaving space for only an index finger snugly under tie).
E. Secure with square knot.

9. Check for proper placement of new tracheostomy cannula.
A. Auscultate breath sounds.
B. Assess oxygenation and ventilation.
C. Obtain chest radiograph to check distal tip placement.

CLINICAL TIPS

1. Have equipment set up before elective procedure.
2. In critical airway obstruction, most children can be oxygenated by bag-valve-mask from the natural airway.

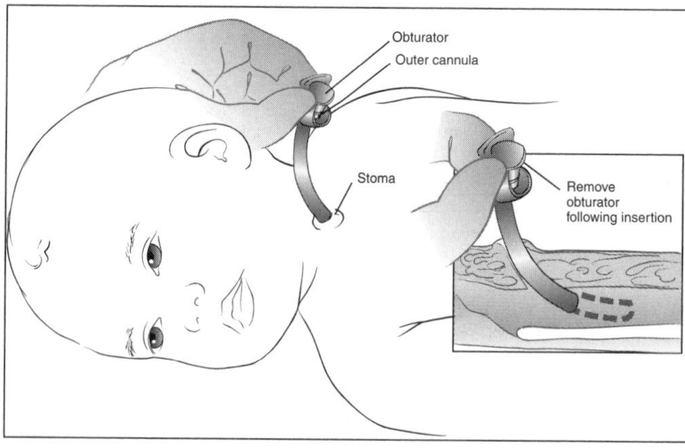

FIGURE 41.1 Inserting a tracheostomy cannula through a tracheal stoma. Ideally, a new tracheostomy cannula of same size and model should be used to replace one that has accidentally dislodged (see Table 41.1). The obturator should be placed in the outer cannula before insertion, removing the inner cannula first, if present. If time allows, lubrication of the cannula tip with gel or saline may aid passage. The cannula is most easily manipulated by holding it with the dominant hand like a pencil, or by the flange. It is gently inserted in a posterior and then caudal direction in a single sweeping motion. Once the tracheostomy tube is in place, the obturator is removed and the inner cannula (if needed) is reinserted. A bag should then be attached with high-flow oxygen and manual breaths provided to check for patency and hyperoxygenation. If resistance is met when reinserting, care must be taken not to force the tube in place, creating a false passage in the subcutaneous tissues of the neck. Notably, the stoma may close after decannulation, even if the tube has been out for only a few hours. A smaller tracheostomy cannula or an endotracheal tube may be attempted in this context. When using an endotracheal tube, it is advisable first to compare its length to the tracheostomy tube to assist in determining the proper depth of insertion.

3. To open the tracheostomy stoma maximally, hyperextend the child's neck by placing towel rolls under it.
4. Choose equipment of appropriate size. When it is unavailable, remember that patients may have a spare tracheostomy tube.
5. If tracheostomy is unavailable, use endotracheal tube of same or smaller diameter through the stoma (Table 41.1).

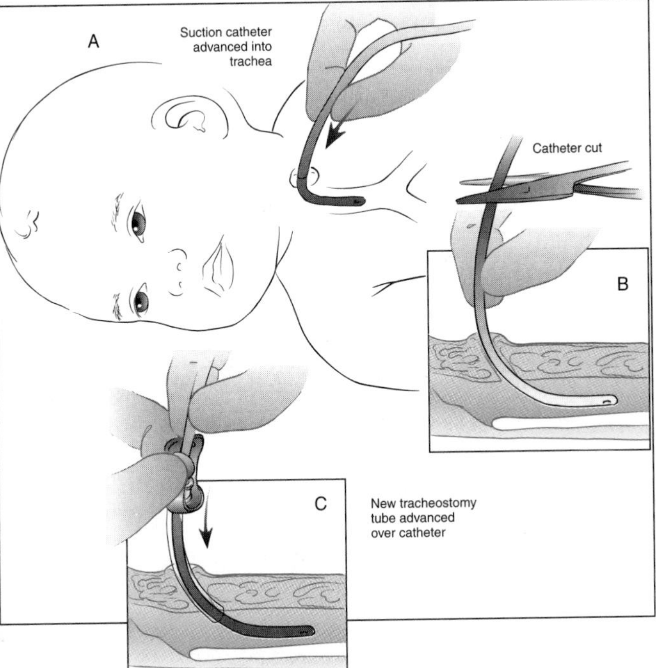

FIGURE 41.2 Replacing a tracheostomy tube over a catheter. Another aid to reinsertion for a difficult recannulation involves the passage of a small suction catheter attached to an oxygen source (0.5 to 1.0 L/minute) a short distance into the trachea. After oxygenation through the catheter, it is necessary to cut the catheter proximally, leaving a length of it outside the stoma to thread through a tracheostomy or endotracheal tube. Care should be taken not to let go of the catheter, which is then used as a stylet for the advancement of the new tracheal tube over it to avoid creating a false passage. If all attempts at recannulation fail, the patient can usually be ventilated through nose and mouth with a bag and mask while the stoma is occluded with a gloved finger and further airway management is undertaken.

CHAPTER 42 •

Thoracentesis

OVERVIEW

1. Identify effusion and whether it is flowing with posteroanterior and lateral decubitus chest radiographs.
2. Monitor with pulse oximetry and frequent vital signs.
3. Consider pharmacologic sedation as necessary.
4. Position child in sitting position leaning forward over chair.
5. Identify insertion site—frequently seventh intercostal space in posterior or posterior axillary line.
6. Prepare sterile field and anesthetize skin and tissue to pleura.
7. Attach needle or angiocatheter to three-way stopcock and syringe and walk needle over top of rib while applying negative pressure to syringe.
8. Once fluid is obtained, thread angiocatheter into pleural space.
9. Reattach syringe and stopcock to catheter and remove pleural fluid.
10. Remove catheter and cover with dressing.
11. Obtain chest radiograph to check for for iatrogenic pneumothorax.
12. Send pleural fluid for protein and lactate dehydrogenase (LDH). Send patient's serum for protein and LDH. Hold other samples in appropriate containers.
13. If a transudate is identified, treat underlying cause.
14. If an exudate is identified, consider further laboratory analysis relative to presenting history and physical examination.

CLINICAL TIPS

1. A lateral decubitus chest radiograph identifies free-flowing pleural fluid.
2. A loculated effusion is best approached with an ultrasound-guided thoracentesis.
3. The neurovascular bundle lies along the inferior border of the rib.
4. The seventh intercostal space posteriorly is a safe landmark to attempt a thoracentesis and is located at the tip of the scapula when the arm is completely abducted.

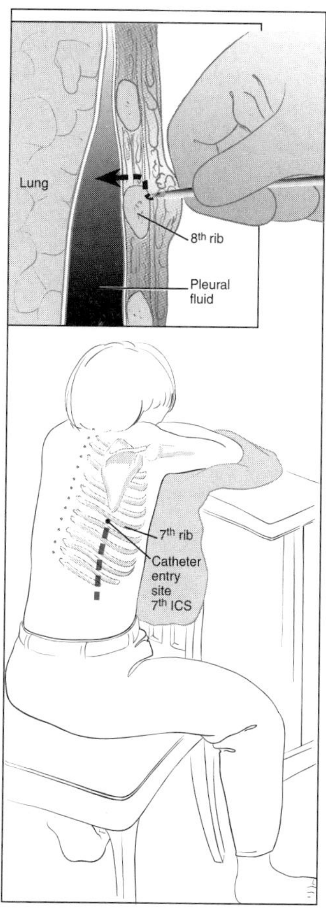

FIGURE 42.1 Thoracentesis. For sampling of free-flowing pleural fluid, the following method is recommended. The patient should have intravenous access and be appropriately monitored, with supplemental oxygen available if needed. Short-acting conscious sedation may be considered for younger or anxious patients. The procedure is usually performed sitting if the patient can tolerate this position, otherwise in the lateral decubitus position. The level of dullness and chest radiograph are used to determine the best location for thoracentesis, although the mid-scapular or posterior axillary lines in the seventh intercostal space are appropriate for most cases. The level of the seventh intercostal space in the posterior axillary line is just below the tip of the scapula when a child's arms are raised. The area is widely prepared with antiseptic. Sterile towels are used to drape the area. A small wheal of anesthetic is raised over the eighth rib, just beneath the intended insertion site, with a small-gauge needle. The needle is removed and changed to a 22-gauge needle attached to a 5-mL syringe. Entering directly through the wheal, and by slowly advancing and injecting, anesthetic is placed to the rib periosteum. Then, the clinician should "walk" the needle over the superior margin of the rib, infiltrate, and proceed to aspirate while advancing the needle. The needle must be kept perpendicular to the skin surface to minimize risk of injury to the intercostal vessels. Once fluid is aspirated, the physician stops infiltrating and marks the depth of the needle (e.g., with a hemostat), and then removes the needle, hemostat, and syringe together. A 15- or 30-mL syringe and an over-the-needle catheter are now attached to a three-way stopcock. The previously identified depth of insertion is "transferred" to this needle by grasping the needle at this level with thumb and index finger. The needle insertion procedure outlined previously is repeated. Once fluid is obtained, the needle is advanced slightly to ensure that the catheter tip is in the pleural space. The catheter is advanced over the needle. The physician should withdraw the needle and place one finger over the open end of the catheter to prevent aspiration of air. The syringe and stopcock are reattached and fluid withdrawn. If the fluid is not free flowing, the child may lean back or to one side. At completion of fluid withdrawal, the catheter is removed, a sterile dressing applied, and an upright chest radiograph obtained to check for iatrogenic pneumothorax.

5. If the pleural fluid does not flow freely, try having the child lean back or to the side. If using the needle approach, care must be taken to prevent accidental puncture of the underlying lung. Commercial thoracentesis needles with side ports may ease fluid retrieval.
6. Empyemas and hemothorax require tube thoracostomy.

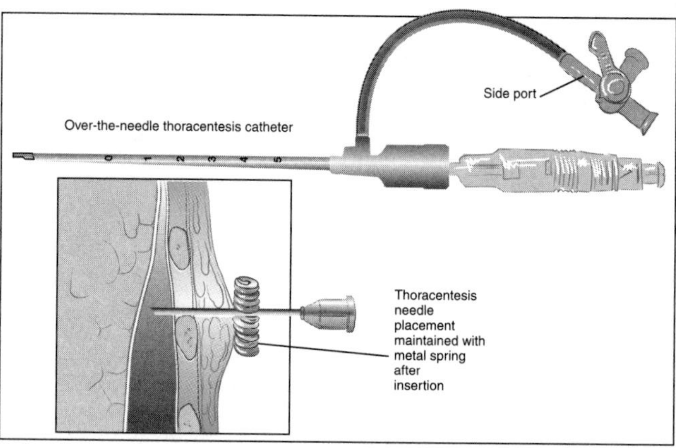

FIGURE 42.2 Thoracentesis with side port catheter or straight needle. Some commercial, over-the-needle thoracentesis catheters have side ports, which may make fluid retrieval easier. Another variant on the thoracentesis procedure described in Fig. 42.1 is that of using a straight needle instead of an over-the-needle catheter. In this context, after the proper depth of insertion is identified during anesthetic infiltration, this depth is transferred to the thoracentesis needle by placing a hemostat or metal spring across the needle at the appropriate site.

CHAPTER 43

Gastric Intubation and Lavage

OVERVIEW

Gastric Intubation

1. General considerations
   A. Fully discuss procedure with patient and family to limit anxiety.
   B. Have necessary equipment and assistants available.
   C. Position patient and protect airway when indicated.
   D. Stabilize neck if any question of cervical spine injury.
   E. Suction patient clear of secretions.
   F. Use well lubricated, size-appropriate tube.
   G. Apply topical anesthetic for nasogastric placement.
   H. Estimate desired length: tip of nares to earlobe and nose to xiphoid, or nostril back around ear and down just below left costal margin.
   I. Gently pass tube into desired position in caudally directed manner, going straight into the nostril, not up.
   J. Check placement with infusion of air; confirm placement with radiograph as needed.

Specific considerations in the unconscious patient
   A. Consider head-down, decubitus positioning and endotracheal intubation before gastric intubation in comatose patients to reduce risk of aspiration.
   B. All unconscious patients should have radiographic confirmation of positioning.

Gastric Lavage

1. Ensure airway protection. Restrain and position patient in left lateral decubitus, head down position. Have suction on at bedside.
2. Measure tube insertion distance and mark tube.
3. Lubricate tube and insert gently through mouth to predetermined distance.
4. Confirm tube placement by auscultation of insufflated air over stomach and by eventual return of gastric contents.
5. Lavage patient using 10 mL/kg aliquots of saline (up to 150 mL) until return is clear.
6. Instill activated charcoal/cathartic before withdrawing tube.

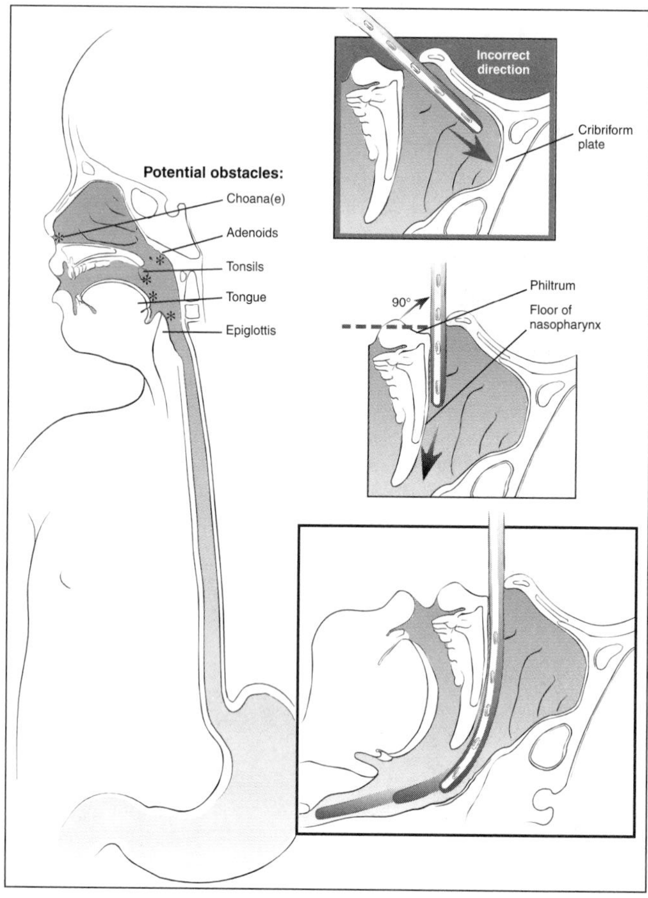

FIGURE 43.1 Even when proper technique is used, there are several potential obstacles in the oropharynx that can cause a gastric tube to "hang up" during insertion. These can usually be overcome by withdrawing the tube slightly and reattempting insertion along the proper path. The site of impedance often can be palpated in the neck and help guide further efforts. A common mistake among novice practitioners is inserting the tube "upward" (i.e., parallel to the nasal bone) rather than "straight in" along the floor of the nasopharynx. A tube that is inserted superiorly impinges on the turbinates or the cribriform plate, often resulting in epistaxis due to mucosal injury. When the tube is inserted perpendicular to the face, it usually follows the normal orientation of the turbinates to the posterior pharynx.

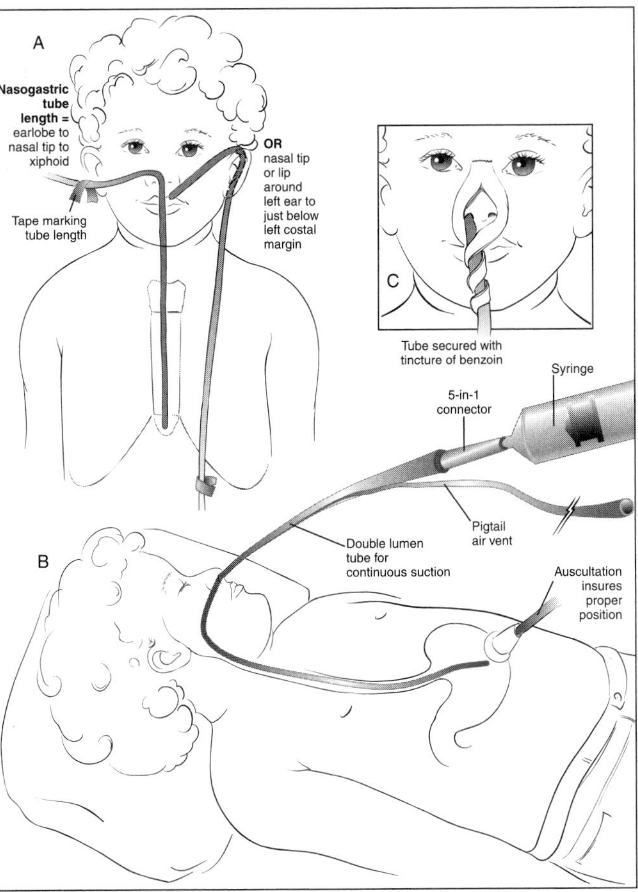

FIGURE 43.2 Technique for gastric intubation. **A:** The appropriate length of tube should be estimated before insertion. This can be done in one of two ways. For the nasogastric route, a good approximation of proper tube length can be obtained by measuring (using the tube) the distance from the earlobe to the tip of the nose and from there to the xiphoid. Alternatively, the length of tube can be measured by externally placing it from the tip of the nose or from the lip (depending on the approach used) back to the ear and down to a point just inferior to the costal margin. The proper length of the tube can then be marked with adhesive tape. **B:** After the tube is inserted, proper placement is confirmed by injecting 3 to 10 mL of air (depending on the size of the child) through a catheter-tipped syringe attached to the tube. Auscultation over the epigastric region should reveal a rumbling sound as evidence of correct positioning. **C:** Although several methods of securing the tube have been described, the basic approach involves securing a small piece of tape with tincture of benzoin to the nasal bridge. The distal end of the horizontally cut tape is wrapped around the segment of the tube extending from the nostril. Orogastric tubes can be secured in a similar manner to the lateral cheek.

CLINICAL TIPS

Gastric Intubation

1. Topical anesthetic jelly (nasogastric tube) or topical anesthetic spray (orogastric tube) limits the discomfort of the procedure.
2. If excessive choking or gagging occurs, the tube should be removed.
3. Talking or crying during the procedure is a good indication that the gastric tube has not been inadvertently placed in the trachea.
4. If difficulty is encountered, palpation of the neck may reveal the site of impedance.
5. Gentle downward displacement of the tongue with a tongue blade may facilitate passage of a nasogastric tube in the young child or infant.
6. If unable to advance the tube, congenital malformations such as choanal atresia, esophageal atresia, and esophageal strictures should be considered.
7. Excess force must never be used in passing a nasogastric tube.

Gastric Lavage

1. Gastric lavage is unpleasant for the patient and clinicians. All equipment and materials should be ready to facilitate rapid completion of the procedure. The patient should be restrained so that the tube cannot be pulled out.
2. Proper positioning (left side, head down) is vital to reduce the risk of complications.
3. Adequate airway protection must be ensured.
4. When lavage fluid is not draining well, repositioning the tube or gently flushing it may restore its function.
5. It may not be possible safely to lavage an awake, screaming child who is forcefully gagging or vomiting around the tube. The procedure should be discontinued because the risk of aspiration is unacceptable.

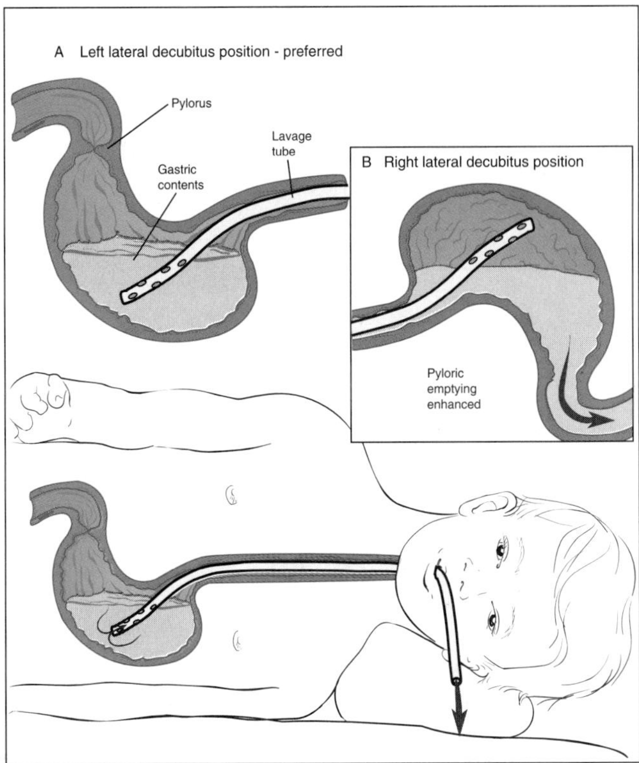

FIGURE 43.3 Gastric lavage should normally be performed with a larger tube (24 to 50 French) because these are most effective for recovering solid fragments. For this reason, the oral route is preferred in almost all instances. **A:** The conscious child should be in the left lateral decubitus position to minimize pyloric emptying. Mild Trendelenburg positioning (head lower than feet) decreases the risk of aspiration. **B:** A child in the right lateral decubitus position has reduced gastric emptying through the tube and increased pyloric emptying into the gastrointestinal tract.

Gastrostomy Tube Replacement

OVERVIEW

1. Assess child's condition. Restrain if necessary. Consider using sedation or analgesia.
2. Obtain replacement tube and check for proper functioning.
3. Remove any clamps from malfunctioning tube and
   A. Withdraw liquid balloon contents
   OR
   B. Insert stylet or obturator.
4. Have child take a deep breath and gently pull out old tube.
5. Lubricate replacement tube and stoma site generously.
6. Insert replacement tube perpendicularly into stoma site.
7. Advance with continuous, steady pressure.
8. Fill balloon with saline/water

   OR

   Remove obturator/stylet.
9. Aspirate stomach contents and listen over stomach while injecting air through replacement tube.
10. Secure tube and cover distal end.

CLINICAL TIPS

1. Water or saline is best for inflating catheter balloons.
2. Prompt opening of fistulous tract of a recently dislodged tube is the most effective way to maintain patency.
3. When inserting the tube, continuous and steady pressure rather than intermittent poking or jabbing is more helpful.
4. Fluid-filled replacement tubes may have more stability during replacement.

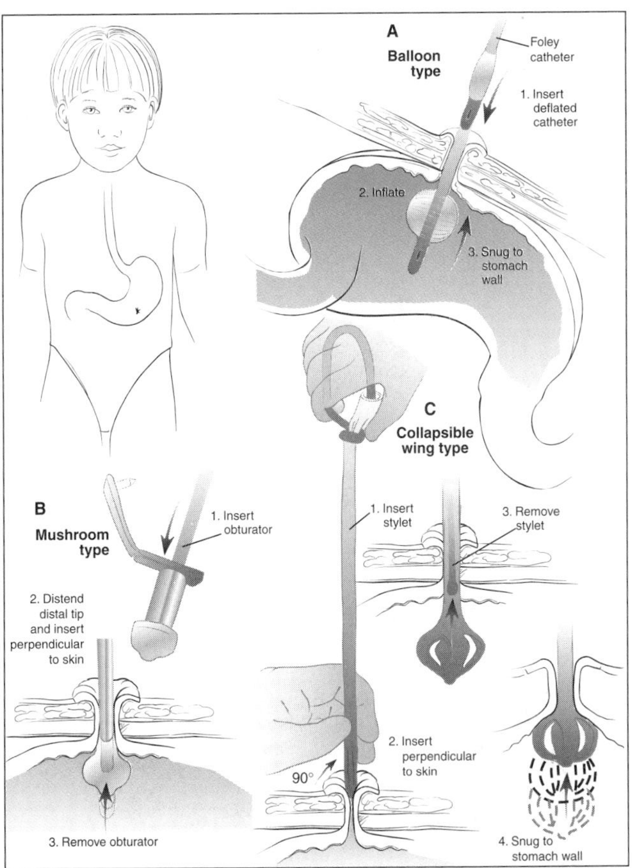

FIGURE 44.1 Techniques for gastrostomy tube replacement vary based on the characteristics of the tube that is used. For all methods, insertion should be performed using slow, steady pressure. Improper technique can result in the formation of a false lumen. Insertion usually is easy when the existing tube is removed immediately before replacement (e.g., a clogged tube). However, if the tube is out for a significant time before insertion of a new tube, the stoma may be partially or completely closed. If the stoma is completely closed, tube replacement should be performed by a surgeon or gastroenterologist. **A:** Foley catheter insertion is the most common temporizing measure for replacing gastrostomy feeding devices. Before insertion, the balloon of the catheter should be inflated to ensure proper function. With the balloon again deflated, the tip of the Foley catheter is inserted through the stoma and into the stomach. If the catheter does not easily go through the stoma, a smaller catheter should be used. If necessary, a cotton-tipped swab inserted into the distal hole of the Foley catheter can be used like a stylet to aid passage of the tube. **B:** With a mushroom or button-type device, an obturator is used to collapse the tip of the tube during insertion. **C:** A similar approach is used with a collapsible wing device, which regains its normal shape after insertion when the stylet is removed.

CHAPTER 45

Paracentesis

OVERVIEW

1. Prepare patient under sterile conditions after placing in restrained sitting, semisupine, or lateral decubitus position.
2. Catheterize the bladder and consider nasogastric intubation to relieve gastric distention.
3. Anesthetize area of choice with 1% lidocaine.
4. Insert intravenous catheter with syringe attached while retracting the skin overlying the site caudally.
5. Advance intravenous catheter with negative pressure applied to syringe until pop is felt and fluid fills syringe. Advance catheter, remove needle, and reattach syringe.
6. Remove enough fluid for therapeutic results or diagnostic tests.
7. Remove catheter when finished and apply clean gauze dressing.

CLINICAL TIPS

1. The sitting or semisupine position is more comfortable for patients in respiratory distress.
2. Formation of the Z-track with caudal traction of overlying skin while placing the needle seals the defect in the peritoneum and prevents leakage when the catheter is removed.
3. Repositioning the patient may improve flow of ascitic fluid through the catheter.
4. Controlled flow of ascitic fluid may be accomplished by a three-way stopcock or intravenous tubing with a flow gauge.
5. Large amounts of ascites fluid may be safely removed if albumin replacement is given intravenously (8 g albumin/1 L peritoneal fluid removed).

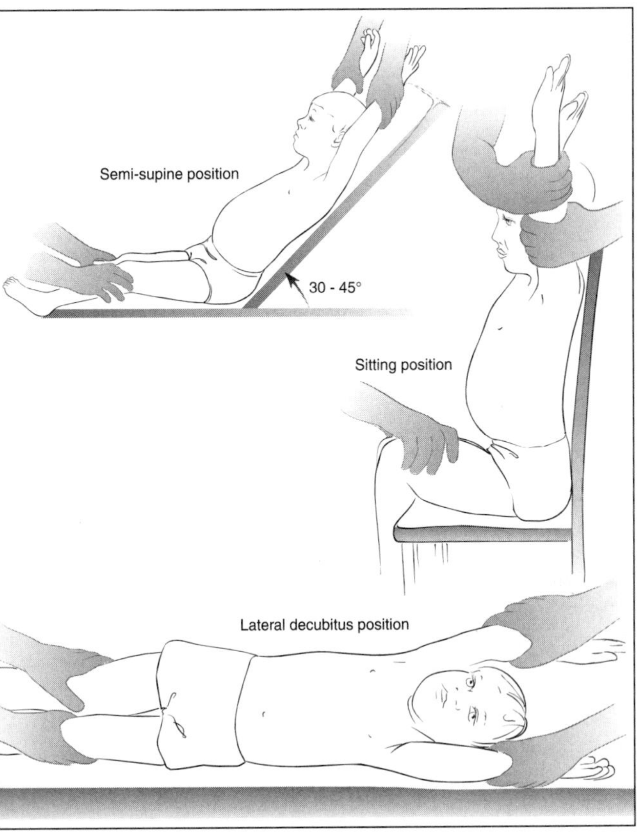

FIGURE 45.1 Patient positions for paracentesis.

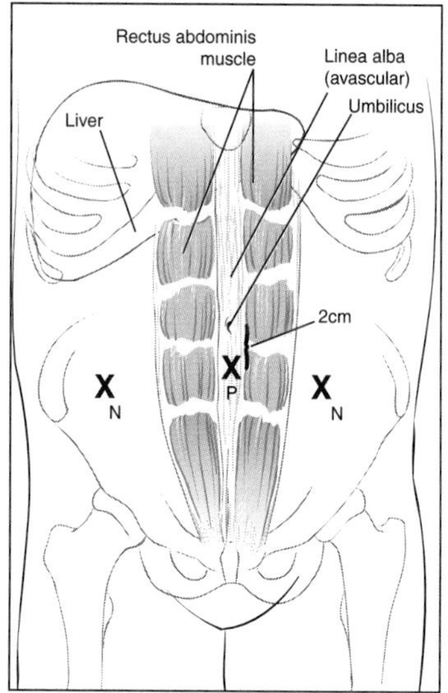

FIGURE 45.2 Neonatal insertion site (N) below the umbilicus, lateral to the rectus abdominis muscle. Pediatric insertion site (P) along the midline at the avascular linea alba 2 cm below the umbilicus.

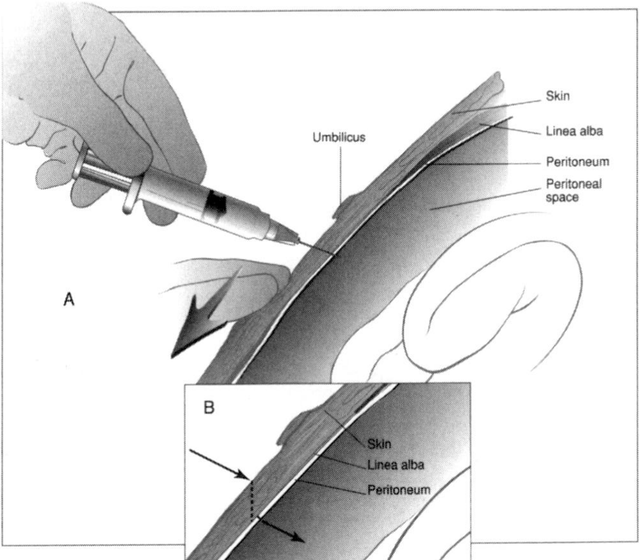

FIGURE 45.3 Technique for paracentesis. **A:** The clinician inserts an intravenous catheter on a syringe at a 30- to 45-degree angle through the wheal of anesthesia while one hand pulls the skin caudally. The clinician applies negative pressure to the syringe as the needle is advanced until a pop is felt. Fluid should then begin to fill the syringe. The needle is inserted no further, and the catheter is advanced into the peritoneal cavity. The needle is removed and the syringe is reapplied to the catheter for collection and removal of fluid. **B:** By pulling the skin caudally during needle insertion, a Z-track is formed after the catheter is removed. This allows for sealing and prevention of a leak.

CHAPTER 46 •

Hernia Reduction

OVERVIEW

1. Confirm the presence of a true hernia before attempting reduction.
2. Ensure that peritoneal signs are not present, and, to the extent possible, that the bowel is not ischemic. If either finding is questionable, seek immediate surgical consultation.
3. Consider sedation.
4. Warm hands before contacting patient.
5. Apply gentle, firm bimanual pressure along entire inguinal canal, using hand most distal to milk out contents or gas within incarcerated bowel.
6. After reducing contents of incarcerated bowel, apply increased pressure over distal as compared with proximal inguinal canal.
7. If bowel fails to reduce after 5 minutes of continuous pressure, try sedation if not used on first attempt. Place patient in Trendelenburg position, apply ice pack to groin, and repeat procedure.
8. Contact surgeon for all incarcerated hernias to arrange admission and semi-elective or emergent surgery.

CLINICAL TIPS

1. Femoral hernias and direct inguinal hernias are rare in children.
2. An indirect inguinal hernia presents with a mass at the internal ring of the inguinal canal.
3. A hydrocele is usually smooth, nontender, and mobile, has brilliant transillumination (bowel can also transilluminate), and does not extend into internal ring of the inguinal canal.
4. Communicating hydrocele often has a history of shrinking during the night.
5. When parents give a reliable history for an inguinal hernia, provocative maneuvers may cause the inguinal hernia to protrude.
6. Even with irreducible incarcerated inguinal hernias, bowel necrosis is rare in children.

7. Most attempts at reduction of an incarcerated inguinal hernia are successful.
8. Irreducible inguinal hernias in girls are more likely to be an incarcerated ovary.
9. Evidence of bowel obstruction is not a contraindication to manual reduction of an inguinal hernia.

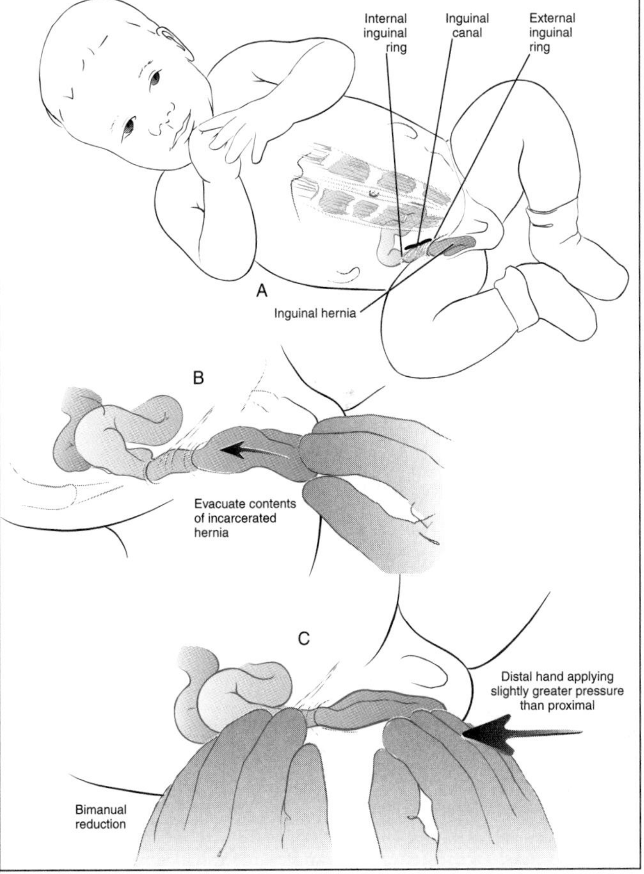

FIGURE 46.1 Bimanual reduction of an inguinal hernia. **A:** Anatomy of an inguinal hernia. **B:** Gas and stool are first milked out of the bowel to reduce its size. **C:** Constant pressure is applied for up to 5 minutes (distal to proximal) to reduce the bowel itself.

CHAPTER 47

Umbilical Granuloma Removal

OVERVIEW

Large Nonpedunculated Granuloma

1. If granuloma appears dry, wet silver nitrate applicator with water.
2. Apply silver nitrate to granuloma for 2 to 3 seconds until mucosa turns gra or black.
3. Apply repeatedly with single stick, taking care to avoid healthy skin o spillage of silver nitrate.
4. Blot excess silver nitrate off the granuloma and surrounding skin.
5. Repeat application in 3 to 5 days as needed.

Large Pedunculated Granuloma

1. Tie off base of granuloma using thick (1-0 to 3-0) silk or nylon surgical tie
2. In 1 week, remove remnant of granuloma, if necessary, and cauterize bas of granuloma using technique described.

CLINICAL TIPS

1. If the umbilical mass is bright red, flesh colored, or excessively moist cautery should not be performed until further evaluation is made becaus this may represent a process other than umbilical granuloma (omphalitis umbilical polyp, patent urachus, or a small omphalocele).
2. Fever and periumbilical redness suggest omphalitis and should preclud any attempts at umbilical cautery.
3. No more than one applicator stick should be used when performing um bilical granuloma cautery.

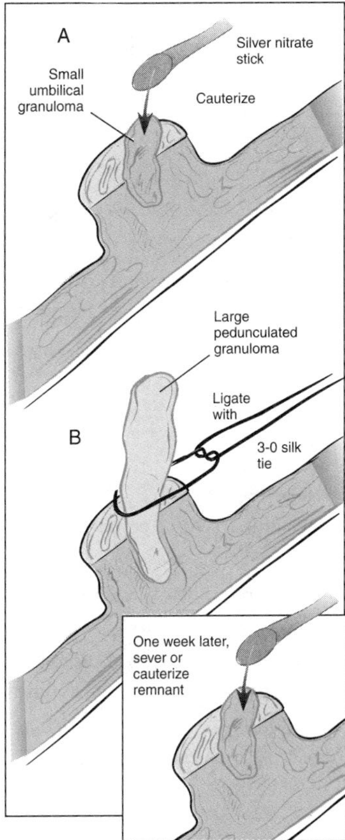

IGURE 47.1 Technique for umbilical granuloma removal. **A:** The tip of a silver nitrate tick is applied for 2 to 3 seconds to the umbilical granuloma, avoiding surrounding tisue. Cautery is indicated by a change in color from red to gray or black. If the surface of he lesion is dry, the tip of the silver nitrate stick should be moistened with tap water beore the procedure. With larger granulomas, multiple applications may be necessary. Caution must be exercised to prevent contact of the silver nitrate with adjacent skin. Any xcess silver nitrate should be wiped with gauze or cotton at the end of the procedure. Applications may be repeated every 3 to 5 days until the umbilical granuloma has reolved. **B:** Large pedunculated granulomas may be tightly ligated at the base with a nonbsorbable stitch. The granuloma subsequently falls off (or is cut off) approximately 1 veek after ligation. The base is then cauterized with silver nitrate as previously described.

CHAPTER 48

Reducing a Rectal Prolapse

OVERVIEW

1. Sedate child as needed.
2. Position child prone in knee-chest position.
3. Generously lubricate prolapsed mucosa with water-soluble lubricant.
4. With gloved hands, apply circumferential pressure on prolapsed mucosa while guiding rectum internally with finger placed in central orifice.
5. Apply a pressure dressing with petroleum jelly–impregnated gauze, dry gauze, and tape.

CLINICAL TIPS

1. The protruding rectal mass should be carefully examined to ensure that the patient does not have hemorrhoids, a prolapsed polyp, or a prolapsed intussusception before attempting reduction.
2. The diagnosis of cystic fibrosis should be considered in an otherwise well child with noninfectious diarrhea and rectal prolapse.
3. Sedation and careful manual compression of the mucosa to decrease edema may help when reduction of the rectal prolapse is difficult.
4. Parents should be informed that the rectal prolapse is likely to recur and prophylactic treatment should be provided for potential underlying causes.

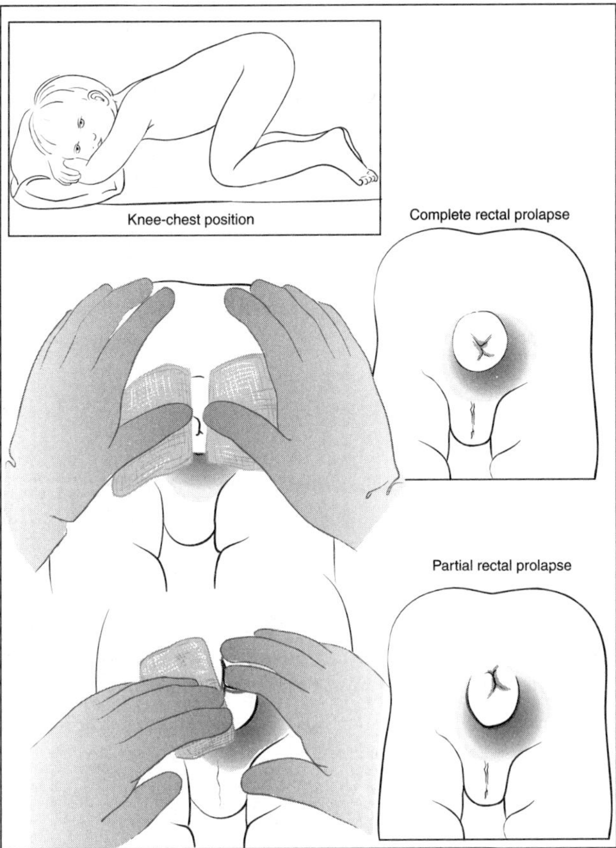

IGURE 48.1 Rectal prolapse reduction is performed with the child prone in the knee-hest position on the parent's lap or on the examination table. With gloved hands, the linician should place gentle but firm pressure on the prolapsed mucosa. A finger may be laced in the rectum to guide reversal of the prolapse. Unlike an inguinal hernia, a rec-al prolapse rarely becomes incarcerated. However, emergent surgical consultation is in-icated if the prolapse cannot be reduced. Emergent surgical consultation is also required f a prolapsed intussusception, rather than a rectal prolapse, is suspected. Distinguishing eatures of a prolapsed intussusception include ill appearance of the child, abdominal ain, inability to pass a finger between the prolapsed bowel and the anal sphincter, and lood in the stool.

CHAPTER 49

Prepubertal Genital Examination and Vaginal Foreign Body Removal

OVERVIEW

Prepubertal Genital Examination

1. Explain how examination will be performed before patient disrobes; answer any questions.
2. Begin with general physical examination and Tanner staging.
3. Have child assume supine frog-leg position—parent may sit on the examining table at child's head for support.
4. Examine labia majora, perineum, and buttocks for abnormalities.
5. Grasp labia majora between thumbs and index fingers and pull laterally, downward, and outward; inspect vulva.
6. Identify clitoris, urethra, and hymen and assess hymenal patency.
7. If necessary, examine child further in knee-chest position.
8. If indicated, obtain specimens for culture by separating labia majora, pausing so hymenal orifice widens, and passing small swab into vaginal vault.
9. Perform bimanual examination using rectoabdominal approach to locate uterus and assess for any abnormal masses.
10. Allow patient to dress privately and then discuss findings of examination and any necessary follow-up.

Vaginal Foreign Body Removal

1. Explain procedure to child.
2. Set up equipment: fill 60-mL syringe with saline and firmly attach to 8-French feeding tube; prime feeding tube with saline.
3. Visualize hymenal orifice using labial traction; allow child to relax before inserting feeding tube.
4. Apply viscous lidocaine to hymen with cotton swab if needed.
5. Gently pass distal end of catheter through hymenal orifice into vaginal vault until slight resistance is felt.

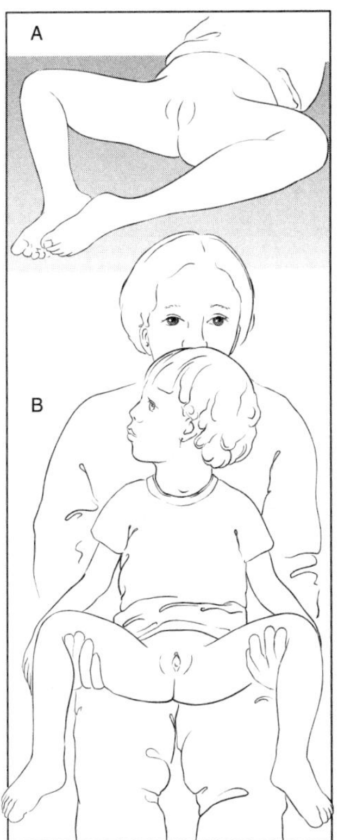

FIGURE 49.1 In contrast to the three stages of the adolescent pelvic examination, a careful external examination is all that is usually required for the prepubertal patient. Few prepubertal girls can tolerate a speculum examination while awake. The external examination can be done on an examining table, on a gynecologic table with stirrups, or with the patient sitting in the parent's lap. **A:** Most examinations begin with the child in the supine frog-leg position because this position is usually less intimidating for the patient. To place the child in the frog-leg position, the clinician should ask the child to lie on her back, bend her knees and "flop her legs out like a frog" or "open them like a book." The child should be encouraged to place the bottoms of her feet together and to abduct her knees completely. **B:** Because the examination is difficult to perform if the parent and child are sitting in a chair, the clinician should instead suggest that the parent sit on the examining table near the patient's head during the examination. Only children who are very uncooperative require examination in the parent's lap.

6. Tell child she may feel cold water "at her bottom."
7. Irrigate vagina until effluent is clear.

CLINICAL TIPS

Prepubertal Genital Examination

1. An unhurried and sensitive approach saves time and makes the examination more pleasant for both the clinician and the patient.
2. Talking to the child during the examination helps the patient relax.
3. Having a third person in the room can provide support to the patient and can protect the clinician from allegations of impropriety.

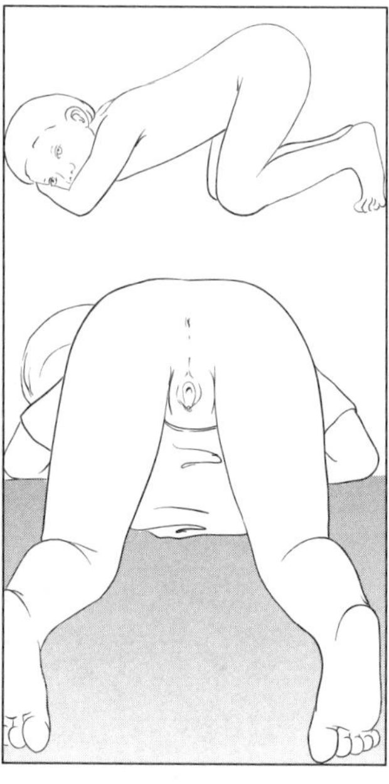

FIGURE 49.2 Using the knee-chest position subsequent to the frog-leg position provides the physician with better visualization of the vaginal vault because the anterior hymenal tissue falls forward in this position. The knee-chest position may be used for better evaluation for a vaginal foreign body, or when the edges of the hymen need to be carefully assessed (as in the case of suspected sexual abuse) and cannot be seen well in the supine position. To place the child in the knee-chest position, the clinician should ask the child to lie on her belly, with her buttocks in the air. Her head and chest should rest on the examining table. Most of her weight should rest on her bent knees, which should be 6 to 12 inches apart to allow for the best visualization. An assistant (or the child's mother) should spread the buttocks by gently pulling them laterally and slightly apart. It should be emphasized that the knee-chest position is often perceived as a vulnerable position for the child because she cannot see what is happening.

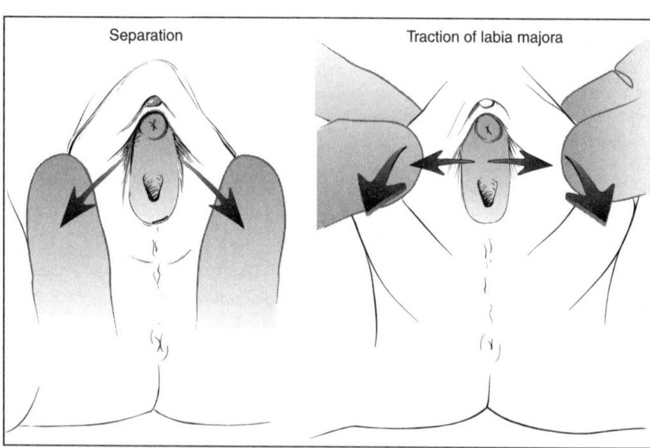

FIGURE 49.3 The vulva is visualized using either the separation or the traction method. The separation method involves placing the thumb or index finger of each hand on the labia majora and displacing them laterally. In the labial traction method, the lower portions of the labia majora are held between the thumb and index finger of each hand, and the labia are pulled laterally, downward, and outward. This should be performed gently in a way that does not hurt the patient. The labial traction method usually allows for better visualization of the vulvar structures than simply separating the labia.

4. Labial traction, accomplished by gently pulling the labia major laterally, downward, and outward allows for better visualization.
5. Pausing before inserting a swab lets the hymenal orifice enlarge to allow passage of the swab without touching the hymen.

Vaginal Foreign Body Removal

1. An unhurried approach ultimately saves time.
2. Examination in the knee-chest position improves the vision into the vagina.
3. Allowing the child to relax after separating the labia enlarges the hymenal orifice. Avoiding contact with the hymenal tissue decreases discomfort.
4. Application of viscous lidocaine to the hymen may improve cooperation.
5. Warmed saline is more comfortable for the child.

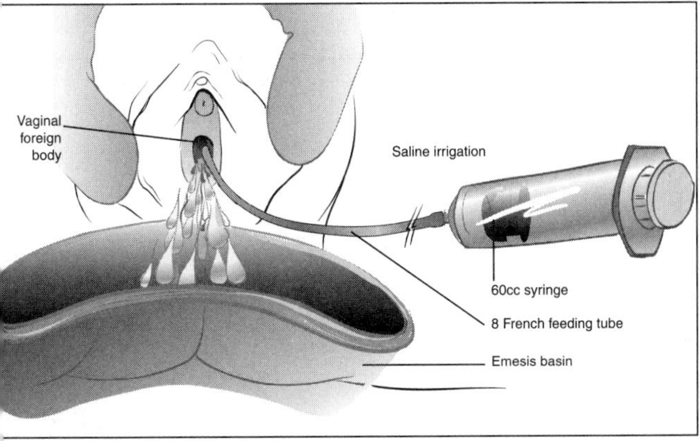

FIGURE 49.4 In prepubertal girls, a vaginal foreign body can sometimes be removed by irrigation of the vagina with saline. This is particularly effective for removing friable material (e.g., toilet paper), but smooth, solid objects such as small beads may also be removed using this technique. The child is placed in the supine position and the labia majora are separated with "down and out" traction. The child is then given time to relax so that the hymenal orifice will open. For a material like toilet paper, which may come out in pieces, irrigation should continue until the effluent is clear. It is unlikely that continued irrigation will successfully remove a foreign body after two or three unsuccessful attempts.

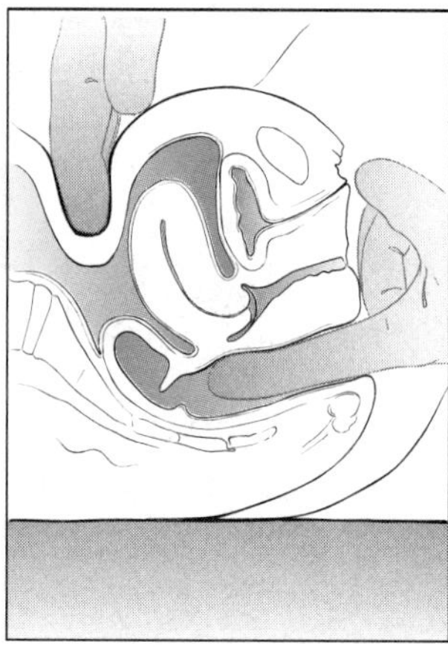

FIGURE 49.5 The bimanual examination of the prepubertal child is done with a finge in the rectum as opposed to the vagina. Adequate lubrication of the gloved finger is es sential to limit discomfort. The smallest finger possible should be used for the rectal ex amination of an infant. Gentle pressure on the abdomen and palpation with the finge that is inserted into the rectum are usually sufficient to locate the uterus. In general, th adnexa are not palpable in the prepubertal child, and therefore a mass detected in thes areas should be further investigated.

CHAPTER 50

Adolescent Pelvic Examination

OVERVIEW

1. Tell patient what will be done and what she will feel.
2. Respect patient's modesty—use drapes and gown.
3. Begin with abdominal examination and Tanner staging.
4. Separate labia majora and inspect vulva.
5. Use speculum warmed and lubricated with water.
6. Insert gloved finger to determine location of cervix and relax posterior musculature.
7. Be careful not to apply pressure anteriorly as speculum is inserted.
8. Insert speculum at 45-degree angle with blades oriented vertically, then rotate speculum to horizontal position.
9. If cervix is not seen, close blades and reposition speculum.
10. Obtain specimens for Papanicolaou smear; fix immediately.
11. Obtain culture specimens for sexually transmitted infections.
12. Used gloved, lubricated finger(s) for bimanual examination.
13. Rectoabdominal examination may be useful if bimanual examination is not tolerated.
14. Discuss findings and arrange for follow-up.

CLINICAL TIPS

1. An unhurried and sensitive approach, and talking the patient through the procedure, saves time and makes the examination more pleasant for both the clinician and the patient.
2. A chaperone should always be present during a pelvic examination (regardless of the sex of the clinician) in addition to the patient's support person to protect the clinician from allegations of impropriety.
3. A speculum appropriate for the age and size of the patient should be selected.

4. When inserting and removing the speculum, the clinician should be careful both to avoid putting pressure anteriorly (against the urethra) and not to trap pubic hairs.
5. Rectoabdominal examination is especially helpful when the vaginal bimanual examination cannot be tolerated, when the uterus is retroverted or retroflexed, or when the patient has complaints specific to the rectum or anus. However, it is not mandatory for all adolescent patients.

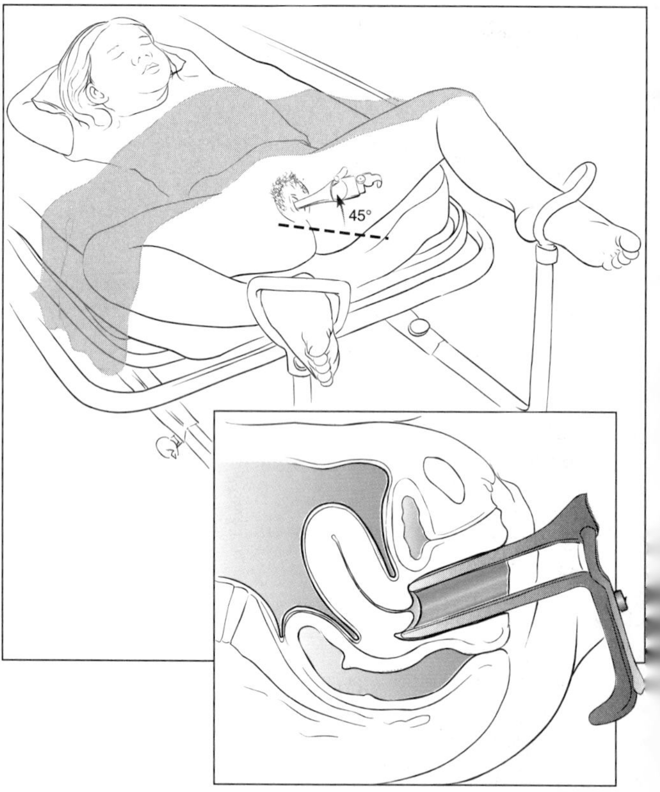

FIGURE 50.1 The speculum is inserted at a 45-degree angle with the blades oriented vertically and rotated into a horizontal position. Pressure on the sensitive periurethral tissues anteriorly is avoided.

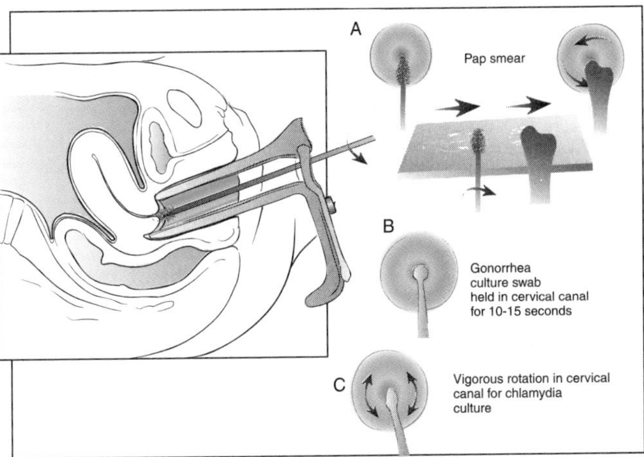

FIGURE 50.2 Specimen collection during a pelvic examination involves obtaining material from the cervix and from the vagina. **A:** If indicated, a Papanicolaou smear should be obtained before other cervical specimens, before the cervical cells are disturbed. Cells from the endocervix and the cervical os are sampled. A cotton-tipped swab or cytobrush is rotated in the endocervical os in one direction. The swab is removed and rotated in the opposite direction on one half of a glass slide. Next, an Ayre wooden spatula is used to scrape the cervix. The spatula is rotated 360 degrees to sample the entire surface of the cervix and smeared on the second half of the glass slide. Fixative is immediately applied to preserve the sample. **B:** Cultures for gonorrhea are obtained by inserting a swab 1 to 2 cm into the cervical canal for 10 to 15 seconds (to allow the swab to absorb secretions). The specimen is applied to a culture plate with medium specific for identification of *Neisseria gonorrhoeae*. **C:** Chlamydial cultures are obtained by inserting a swab with either a plastic or metal stick (wood inhibits chlamydial growth) into the cervical canal and rotating the swab vigorously to pick endocervical cells. Sampling of the vaginal secretions (not shown) is necessary to diagnose trichomoniasis, bacterial vaginosis, or candidiasis. A wet preparation or potassium hydroxide (KOH) preparation is performed by collecting a sample of vaginal secretions from the posterior fornix using a swab. The swab is mixed with a few drops of normal saline in a container, or slides are prepared directly after collection.

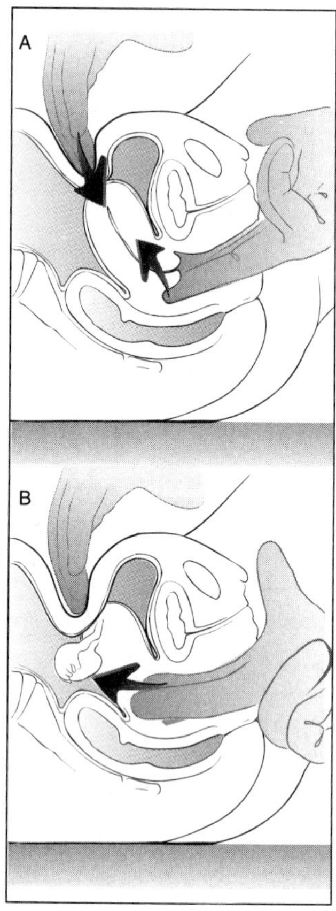

FIGURE 50.3 The last part of the pelvic examination is bimanual palpation, which allows for assessment of the size, position, and configuration of the internal pelvic organs. **A:** The index and middle fingers of the clinician's gloved, dominant hand are lubricated with a water-soluble lubricant gel. One or two fingers are gently inserted into the vagina. When the patient is relaxed, external pressure is applied to the abdomen with the other hand. As the internal hand lifts and supports the uterus, the external hand palpates for size and position. Cervical motion or uterine tenderness is noted. **B:** The adnexa are palpated by placing the internal fingers laterally to one side of the fornix and pressing deeply on the ipsilateral lower abdominal wall. Finding the pulsations of the ovarian artery in the lateral vaginal recess and then sliding the fingers medially to locate the adnexa can sometimes be helpful. The adnexa is a smooth, walnut-size mass (normal ovary size is approximately 3 cm in diameter). Both sides must be examined.

CHAPTER 51

Bladder Catheterization and Suprapubic Bladder Aspiration

OVERVIEW

Bladder Catheterization

1. Provide careful explanation of relevant anatomy and procedural technique to patients and families, and seek history of latex or iodine allergy.
2. Maintain strict adherence to sterile technique.
3. Inspect and test catheter tip (and balloon) before insertion.
4. In boys, gently retract the foreskin as necessary and pull back over glans after completing procedure.
5. In boys, hold penis with gentle traction away from and perpendicular to lower abdomen while advancing catheter.
6. In girls, achieve visualization of urethral meatus with gentle traction on labia or downward displacement of cephalad aspect of vaginal introital fold with cotton-tipped applicator.
7. With an indwelling catheter, it is important to advance catheter well into bladder before balloon inflation to avoid urethral injury if balloon is inadvertently placed in proximal urethra.

CLINICAL TIPS

Bladder Catheterization

1. The physician should anticipate some patient and family anxiety around social and psychological issues related to manipulating the child's genitalia.
2. It is often convenient to have an extra pair of gloves and catheter available before beginning the procedure, so that the patient need not remain "exposed" while the clinician searches for these in the event of an inadvertent contamination.
3. Latex allergy is common in patients with spina bifida and may be anticipated.
4. An assistant usually should be available to help restrain and position female infants and young children of either sex.

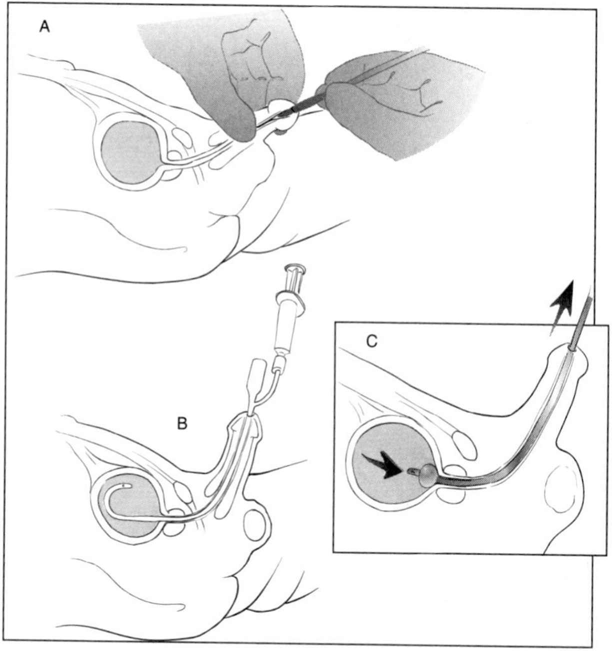

FIGURE 51.1 When performing bladder catheterization in boys, the urethral meatus is usually easy to locate, but the long course of the urethra and its relative fixation at the level of the pubic symphysis can sometimes make passage of the catheter somewhat difficult. For circumcised boys, the clinician holds the penis using the nondominant hand and swabs the glans and urethral meatus with povidone-iodine–saturated cotton held in tweezers or forceps. The dominant hand is maintained in a sterile condition. With an uncircumcised boy, the foreskin is gently retracted, if possible, for cleaning and visualization of the meatus. If the foreskin is tight, the clinician should aim for the center of the glans. It is important to pull the retracted foreskin forward over the glans on completion of the procedure to avoid paraphimosis. **A:** The penis is held with gentle traction perpendicular to the lower abdomen to straighten the course of the urethra. The catheter is inserted using the dominant hand. **B:** If an indwelling catheter is placed, it must be fully advanced into the bladder before any attempt is made to inflate the balloon. **C:** The catheter is withdrawn slowly after balloon inflation until it lodges against the trigone.

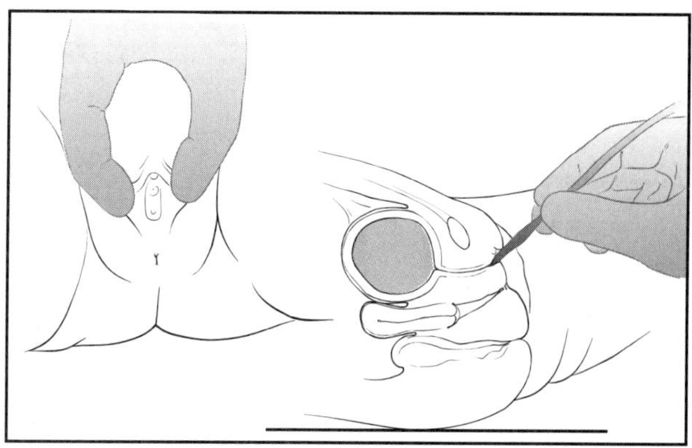

FIGURE 51.2 With girls, the urethra is short, allowing easy passage of a bladder catheter, but the urethral meatus is more difficult to visualize. The meatus of a girl is close to the vaginal introitus, so that the catheter may be mistakenly passed into the vagina. The mucosa of the introitus may also cover the urethral meatus. If the vagina is unintentionally catheterized, leaving the catheter in place may serve as a useful landmark during further attempts at locating the urethra.

5. If resistance is met in attempting to pass the catheter in a boy, slow, gentle pressure with accentuation during inhalation and plantar flexion of the toes may help.
6. If the vagina is inadvertently entered when attempting catheterization of a female infant, leaving the vaginal catheter transiently in place may facilitate visualization of the anteriorly located urethral meatus.
7. A nondeflating balloon may be remedied by removing the adapter plug, attempting to overcome a flap valve defect by insertion and rotation of a guide wire in the inflating channel, or cutting the catheter a few cm from the urethra. Additional approaches probably warrant urologic consultation.

OVERVIEW

Suprapubic Bladder Aspiration

1. Securely restrain child on his or her back in frog-leg position.
2. Prepare skin from the urethra to the umbilicus with povidone-iodine solution.
3. Identify insertion site 1 to 2 cm superior to pubic symphysis in the midline and drape site.

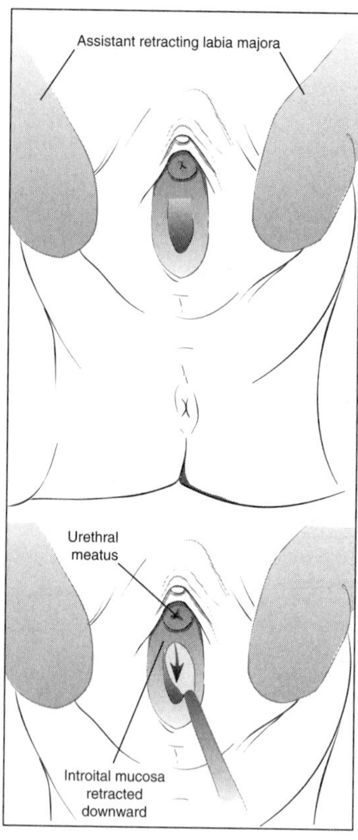

FIGURE 51.3 Applying gentle lateral traction to the labia with simultaneous downward traction applied to the introital mucosa may better expose the female urethral meatus.

4. Infiltrate lidocaine locally at insertion site (optional).
5. To prevent patient from urinating during the procedure, occlude urethral opening by squeezing the penile urethra in boys or applying pressure to the urethral meatus in girls.
6. Insert needle through the abdominal wall in a slightly cephalad direction approximately 20 degrees from vertical and apply negative pressure to syringe as needle is advanced.
7. If unsuccessful, withdraw needle and reinsert it at the same site oriented perfectly upright (vertical).
8. If still unsuccessful, hydrate the child for at least 1 hour before reattempt-

ing procedure. Alternatively, use ultrasound after hydration to identify a full bladder.

9. When urine is obtained, place it in a sterile container for transport to the laboratory.

10. Clean remaining povidone-iodine from the site and place an adhesive bandage over puncture wound.

CLINICAL TIPS

Suprapubic Bladder Aspiration

1. The best use of suprapubic bladder aspiration is for a struggling infant who requires a sepsis evaluation. In such cases, this procedure facilitates the important task of obtaining an uncontaminated urine specimen.
2. Lidocaine may be infiltrated locally at the planned puncture site, but this is probably more painful than inserting the needle and obtaining the urine specimen.
3. Although intestinal penetration can occur when a loop of bowel overlies the bladder, the small puncture created by the needle rarely leads to peritonitis.

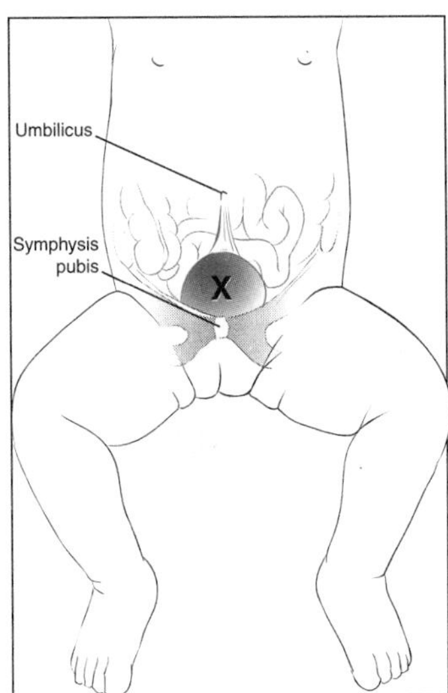

FIGURE 51.4 The child who undergoes suprapubic bladder aspiration should be securely restrained on his or her back in the frog-leg position, which facilitates stabilization of the pelvis. The skin from the umbilicus to the urethra is prepared with povidone-iodine solution and the insertion site is identified. The appropriate site of needle insertion is in the midline 1 to 2 cm above the pubic symphysis on the abdominal wall.

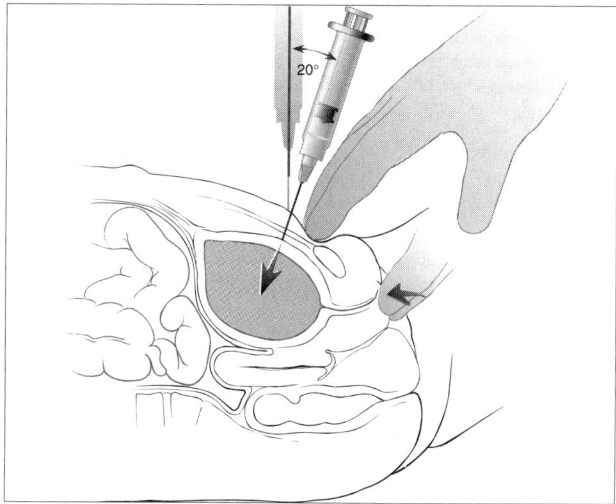

FIGURE 51.5 Before needle insertion, the urethral opening should be occluded by squeezing the penile urethra in the boy or applying urethral pressure to the meatus in the girl. Infants frequently urinate when they feel pressure on the lower abdomen, making occlusion of the urethra necessary to avoid losing the specimen. The skin is punctured and the needle is advanced in a cephalad direction angled approximately 20 degrees from the vertical while applying mild negative pressure to the syringe. In this way, the needle punctures the center of a full bladder. When the needle enters the bladder cavity, urine is aspirated. If the bladder is partially empty, however, this angle of entry may result in passing the needle over the top of the bladder and unsuccessful aspiration. In such cases, the needle is withdrawn and a second attempt is made at the same site with the needle oriented vertically.

CHAPTER 52

Manual Detorsion of the Testes

OVERVIEW

1. Triad of acute scrotal pain, high-riding testis, and absent cremasteric reflex suggest testicular torsion.
2. Always seek urologic consultation for initial assessment and follow-up.
3. Manual detorsion may be successful and of value in first 8 to 12 hours of symptoms.
4. Administer intravenous conscious sedation or perform spermatic cord block as indicated.
5. Torsion almost always occurs with inward or internal rotation—rotate testis within scrotum in outward direction one or two 360-degree turns.
6. Prompt relief of pain and return to normal position in scrotum suggest successful detorsion.
7. After successful detorsion, surgical exploration and orchiopexy should proceed as soon as possible.

CLINICAL TIPS

1. Torsion involves an average of two 360-degree inward twists.
2. A positive cremasteric reflex excludes testicular torsion. An absent cremasteric reflex does not rule it in.
3. Detorsion results in relief of pain and a normal configuration of the scrotum.
4. Urologic consultation is vital and urgent for patients with testicular torsion. Scrotal exploration is always indicated after manual detorsion.

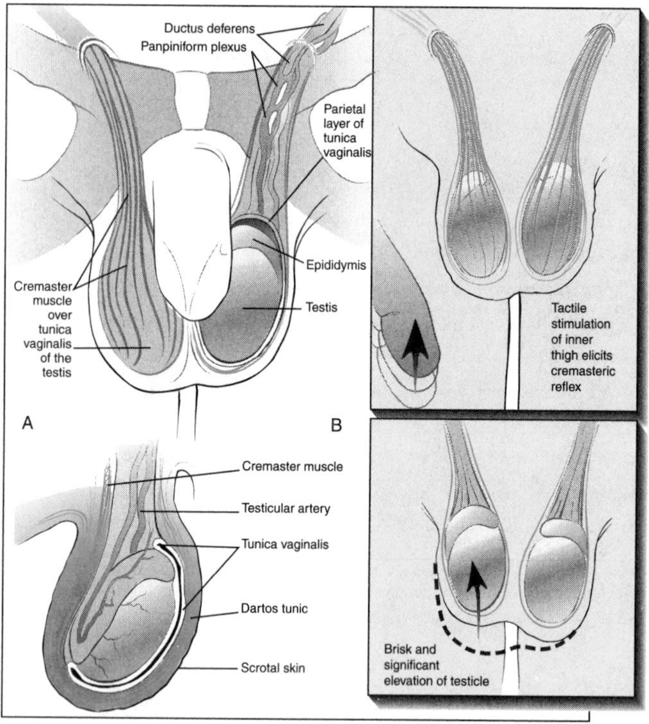

FIGURE 52.1 Normal scrotal anatomy and the cremasteric reflex. **A:** The testes and epididymis are enveloped in the tunica vaginalis. Attached to the testes and epididymis are the gonadal artery and vein within the cremaster muscle fibers. **B:** Stroking the inner thigh produces shortening of the cremaster muscle with upward excursion of the gonad. This shortening should be significant (1 to 2 cm) so as to not be confused with simple wrinkling of the dartos muscle.

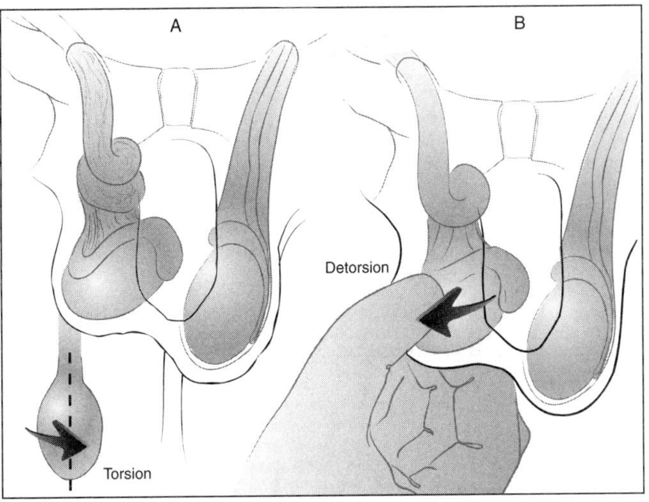

FIGURE 52.2 Manual detorsion. **A:** Torsion of the testes with two inward twists has resulted in a new high-lying position. **B:** The testis is grasped with the fingers and rotated outwardly with two full 360-degree twists.

CHAPTER 53

Paraphimosis Reduction

OVERVIEW

1. Remove urinary catheter if present.
2. Attempt gentle reduction if swelling is mild.
3. Consider sedation or dorsal penile nerve block if paraphimosis is not quickly and easily reduced.
4. Reduce swelling with manual compression, compression dressing, or ice.
5. Repeat manual reduction technique after swelling has diminished.
6. Recommend follow-up to urologist for possible circumcision.

CLINICAL TIPS

1. Prompt reduction of paraphimosis obviates later difficult reduction of the extremely swollen foreskin and glans penis.
2. Prolonged and painful attempts at reduction must be avoided. With more difficult cases, urologic consultation should be sought early.
3. Parents of uncircumcised boys should be cautioned not to retract the foreskin forcibly. Uncircumcised boys with retractable foreskin should be taught to return it to the normal (unretracted) position after cleaning.

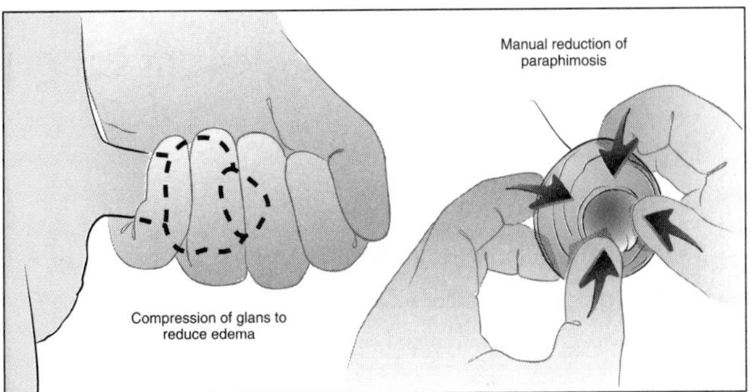

FIGURE 53.1 When a paraphimosis has resulted in significant swelling, it may be necessary to reduce the swelling before a successful reduction can be achieved. The clinician can accomplish this by gently compressing the penis for approximately 5 minutes to remove the edematous fluid from the foreskin. Reduction should then be attempted before the edema reaccumulates. With the thumbs on the glans penis and the fingertips on the tight band of foreskin, the glans is pushed as the foreskin is pulled over the glans.

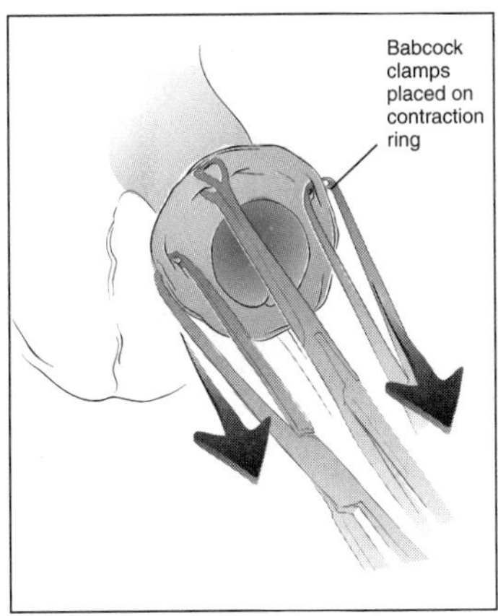

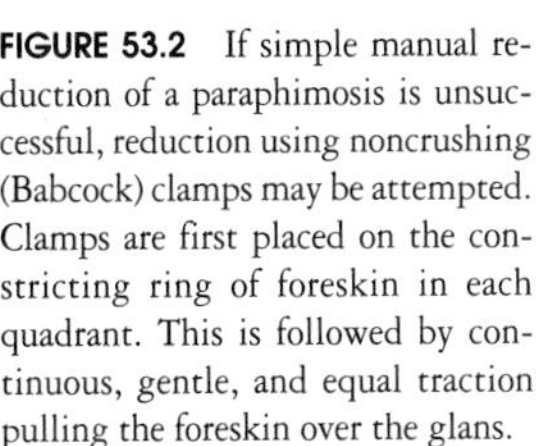
FIGURE 53.2 If simple manual reduction of a paraphimosis is unsuccessful, reduction using noncrushing (Babcock) clamps may be attempted. Clamps are first placed on the constricting ring of foreskin in each quadrant. This is followed by continuous, gentle, and equal traction pulling the foreskin over the glans.

CHAPTER 54 •

Management of Zipper Injuries

OVERVIEW

1. Restrain child and prepare entrapped tissues with antiseptic solution.
2. Use local or regional anesthesia if extrication is difficult.
3. Place mineral oil on involved area and apply gentle traction.
4. Cut median bar with wire or bone cutters if traction fails.
5. Separate rows of teeth and free entrapped tissue.
6. Provide local wound care.
7. Instruct patients to observe at home for complications of wound infection or urethral obstruction.

CLINICAL TIPS

1. Conscious sedation may be necessary with an anxious patient.
2. Ice may reduce the swelling and facilitate the extrication of the entrapped skin.
3. Cutting the zipper out of the pants or pajamas makes it easier to cut the median bar.
4. If the previously described techniques are unsuccessful, a urologist may need to perform a circumcision under general anesthesia.
5. Urethral obstruction with urinary retention may result from posttraumatic edema and can occur up to 8 hours after the procedure. This may require temporary placement of a Foley catheter.

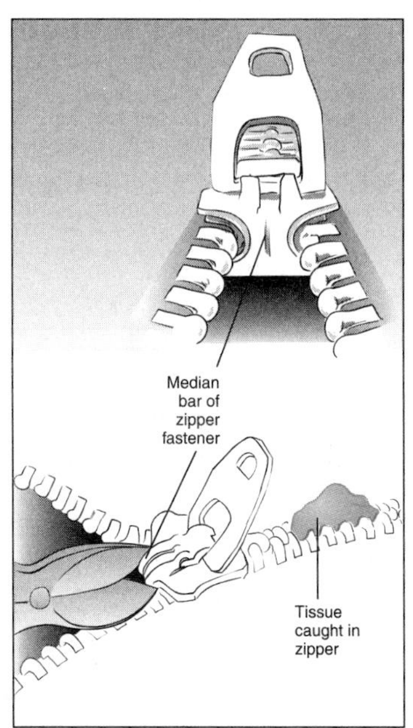

FIGURE 54.1 After appropriate anesthesia is undertaken and the child is restrained appropriately for age, mineral oil may be applied liberally to the surface of the involved area and, after a few minutes, gentle traction applied to the zipper. At this point, the tissue may slide out of the zipper mechanism without further injury. If gentle traction does not free the tissue, then the median bar (or "diamond") of the zipper fastener should be cut with wire cutters or a bone cutter. With the median bar cut, the side plates of the zipper fastener separate and the teeth fall apart.

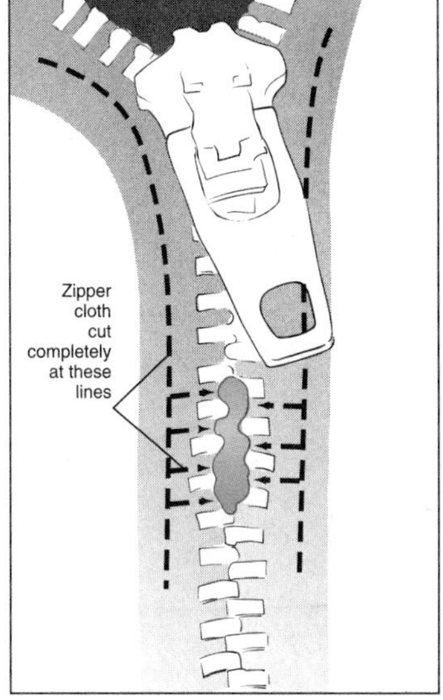

FIGURE 54.2 If the alignment of the interlocking teeth in a zipper is not maintained in a two-dimensional plane, the teeth edges fall apart. This can be accomplished by cutting the zipper cloth around the area of injury as shown. A bandage scissors is used first to cut the zipper cloth along both sides of the interlocking teeth. Several cuts are then made completely through the cloth (between the teeth) above and below the entrapped skin. The side plates easily separate, freeing the tissue. In general, assuming that the appropriate tools are available, the median bar method is easier to perform.

CHAPTER 55

Obstetric Procedures

OVERVIEW

1. Perform brief assessment of mother, including vital signs and fetal heart tones.
2. If mother is in early labor, transfer her to delivery suite.
3. If contractions are 2 to 3 minutes apart and infant's head is distending perineum, prepare for emergency delivery.
4. Notify obstetrician that assistance is needed immediately.
5. Assign one person for mother and one for infant; set up equipment for delivery and newborn resuscitation.
6. Position mother on her back with hips flexed and abducted and knees flexed; mother's support person should be at head of bed.
7. Clean perineum with povidone-iodine solution and drape abdomen and legs.
8. As head emerges, apply one hand to head to control speed of delivery; other hand exerts upward pressure on perineum.
9. Check neck for loop of umbilical cord—if present, slip over infant's head; if cord is tight, clamp in two places and cut between clamps.
10. After head is delivered, wipe face and suction nose and mouth.
11. Deliver shoulders and rest of body.
12. Clamp umbilical cord in two places and cut between clamps within 1 minute.
13. Assess infant and provide resuscitation as needed.
14. Wait for placenta to separate. Assist mother in delivering placenta with downward pressure on abdomen; do not pull on umbilical cord. Save placenta for inspection.
15. Massage uterus to stimulate contractions and prevent further bleeding; oxytocin (20 to 40 U/L at 200 mL/hr) can be given intravenously.
16. Check cervix and perineum for lacerations.

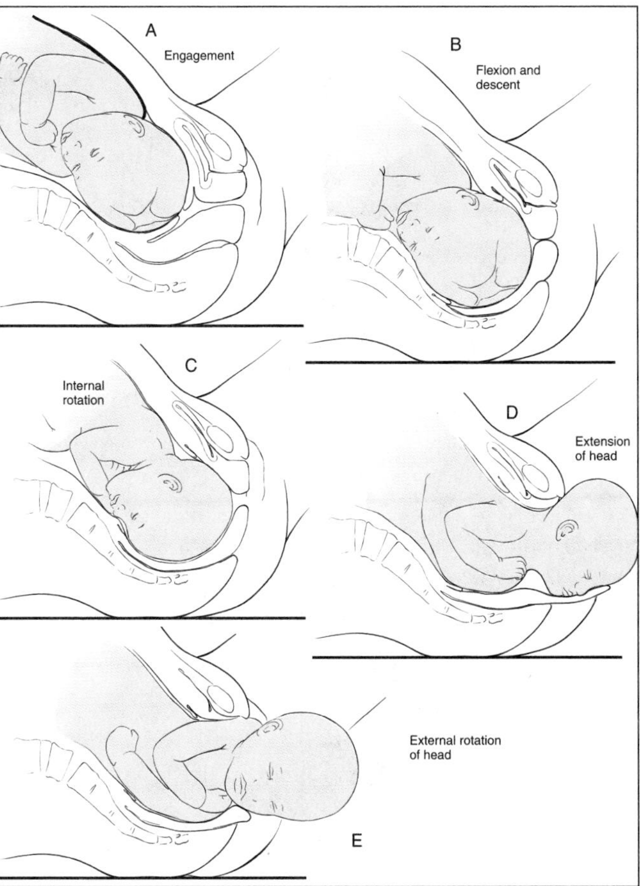

FIGURE 55.1 Sequence of events in vertex presentation. **A:** Engagement refers to the passage of the head through the pelvic inlet. This usually occurs in the last 2 weeks of pregnancy in the primiparous patient and at the onset of labor in the multiparous patient. **B:** Flexion of the neck is necessary for passage of the smallest diameter of the head through the bony pelvis. Descent of the head into the lower pelvis occurs gradually as a result of uterine contractions. **C:** Internal rotation of the head is necessary for the presenting part to traverse the ischial spines. **D:** Extension occurs after the head has begun to pass through the introitus. **E:** External rotation occurs after delivery of the head as it rotates to the position it occupied at engagement. The shoulders then descend along the same pathway as the head, and the remainder of the fetus is delivered.

CLINICAL TIPS

1. The clinician should remain calm, even though this procedure is not commonly performed. Most deliveries proceed spontaneously without difficulty.
2. Universal precautions should be observed.
3. Neonatal resuscitation equipment should be ready to use.
4. An isolette should be turned on before delivering the baby.
5. A support person who can help the mother focus on the delivery should be included.

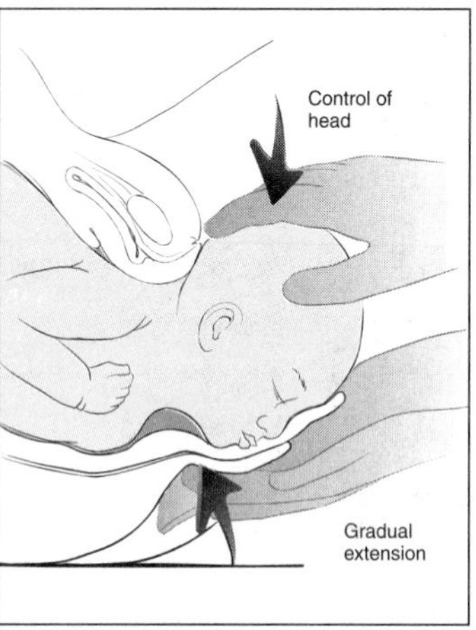

FIGURE 55.2 A gentle, gradual delivery is best for the mother and infant. As the head advances, the clinician places one hand over the occiput to control delivery. The second hand, draped with a sterile towel to avoid fecal contamination, may apply gentle pressure on the perineum from the coccygeal region upward (modified Ritgen maneuver). This maneuver helps extend the head at the proper time, thus protecting the maternal perineal musculature.

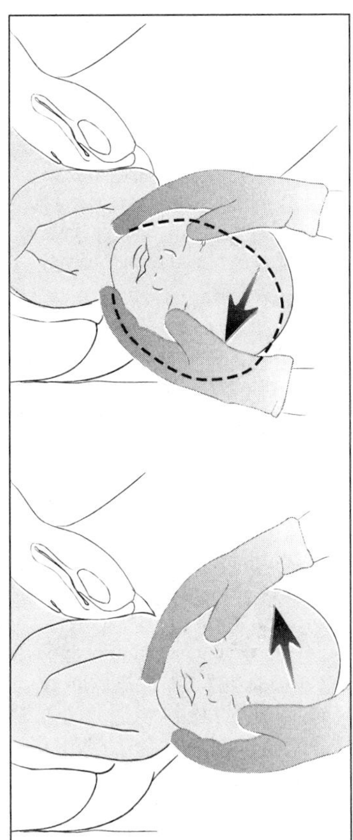

FIGURE 55.3 Delivery of the shoulders should also proceed gradually. Gentle downward traction on the head helps deliver the anterior shoulder, followed by gentle upward traction, which delivers the posterior shoulder. Forceful traction, especially with rotation, can injure the infant's brachial plexus and great vessels.

CHAPTER 56

Splinting Procedures

OVERVIEW

Basic Splint Assembly

1. Most splints incorporate four layers: stockinette for skin protection; Webril for padding; a firm layer of plaster or fiberglass for immobilization; and an elastic bandage to secure the splint to the limb and protect the firm layer (Fig. 56.1*A*).
2. Steps for general application of splints include the following:
   A. Plaster or fiberglass preparation (cut dry plaster or fiberglass and stockinette to fit area to be splinted, use opposite extremity to measure materials if possible, areas where splint may have to bend around joints can have notches cut laterally to minimize folding of the plaster or fiberglass).
   B. Slide stockinette on extremity and roll Webril around stockinette (see Fig. 56.1*B*);
   C. Position child's extremity for optimal plaster or fiberglass application, wet plaster or fiberglass and apply using cool to tepid water, and perform initial splint shaping at large joints (see Fig. 56.1*C*).
   D. Overwrap plaster or fiberglass with elastic bandage, shape splint contours to final form, and maintain splint position until plaster or fiberglass has hardened (see Fig. 56.1*D*).
   E. Discharge plans for splinted patients include elevation of injured limb and application of ice often for 36 hours; keeping the splint dry; provision for pain management; instruction to return to emergency department for pain or sensory changes distal to the splint; and provision for orthopedic follow-up as needed.

CLINICAL TIPS

1. If in doubt as to whether a fracture is present in a child, place a splint until a follow-up radiograph is obtained.
2. Measure splint materials carefully using the child's opposite, unaffected limb.
3. Plan ahead! Proper positioning of the patient, molding of the plaster or fiberglass, and adequate drying time for hardening of the plaster or fiberglass are crucial for a functional and durable splint.
4. Always provide the patient or parents with discharge instructions and plans for follow-up care.

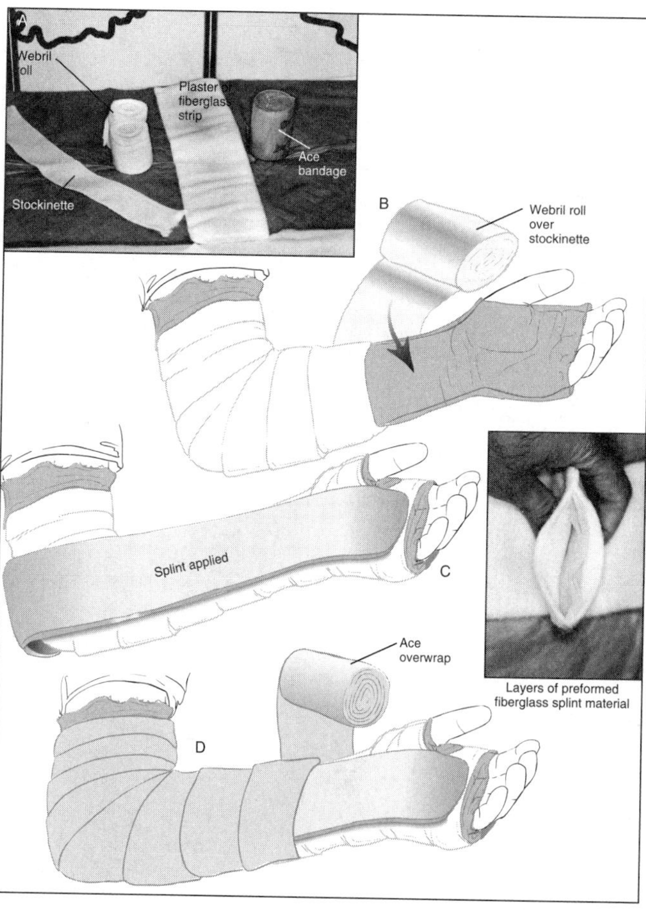

FIGURE 56.1 Distal sugar tong splint. This splint has a broad range of uses, particularly for stable forearm and wrist fractures. The width of the distal splint should slightly overlap the radial and ulnar edges of the arm. The length should extend from the dorsal aspect of the knuckles, around the elbow, to the volar palmar flexion crease. The arm is splinted with the elbow held in 90 degrees of flexion and the wrist and hand in the neutral position of function (wrist slightly extended, thumb abducted, metacarpophalangeal joints flexed, and interphalangeal joints slightly flexed, as if grasping a softball). The splinted arm should be supported with a sling.

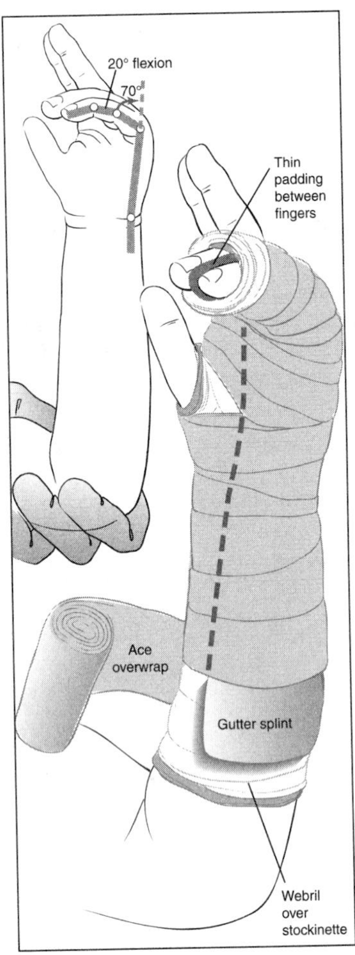

FIGURE 56.2 Ulnar gutter splint. Gutter splints are indicated to immobilize metacarpal and proximal phalangeal fractures. The ulnar gutter splint (illustrated) immobilizes the plane of the fourth and fifth digits. A radial gutter splint immobilizes the plane of the second and third digits, with a hole cut for the thumb to pass through. The gutter splint's width should be enough to wrap to the midline of the hand on the dorsal and volar surfaces, and its length should extend from the nail base to proximal forearm. The patient is positioned with the forearm vertically erect. The splint is shaped with the wrist in neutral position, metacarpophalangeal joints in 70 degrees of flexion, and proximal interphalangeal joints in 20 to 30 degrees of flexion. An extra layer of padding may be added between the splinted fingers to make the splint more comfortable.

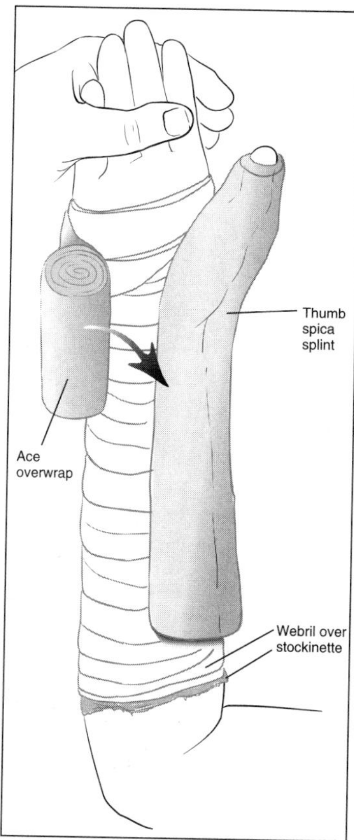

FIGURE 56.3 Thumb spica splint. This is a gutter splint adapted for the thumb, and is useful for nondisplaced fractures of the scaphoid, first metacarpal, and proximal phalanx. The dimensions for the thumb spica are the same as for the gutter splints, as is the position in which the child is held. The splint is shaped with the wrist in neutral position, and the thumb abducted and in slight flexion at the metacarpophalangeal and interphalangeal joints ("wine glass" thumb position).

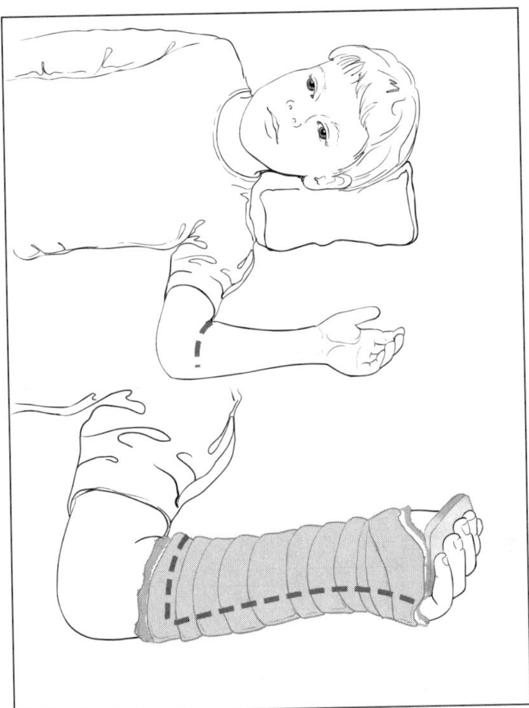

FIGURE 56.4 Colles' splint. A Colles' splint provides volar support and can be used in older children for distal forearm and wrist fractures as an alternative to the sugar tong splint, which provides both volar and dorsal support and is thus preferred in young children. The Colles' splint is wide enough to cover fully the volar forearm, and long enough to extend from the proximal fingers to the proximal forearm. The child is typically positioned on his or her side, with the dorsal aspect of the affected arm against the stretcher, and held at the elbow and fingers as tolerated. The splint is shaped with the wrist in neutral position and digits slightly flexed at all joints.

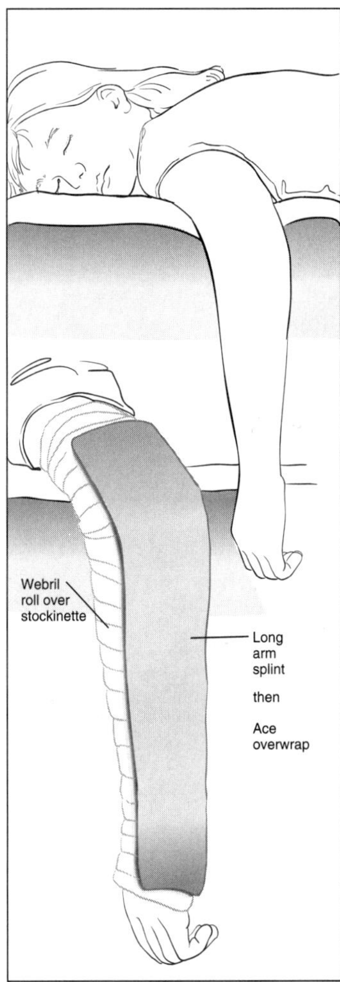

FIGURE 56.5 Long arm splint. A long arm splint is used for stable injuries in the elbow area. Its dimensions are width to cover one half of the arm circumference, and length to extend from the dorsal aspect of mid-upper arm, over the olecranon, and down the ulnar aspect of the forearm to the distal palmar flexion crease. The child is positioned prone with the injured arm at the stretcher's edge, the forearm hanging down, and elbow flexed 90 degrees. The elbow is maintained in 90 degrees of flexion and the forearm and wrist in neutral position. A sling is used to help support the splint.

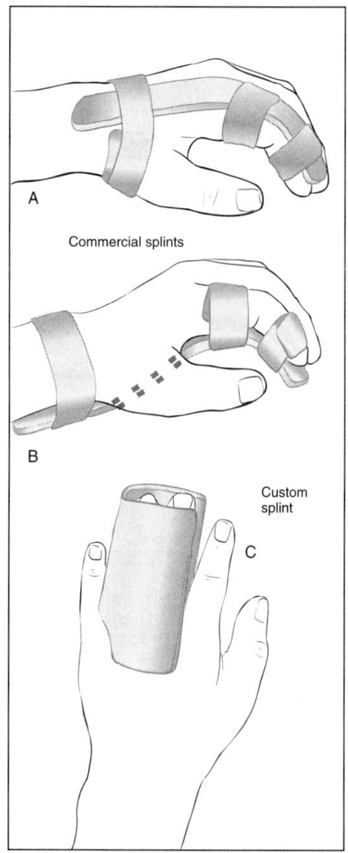

FIGURE 56.6 Finger splints. Finger splints come as commercially available padded metal strips (**A,B**), or can be custom made from plaster or a fiberglass splinting roll (**C**). These are used for simple fractures of the middle or distal phalanx. The splint should be shaped to hold the metacarpophalangeal joint flexed 50 degrees and the interphalangeal joints flexed 15 to 20 degrees.

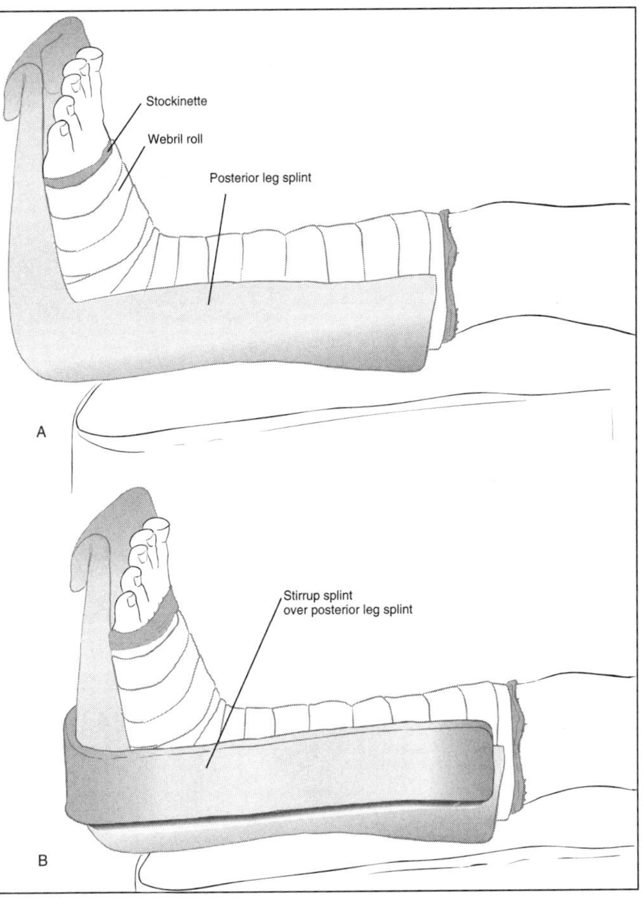

FIGURE 56.7 Posterior leg splint (**A**) and splint with stirrup for added lateral stability (**B**). A posterior leg splint provides support for injuries of the distal tibia or fibula, the ankle, and foot. The stirrup splint is often combined with a posterior splint to stabilize ankle injuries. The splint width should cover at least one half of the leg circumference and the length should extend posteriorly from the level of the fibular neck, over the heel to the base of the digits. The child is positioned prone on the stretcher or parent's lap. The splint is shaped with the foot in neutral position at 90 degrees to the leg. Added padding at bony prominences may enhance comfort. The splint should not compress the region of the fibular neck to avoid peroneal nerve injury. Crutches are recommended for ease of ambulation in children older than 6 years of age. The stirrup splint (sugar tong) provides lateral support to the ankle. It may be used in combination with posterior splints to stabilize ankle fractures. The stirrup splint is fashioned wide enough to cover at least one half of leg circumference and long enough to extend from just below the fibular head, around the heel, and end just below the medial aspect of the knee. Patient positioning is the same as for a posterior splint.

TABLE 56.1 Summary of Splint Types and Indications

Splint	*Fracture Indications*	*Comments*
Upper Extremity Splints		
Colles'[a]	Distal forearm Wrist	Alternative to sugar tong; not for young children
Digits'[a]	Phalanx	
Long arm	Elbow	Must use sling
Gutter	Metacarpal or proximal phalanx	*Radial* for second/third digits *Ulnar* for fourth/fifth digits
Sugar tong	Humerus = proximal Forearm and wrist = distal	Useful for most upper extremity fractures; must use sling
Thumb spica	First metacarpal Proximal phalanx Scaphoid	
Lower Extremity Splints		
Long leg	Distal femur Proximal tibia/fibula	Crutches for children older than 6 years of age
Posterior (short leg)	Distal tibia/fibula Ankle Foot	Crutches for children older than 6 years of age
Stirrup	Ankle (including soft tissue injuries)	Allows for weight bearing; fits in a shoe

[a] Prefabricated splints are commercially available.

CHAPTER 57

Short Arm and Leg Casts

OVERVIEW

Short Arm Cast

1. Assemble materials (two rolls of plaster usually are adequate, 2- to 3-inch size for child, 4-inch for adult; with fiberglass, use narrower rolls).
2. Position patient and extremity: supine, should be abducted 90 degrees, elbow flexed 90 degrees.
3. Apply stockinette (optional): thumbhole necessary, avoid wrinkles (Fig. 57.1*A*).
4. Apply cast padding: wrap from proximal palmar crease to approximately 1 inch below flexion crease of elbow. Make transverse tear in padding before wrapping around thumb webspace. Apply additional padding over ulnar styloid (see Fig. 57.1*B,C*).
5. Apply cast material rolls: roll from distal to proximal. Twist 180 degrees when wrapping through thumb webspace. Before second roll, fold over ends of stockinette. A total of four to six layers of plaster, three of fiberglass, is sufficient. Do not begin too distally. Allow for 90 degrees of flexion at metacarpophalangeal joints, for fanning of fingers, and for opposition of thumb to index and little fingers (see Fig. 57.1*D,F*).
6. Smooth and shape: begin rubbing when plaster is the consistency of wet cardboard. Mold to shape of forearm using palms and thenar eminence, not digits. Shape should be cylindrical, not round (see Fig. 57.1*G*).
7. Maintain immobilization during drying. Reassess for pressure points, pain relief, neurovascular compromise. Trim ends of cast as needed to allow for adequate finger and thumb motion (see Fig. 57.1*H*).
8. For thumb spica, use same approach except include thumb in extension in cast. Cut 2-inch cast padding to 1-inch size for use around thumb itself (Fig. 57.2).

Short Leg Cast

1. Assemble materials (three rolls of plaster usually are adequate, 3- to 4-inch size for child, 6-inch for adult; with fiberglass, use narrower rolls).
2. Position patient and extremity—alternatives:
   A. Patient sitting, knee flexed to 90 degrees.

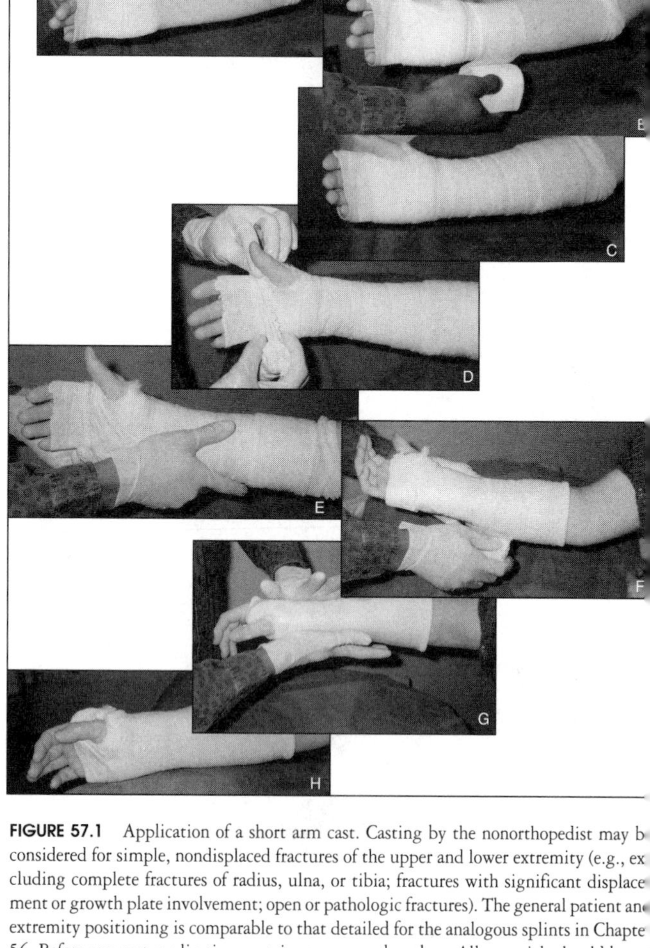

FIGURE 57.1 Application of a short arm cast. Casting by the nonorthopedist may b considered for simple, nondisplaced fractures of the upper and lower extremity (e.g., ex cluding complete fractures of radius, ulna, or tibia; fractures with significant displace ment or growth plate involvement; open or pathologic fractures). The general patient an extremity positioning is comparable to that detailed for the analogous splints in Chapte 56. Before any cast application, certain steps must be taken. All materials should be as sembled. The patient is positioned and draped properly. The skin of the involved ex tremity is washed with soap and water and dried thoroughly. All superficial wound should be carefully cleansed and then covered with thin, sterile dressing. A short arm cas is indicated for torus fractures of the radius and ulna, nondisplaced Salter-Harris type fractures of the distal radius, and nondisplaced, stable metacarpal fractures. **A:** Maintai casting position and apply stockinette. **B,C:** Apply cast padding on to the extremity dis tally to proximally, overlapping each turn. **D:** Beginning distally, apply plaster rolls. **E** Smooth plaster. **F,G:** Fold over ends of stockinette to provide smooth ends for the cast **H:** Maintain positioning of the extremity until cast is hardened.

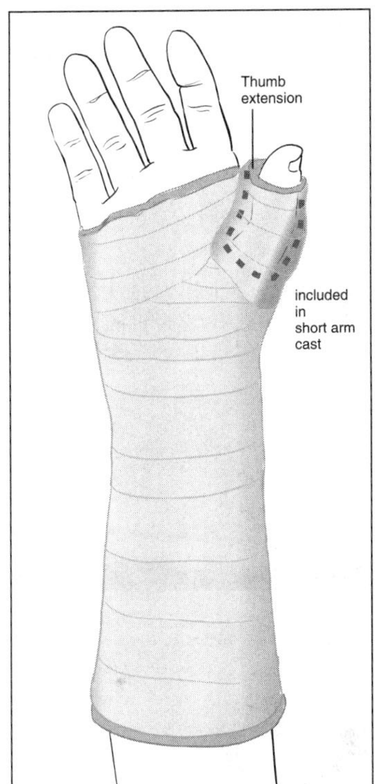

FIGURE 57.2 The thumb spica cast is indicated for clinically suspected scaphoid (navicular) fractures (discuss with orthopedist if overt fracture). Use the same approach as short arm cast, except include thumb in an extension of the cast. Cut 2-inch cast padding to 1-inch size for use around thumb itself.

B. Patient supine, hip and knee flexed to 90 degrees, assistant supporting leg.

C. Patient prone, knee flexed to 90 degrees.

3. Apply stockinette (optional): if single piece, cut away transverse fold in front of ankle; better to apply two short segments at proximal and distal ends of cast (Fig. 57.3*A,B*).

4. Apply cast padding: wrap from level of distal metatarsals to one fingerbreadth below tibial tubercle; apply additional padding over malleoli and heel.

5. Apply cast material rolls: roll from distal to proximal. A total of five to seven layers of plaster, three of fiberglass, is sufficient. If weight bearing is intended for a larger child, reinforcing splints will need to be added when using plaster. Two plaster splints can be incorporated posteriorly, folding

back last 1 to 2 inches at level of distal metatarsals (see Fig. 57.3*C*). Alternatively, fold 4-inch plaster splints in half longitudinally, placing one posteriorly and in a stirrup (U-shape from medial to lateral). Do not begin too distally.

6. Smooth and shape: begin rubbing when plaster is the consistency of wet cardboard. Mold to shape of lower leg using palms and thenar eminence, not digits (see Fig. 57.3*D*). Allow for flexion and fanning of all the toes (see Fig. 57.3*E*).

7. Maintain immobilization during drying. Reassess for pressure points, pain relief, and neurovascular compromise. Fit for cast boot or crutches as needed. There should be no weight bearing for a minimum of 24 hours.

CLINICAL TIPS

Short Arm Cast

1. Always use a clean bucket and water when immersing plaster rolls.
2. Using the widest roll of cast material practical for the size of the extremity speeds application and allows for a more even cast.
3. For thumbs and smaller hands, make 1-inch rolls of padding by cutting 2-inch rolls in half.

Short Leg Cast

1. Always use a clean bucket and water when immersing plaster rolls.
2. Using the widest roll of cast material practical for the size of the extremity speeds application and allows for a more even cast.

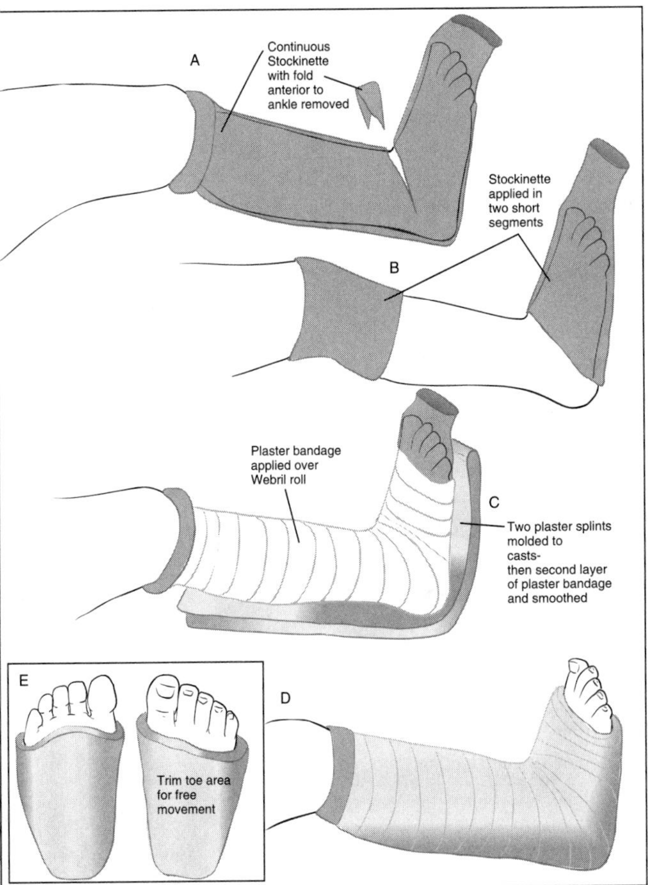

FIGURE 57.3 The short leg cast is indicated for minor fibula fractures (including suspected Salter-Harris type 1 fractures of distal fibula), toddler's fractures, severe ankle sprains, stable metatarsal fractures, and simple fractures of the midfoot and hindfoot. Apply stockinette in either continuous piece (**A**) or in two short segments at proximal and distal ends of cast (**B**). Apply cast material rolls (**C**). Smooth and shape plaster (**D**). Allow for flexion and fanning of all the toes (**E**).

CHAPTER 58

Hand and Finger Injuries

OVERVIEW

Subungual Hematomas

1. Obtain radiographs of any suspect injury.
2. Use restraints as needed.
3. Use anesthesia–digital block if necessary.
4. Prepare antiseptically.
5. Carry out trephination.
6. Apply protective dressing.
7. Warm soaks.
8. Splint fractures 14 days.

Subungual Foreign Bodies

1. Radiographs are unnecessary unless confirming presence of foreign body.
2. Use restraints as needed.
3. Use anesthesia–digital block as needed.
4. Remove the foreign body.
5. Thoroughly clean and irrigate the wound.
6. Apply protective dressing.
7. Warm soaks.
8. Administer antibiotics if indicated.

Nailbed Repair

1. Obtain radiographic evaluation.
2. Use anesthesia.
3. Use restraints as needed.
4. Remove the nail.
5. Irrigate and clean.

6. Apply digital tourniquet.
7. Repair nailbed.
8. Repair skin.
9. Apply nailbed splint (replace nail, Silastic, or mesh gauze).
10. Apply dressing.
11. Ensure fracture stabilization.
12. Ensure hand surgeon follow-up.
13. Administer antibiotics as needed.

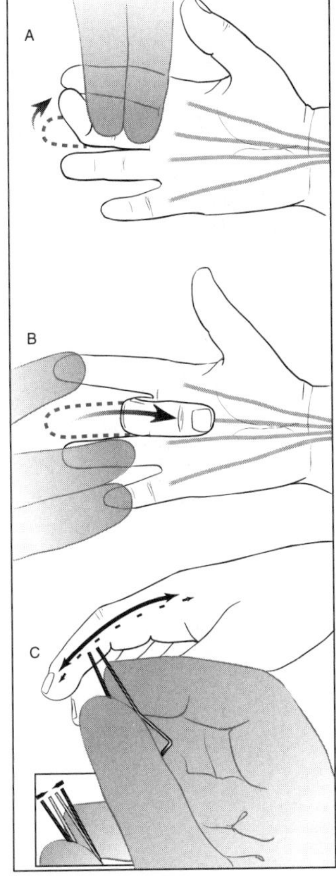

FIGURE 58.1 Basic examination of the digits. Motor function is assessed by testing both muscle strength and tendon function. The child places the affected hand palm up on the examining table. The clinician places two fingers on the involved finger just proximal to the distal interphalangeal joint, holding the finger firmly against the table (**A**). The patient is asked to bend the finger tip, and if he or she is able to, the maneuver is repeated against resistance (testing flexor digitorum profundus integrity). Next, the child's noninjured fingers are held against the table (**B**) and the child is asked to again bend the affected finger first without, and then against, resistance (testing flexor digitorum superficialis integrity). Extensor function is then tested by asking the child to open and close his or her hand, curling and uncurling the affected finger. Significant pain or disability with these maneuvers suggests tendon injury. Sensory function may be tested in cooperative children by two-point discrimination (normal down to 6-mm separation) using a bent paper clip (**C**), or by simple light touch in younger children. In uncooperative children, the affected finger may be placed in a bowl of warm water for a few minutes. Injured fingers with areas of interrupted nerve supply do not wrinkle.

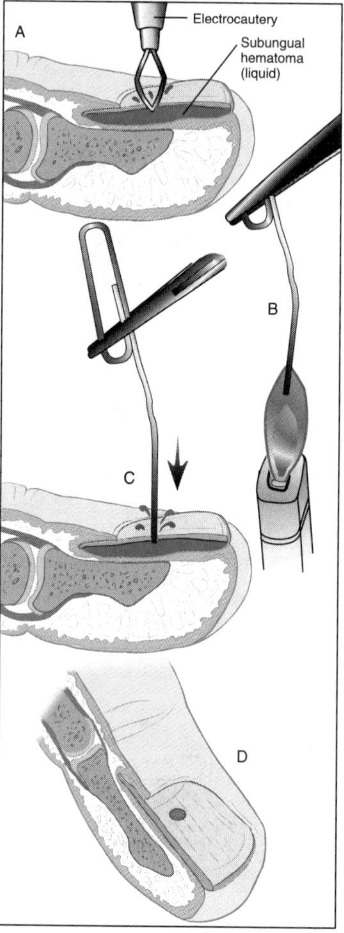

FIGURE 58.2 Nail trephination for subungual hematoma. Nail trephination affords rapid pain relief for most cases of subungual hematoma (SUH) secondary to blunt trauma. However, if the nail plate or margins are disrupted, the nail should be removed and the nailbed explored for possible lacerations requiring repair. Traditionally, some authorities have recommended nail removal also for large SUH (25% to 50% or larger), but many experts believe that such an aggressive approach is unnecessary. A hole 3 to 4 mm in size is usually adequate. A digital block may be necessary for some patients, but the brief, if any, pain associated with electrocautery trephination is usually less than that associated with the block. The nail is cleaned with antiseptic solution (if alcohol is used, it must be allowed to dry completely so as not to ignite when heated!). The electrocautery is held perpendicular to the nail over the SUH and heated, and then gentle downward pressure is used to create the hole (**A**). Blood rapidly exits through the hole, and any remainder may be extruded with gentle pressure on the nailbed. Alternatively, a heated paper clip may be used (**B**). After drainage, a protective dressing can be applied. Any underlying fracture should be splinted, with consideration of orthopedic referral.

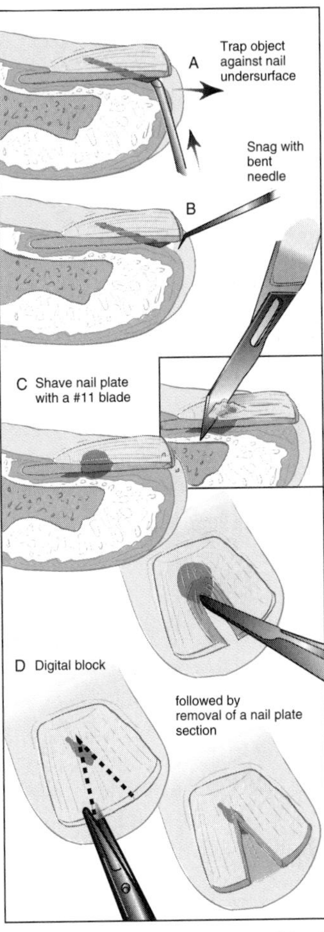
A
Trap object against nail undersurface
Snag with bent needle
B
C Shave nail plate with a #11 blade
D Digital block
followed by removal of a nail plate section

FIGURE 58.3 Subungual foreign body removal. The technique for removing a subungual foreign body depends on the position of the foreign body beneath the nail. If it protrudes beyond the nail edge, it may be grasped with a small forceps. A small protruding stump can be pinned against the undersurface of the distal nail by a scissors tip, needle, or scalpel blade and drawn forward (**A**). Distal foreign bodies that are not easily grabbed or pinned may be snagged with a 25- to 27-gauge needle tip that has been bent 90 degrees with a hemostat (**B**). Alternatively, a no. 11 blade can be held horizontally, nearly parallel to the nail, and used to shave the nail proximally to distally over the foreign body (**C**). This procedure exposes the foreign body, allowing it to be grasped and removed (**D**). Most patients can tolerate these methods without anesthesia. Deeper or firmly embedded foreign bodies and any procedures requiring nailbed manipulation require a digital block (Fig. 17.4). After adequate anesthesia, the nail may be lifted on either side of the foreign body using the sharp point of a pair of iris scissors to separate the nail from the nailbed (see Fig. 58.4*B*). The scissors is held so that the point is angled slightly dorsally and the point is run along the undersurface of the nail to avoid damaging the nailbed. Two or three tracts along the long axis of the finger should release enough of the nail from the nailbed to allow the foreign body to be grasped with forceps and removed. For objects unable to be removed in this fashion, a V-shaped wedge may be cut out of the elevated nail overlying the foreign body to allow access for removal (**D**).

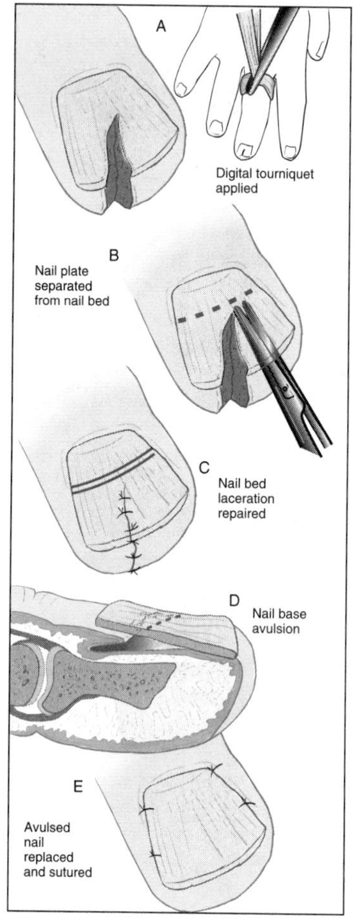
A
Digital tourniquet applied
B
Nail plate separated from nail bed
C
Nail bed laceration repaired
D
Nail base avulsion
E
Avulsed nail replaced and sutured

FIGURE 58.4 Nailbed injury repairs. Initial care of any nailbed injury includes age-appropriate restraint and adequate anesthesia. In some cases, conscious sedation may also be required. After antiseptic preparation of the entire finger, the fingernail is lifted to provide complete access to the nailbed. The nail is gently separated from the nailbed with the sharp end of a scissors tip (**A,B**), beginning as detailed in the discussion for embedded foreign body removal in Fig. 58.3. Then, to lift the nail, the scissors is slowly advanced as it is spread open to lift the nail plate. Similarly, the eponychial and lateral folds are freed from the nail by inserting the scissors tip between the skin folds and the nail itself. For nailbed and plate injuries such as that illustrated here, the nail may need be separated only to the indicated dotted line, and then cut off horizontally, leaving the intact nail plate remnant in place as a stent, while allowing exposure for repair of the nailbed. For more extensive lacerations, complete nail removal is indicated, and the dissection is extended all the way back to the germinal matrix under the eponychium. Once the nail is removed, the nailbed is copiously but gently irrigated with saline. A bloodless field is required and may be effected by using a sterile Penrose drain as a tourniquet (**A**). Alternatively, a sterile glove the patient's size may be used. The tip of the glove finger corresponding to the involved finger is cut off and the glove placed on the hand. The cut rubber finger is rolled back proximally until it reaches the hand, which will provide an evenly compressive tourniquet.

All nailbed lacerations should be repaired with fine absorbable suture on side-cutting needles, such as 6-0 to 7-0 chromic or Vicryl (**C**). If it is suspected that the laceration extends beneath the eponychium, the eponychium is cut back several millimeters, perpendicular to its edges, at the point it curves distally. Retraction of the eponychial skin folds then allows access to the germinal matrix for inspection and repair. The eponychial cuts may be closed with 5-0 nylon suture.

Proximal nailbed base avulsions may occur when the fingertip is crushed, and usually require nail removal to effect complete nailbed inspection and repair of any laceration or tissue avulsion. If small fragments of nailbed tissue adhere to the avulsed nail, these are best left attached and replaced as a unit with the nail. Larger fragments can be gently trimmed off the nail with a no. 15 scalpel blade and sutured into place. Nail avulsions that tear the germinal matrix proximally and pull it out from beneath the eponychium, still attached to the nail, are best referred to a hand surgeon. Lacerations to the lateral or eponychial folds are repaired with 5-0 or 6-0 nylon sutures, with care taken to maintain the folds while carefully approximating skin edges. All nailbeds require splinting, which is best accomplished with the original nail itself. The nail should be gently cleaned, have a center hole for drainage placed, and be replaced into position beneath the eponychium. It can be sutured into place with two 5-0 nylon sutures (**E**). If the original nail cannot be used, a nonadherent splint of Silastic, mesh gauze, or sterile foil cut from a suture packet may be secured beneath the eponychial fold. This is typically left in place for 1 to 2 weeks. A protective dressing and splint may be applied, and a follow-up visit scheduled for 24 hours.

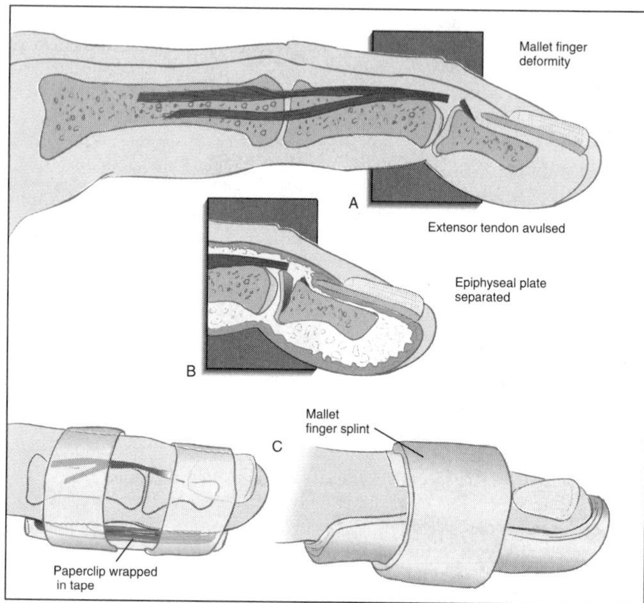

FIGURE 58.5 Splinting of mallet finger deformity. The mallet finger deformity typically occurs when forced flexion results in extensor tendon avulsion from the distal phalanx, as when the extended finger is hit head-on by a blunt object (e.g., a baseball). Tendon laceration due to lacerations of the dorsal finger at the level of the distal interphalangeal (DIP) joint may produce a similar deformity. In adolescents, the tendon pulls off the distal phalanx with or without a portion of the dorsal lip of the distal phalanx itself (**A**). In younger children, the epiphyseal plate separate and the proximal epiphysis remains attached to the extensor tendon (**B**). Mallet finger injuries due to tendon lacerations or those associated with fractures or epiphyseal separations may require operative repair, and should be referred to a hand surgeon. However, a closed mallet finger deformity without fracture typically heals well with splinting. A dorsal foam splint, or one fashioned from a tape-wrapped paper clip, should be applied to hold the DIP joint fully extended and bring the extensor tendon and distal phalanx into juxtaposition (**C**). Full flexion must be allowed at the proximal interphalangeal joint. The splint should be maintained for 6 to 8 weeks. It can be removed transiently when wet or dirty, but the patient should be carefully instructed to maintain constant extension at the DIP joint until the splint is reapplied.

CHAPTER 59

Arthrocentesis

OVERVIEW

1. Discuss procedure with parents and child and obtain informed consent.
2. Review technique for arthrocentesis of specific joint by studying corresponding figure and legend; remember to note joint positioning, insertion sites based on bony landmarks, and direction needle should be inserted.
3. Gather necessary equipment.
4. Consider sedation, immobilization, and need for an assistant.
5. Palpate bony landmarks to find reference points in locating insertion site—may want to mark skin with closed retractable pen.
6. Prepare joint entry site for sterile technique.
7. Anesthetize entry site with local anesthetic or vapocoolant.
8. Place joint in correct position and consider joint distraction.
9. Direct needle as recommended in specific approaches to lessen chance of scoring cartilage.
10. Remember to send synovial fluid for analysis (listed in order of importance): culture and sensitivity, Gram stain, and cell count with differential.
11. Send synovial fluid to laboratory in sterile glass or plastic tube without additives for immediate culture and Gram stain, and ideally a heparinized tube for cell count and differential (50 U heparin/mL synovial fluid).
12. Examine synovial fluid in clear test tube for color and clarity.

CLINICAL TIPS

1. Joints may have more than one route of entry. The preferred route is usually the shortest distance from the point of entry to the joint space and avoids skin lesions or superficial infections, major vessels, tendons, and nerves. An approach on the extensor side of the joint usually accomplishes this goal.
2. The skin over the aspiration site can be marked with a closed retractable pen while the unprepared joint is manually examined.
3. Local anesthetic should not be injected into the joint cavity because it may cause artifact and sterilize septic synovial fluid.
4. Discomfort of arthrocentesis can be decreased sufficiently by a local vapocoolant, such as ethyl chloride.

5. Because joint fluid is so viscous, use the largest needle that can atraumatically enter the joint cavity.
6. Size of the syringe should correspond with the estimated volume of the joint effusion.
7. Remember to loosen the seal on the syringe before aspirating the joint to prevent trauma from undue struggling with the syringe.
8. If synovial fluid stops flowing into the syringe and joint fluid still remains, flow can often be reestablished by repositioning the needle or by reinjecting a small amount of joint fluid.
9. Distraction of the joint may facilitate arthrocentesis of joints in the wrist and the hand.
10. Synovial fluid, like any other body fluid, should be considered infectious.

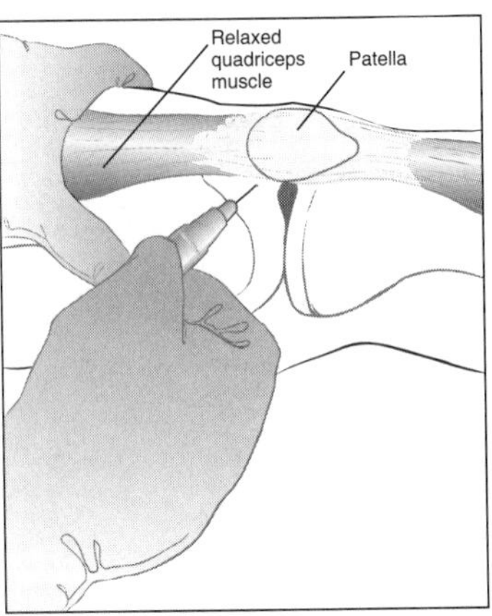

FIGURE 59.1 Arthrocentesis of the knee by superolateral approach. The general approach to joint aspiration is summarized in the accompanying Overview and Clinical Tips sections. A young or uncooperative child may require restraint and judicious sedation to maintain complete joint immobility during the procedure. The overlying skin is prepared with antiseptic solution. Residual povidone-iodine should wiped away to avoid instillation into the joint. In general, the largest needle that can atraumatically aspirate a joint should be used, usually 18 to 20 gauge for the knee and 20 to 23 gauge for smaller joints. Local anesthesia may be used, but again none should be allowed entry into the joint. The needle insertion site may be marked before skin preparation by pressure with the tip of a closed retractable pen. A distinct pop may be felt when puncturing the joint capsule. As the needle advances toward the joint space, the clinician should withdraw slightly on the syringe to aspirate synovial fluid as soon as the joint cavity is entered.

Experts are divided on which approach to the knee joint is optimal. In general, a large effusion with bulging at the superolateral pouch may be treated more easily with the superolateral approach.

Position: Patient's knee should be extended as much as possible.

Insertion: The needle is inserted slightly lateral to the superolateral border of the patella.

Direction: The needle is directed slightly inferiorly and slightly posteriorly to pass underneath the patella, aiming for the intercondylar fossa.

Comments: Relaxation of the quadriceps greatly facilitates needle placement.

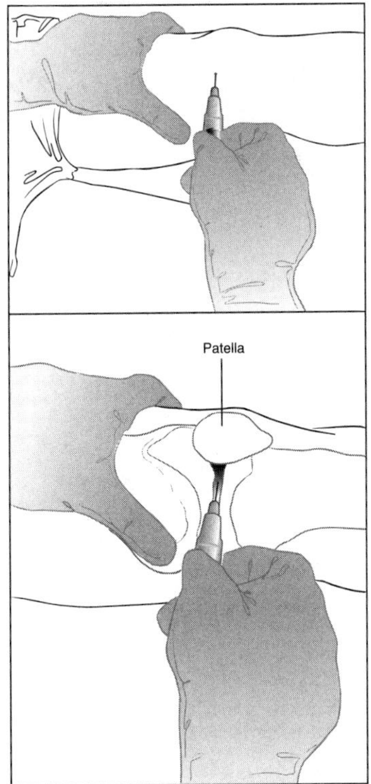

FIGURE 59.2 Arthrocentesis of knee by medial approach.

Position: The knee may be fully extended or flexed to 45 degrees.

Insertion: The needle is inserted at the midpoint of the patella or the superomedial border of the patella.

Direction: The needle is directed underneath the patella aiming for the intercondylar fossa.

Comments: It may be easier to use this approach if the effusion is small.

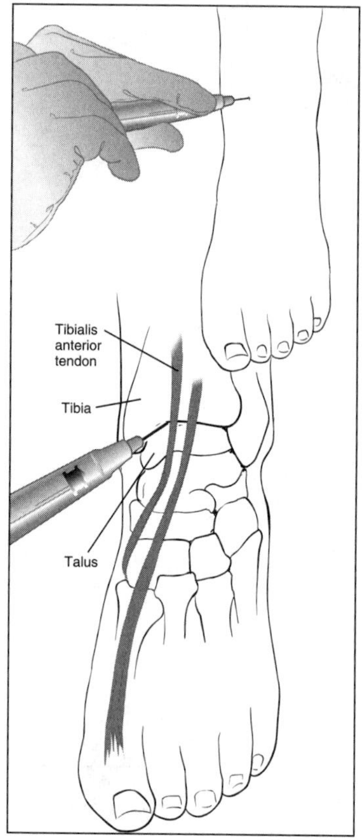

FIGURE 59.3 Arthrocentesis of ankle at tibiotalar joint.

Position: The ankle should be slightly plantar flexed because the joint space is widened.

Insertion: The needle is inserted anterior to the medial malleolus, in a sulcus just medial to the tibialis anterior tendon.

Direction: The needle is directed posterolaterally.

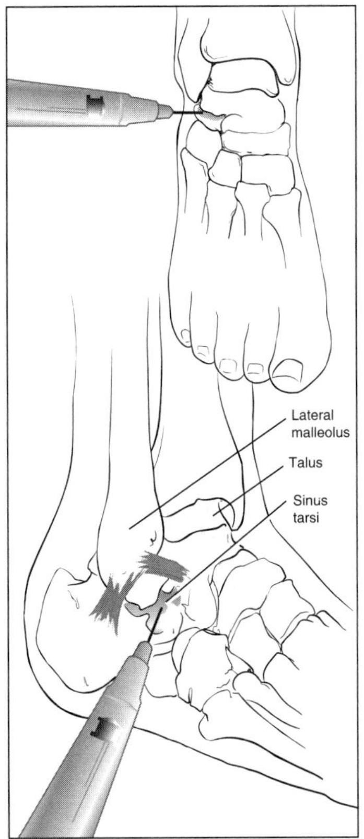

FIGURE 59.4 Arthrocentesis of ankle at subtalar joint.
Position: The ankle is at 90 degrees and slightly inverted.
Insertion: The needle is inserted just distal to the tip of the lateral malleolus.
Direction: The needle is held horizontal to the subtalar joint and is directed medially.
Comments: This can be a difficult joint space to enter.

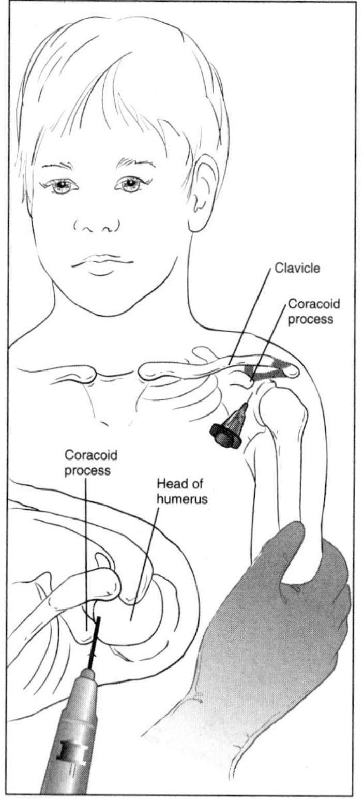

FIGURE 59.5 Arthrocentesis of the shoulder.

Position: The patient is allowed to sit upright with the arm at rest and the hand in the lap.

Insertion: The needle is inserted just inferior and lateral to the coracoid process.

Direction: The needle should be directed posteriorly or posteriorly and slightly superiorly and laterally.

Comments: Arthrocentesis of this joint can be difficult. In an uncooperative child, sedation is encouraged and consultation may be required.

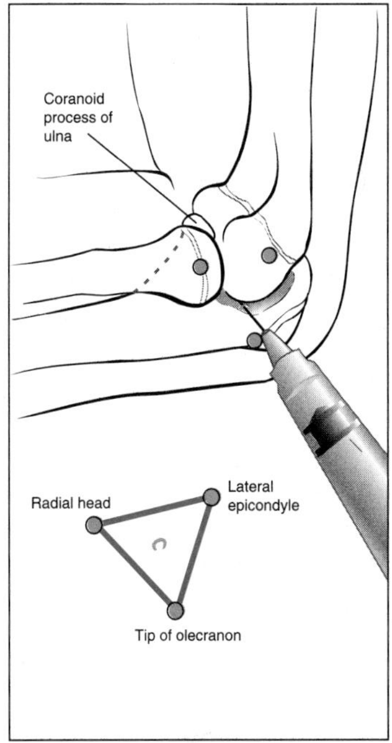

FIGURE 59.6 Arthrocentesis of the elbow.

Position: The patient's elbow is held at 90 degrees, preferably resting on a table or a bed.

Insertion: The needle is inserted in the center of the anconeus triangle, a space between the lateral epicondyle of the humerus, the radial head, and the olecranon process.

Direction: The needle should be directed medially and slightly anteriorly toward the coronoid process of the ulna.

Comments: If a significant effusion is present, this space often bulges outward.

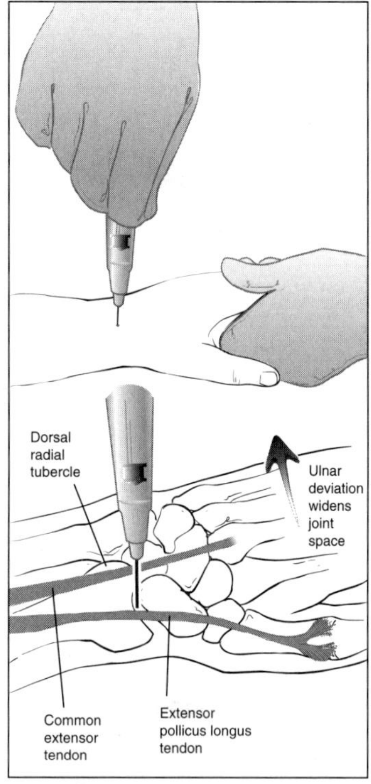

FIGURE 59.7 Arthrocentesis of wrist.

Position: The wrist is flexed 30 degrees and ulnarly deviated.

Insertion: The needle is inserted just distal to the dorsal radial tubercle (of Lister) and in the sulcus between the extensor pollicis longus tendon and the common extensor tendon to the index finger.

Direction: The needle is inserted perpendicular to the skin.

Comments: Application of traction to the hand may facilitate the procedure by widening the joint space.

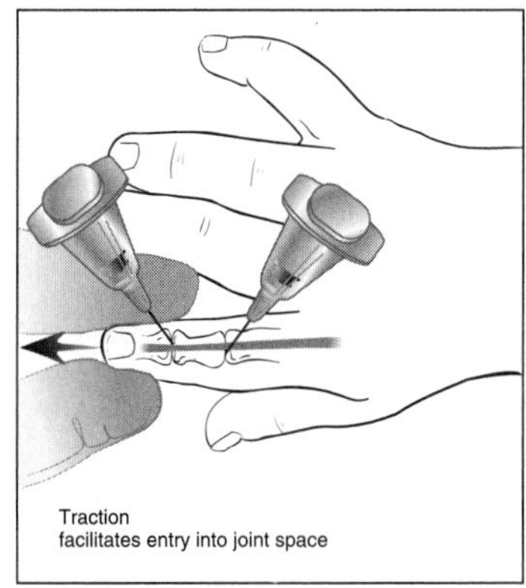

IGURE 59.8 Arthrocentesis of ıetacarpophalangeal and interphaıngeal joints.

Position: The fingers are flexed 15 ɔ 20 degrees.

Insertion: The needle is inserted orsally, just medial or lateral to the xtensor tendon.

Direction: The needle is directed erpendicular to the skin.

Comments: The needle does not ave to enter between the joint suraces. Applying traction may faciliate entry into the joint space.

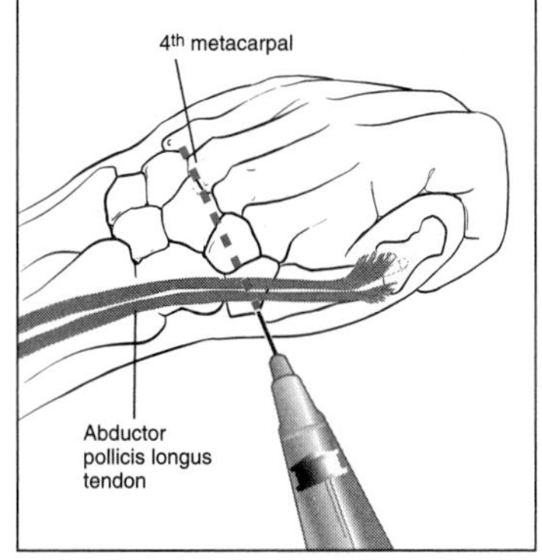

IGURE 59.9 Arthrocentesis of the humb at the carpometacarpal joint.

Position: The thumb should be pposed with the little finger, or laced in the palm of the hand with a losed fist.

Insertion: The needle is inserted roximal to the prominence at the ase of the first metacarpal on the palnar side of the abductor pollicis ɔngus tendon.

Direction: The needle should be irected toward the base of the fourth ıetacarpal.

Comments: The abductor pollicis ɔngus tendon is easiest to palpate vhen the thumb is extended.

CHAPTER 60

Reduction of Joint Dislocations and Subluxations

OVERVIEW

Radial Head Subluxation

1. Have child sit comfortably in caretaker's lap.
2. Support child's arm in nondominant hand, applying moderate pressure on radial head with thumb or fingers.
3. Hold child's wrist in dominant hand, placing fingers on volar aspect of wrist and thumb on dorsal aspect.
4. Apply gentle longitudinal traction to arm.
5. While maintaining traction, in one motion supinate arm then fully flex it.
6. An audible reduction click may be heard.
7. If procedure is successful, child should be using arm within 20 to 30 minutes.
8. If several appropriate attempts fail, radiographs should be obtained.
9. If radiographs are normal, child should be placed in a sling and referred to an orthopedist; spontaneous reduction may occur in a day or two.

Digit Dislocation

1. Remove all rings from affected finger and achieve anesthesia with a digital block.
2. Securely brace affected hand or foot.
3. Apply gentle traction to affected digit.
4. For dorsal dislocation joint is gently hyperextended; for volar dislocation hyperflexed.
5. Push dislocated phalanx into its proper position.
6. Obtain radiographs after reduction and splint digit.

Shoulder Dislocation

1. Reduction by gravity.
   A. Use appropriate analgesia and sedation and monitor patient.
   B. Have patient lie on stretcher in prone position with affected arm dangling over side.
   C. Attach 2- to 5-kg weight to arm.
   D. Allow arm to hang for 20 to 40 minutes.
   E. After reduction, arm swings freely and painlessly in forward position.

2. Reduction by scapular manipulation.
   A. Prone position.
      1) Use appropriate analgesia and sedation and monitor patient.
      2) Have patient lie on stretcher in prone position with affected arm hanging over side.
      3) Attach 2- to 5-kg weight to arm or have assistant apply downward traction to arm.
      4) Gently rotate scapula by simultaneously pushing its tip medially and its superior aspect laterally.
      5) An audible or palpable "clunk" occurs with successful reduction.
   B. Seated position.
      1) Use appropriate analgesia and sedation, if needed.
      2) Have patient sit in chair facing back of chair.
      3) While assistant applies forward traction to affected arm, scapula is rotated as described in 2-A.

3. Reduction by traction–countertraction.
   A. Use appropriate analgesia and sedation and monitor patient.
   B. Patient is placed in supine position with elbow of affected side in slight abduction and 90 degrees of flexion.
   C. Sheet is looped around flexed forearm distal to elbow, then around clinician (clinician should be standing next to hip on affected side).
   D. Have assistant loop second sheet about himself or herself and then around patient's chest under axilla on affected side.
   E. Exert continuous longitudinal traction on affected arm, gradually increasing force until the reduction is achieved; it may be necessary to lean back against sheets to gain mechanical advantage.

Patella Dislocation

1. Use appropriate analgesia and sedation and monitor patient.
2. Place patient in supine position with hips in flexion.

3. Bring knee joint to full extension while gradually applying medial pressure on patella to achieve reduction.
4. Appropriately immobilize knee after examination.

Hip Dislocation

1. Supine position.
   - A. Use appropriate analgesia and sedation and monitor patient.
   - B. Place patient in supine position with both hip and knee in 90 degrees of flexion and hip in slightly internal rotation and adduction.
   - C. Have assistant stabilize pelvis with downward pressure applied to both iliac crests.
   - D. Apply continuous traction to distal femur in line with deformity.
   - E. Use gentle rotary motion of femur gradually to bring femoral head over posterior acetabular rim and into the acetabulum.
2. Prone position.
   - A. Use appropriate analgesia and sedation and monitor patient.
   - B. Place patient in prone position with thigh hanging vertically from stretcher.
   - C. Apply downward vertical traction on distal femur until reduction is achieved.
3. For both techniques, postreduction radiographs should be obtained. Casting may be needed for appropriate immobilization.

Posterior Elbow Dislocation

1. Use appropriate analgesia and sedation and monitor patient.
2. Apply traction to proximal forearm with elbow slightly flexed.
3. Apply forward and downward pressure to olecranon while flexing elbow.
4. Apply appropriate immobilization.

Knee Dislocation

1. Use appropriate analgesia and sedation as needed and monitor patient.
2. Apply longitudinal traction.
   - A. For anterior dislocation, lift femur anteriorly or push proximal tibia posteriorly.
   - B. For posterior dislocation, extend knee while lifting proximal tibia into reduced position.

3. Angiography should be performed after reduction.
4. If no vascular injury is present, immobilize appropriately.

Ankle Dislocation

1. Use appropriate analgesia and sedation as needed and monitor patient.
2. Place patient in supine position.
3. Apply traction to foot while assistant applies countertraction to lower leg; dominant hand should hold heel and nondominant hand the forefoot.
4. For poster dislocation, apply traction with foot in a slight plantar flexion.
5. For posterior dislocation, lift foot anteriorly while gently dorsiflexing it.
6. For anterior dislocation, apply the traction with foot in slight dorsiflexion.
7. For anterior dislocation, further dorsiflex foot then push it posteriorly while plantar flexing it gently.
8. Immobilize ankle appropriately.

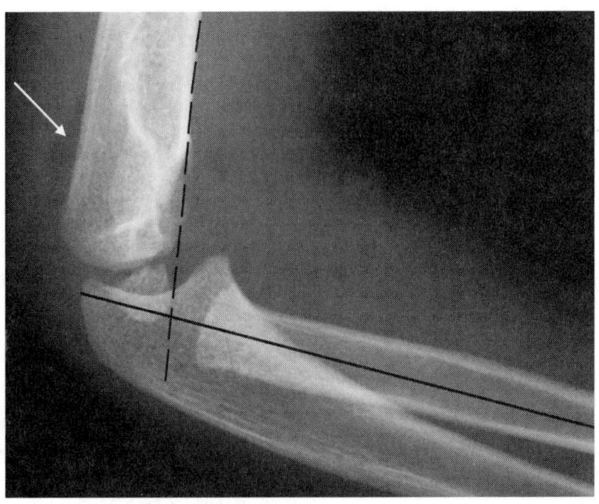

IGURE 60.1 Posterior fat pad sign, anterior humeral line, and radiocapitellar line. Lateral view radiograph of the elbow reveals a posterior fat pad sign (*arrow*) and slight posterior displacement of the capitellum relative to anterior humeral line (*dashed line*) indicative of supracondylar fracture. Subtle abnormalities such as these exclude the diagnosis of radial head subluxation and suggest the need for orthopedic evaluation. The radiocapitellar line (*solid line*) in this patient is normal.

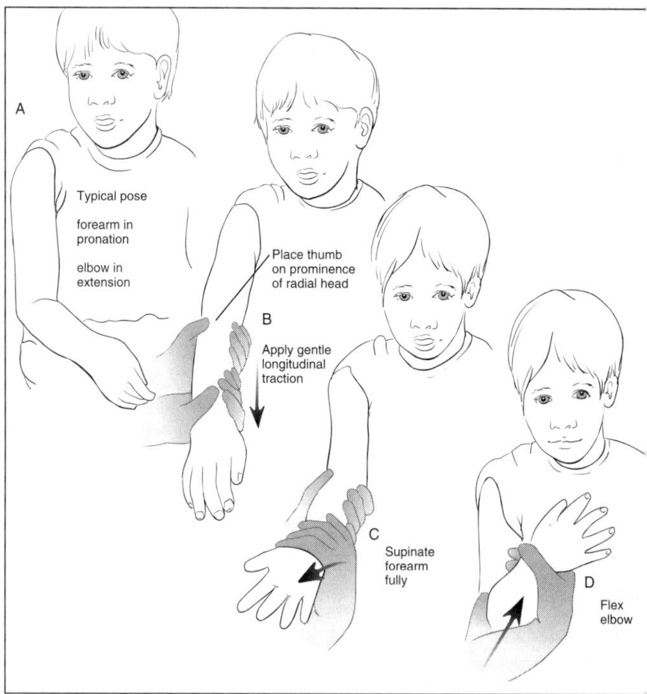

FIGURE 60.2 Reduction of radial head subluxation. The child should sit comfortably i the parent's lap (**A**). The clinician, using the nondominant hand, supports the elbow gen tly with the palm and applies moderate pressure on the radial head with either the thum or fingers. With the dominant hand, the clinician grasps the wrist of the affected arm b placing fingers on the volar aspect of the wrist and the thumb on the dorsal aspect (**B** In one quick, deliberate motion while applying gentle longitudinal traction, the forearr is forcefully and fully supinated (**C**), and the elbow is then flexed (**D**). In 80% to 90% c maneuvers, a palpable or audible click or "clunk" at the radial head area accompanies an indicates a successful reduction. Most patients have return of arm use within 10 to 1 minutes. However, if reduction is delayed more than 8 to 12 hours, full recovery ma take up to 1 to 2 days. In such a case, the arm should be immobilized with a long poste rior splint (see Fig. 56.5) and reevaluated in 24 hours.

CLINICAL TIPS

1. Use analgesia and sedation as needed.
2. Restraint may sometimes be required.
3. Monitor the patient well.
4. Consider the possibility of neurovascular compromise.
5. Seek orthopedic consultation in dislocations with significant potential morbidity *but*, if consultant cannot be available in timely fashion, attempt to reduce the dislocation.
6. After a successful reduction, immobilize the joint appropriately.

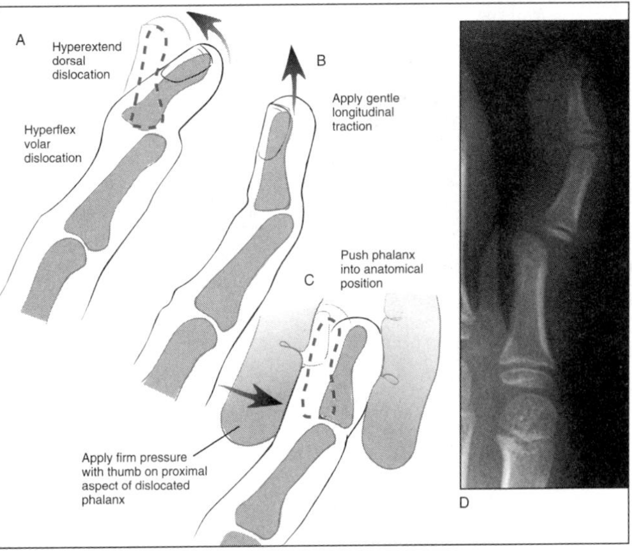

IGURE 60.3 Reduction of dorsal distal interphalangeal joint dislocation (A–C). Ra-iograph of dorsal proximal interphalangeal joint dislocation, which is reduced similarly D). Before performing the reduction maneuver, radiographs are obtained to examine for ssociated fractures or volar plate injury. All rings should be removed and the digit anes-hetized with a digital block (see Figs. 7.4 and 17.6). With the patient's hand or foot se-urely braced, the clinician grasps the dislocated phalanx; dry gauze loosely wrapped round the phalanx may improve grip. The joint is hyperextended (**A**) with gentle lon-itudinal traction for a dorsal dislocation (**B**), or hyperflexed for a volar dislocation. The islocated phalanx is then pushed gradually into its normal anatomic position (**C**). Trac-on should not be vigorously applied in a child because it may result in interposition of ft tissue or an osteochondral fragment into the distracted joint space and prevent re-uction. After reduction, the joint is carefully examined for full range of motion and sta-lity, radiographs taken to confirm correct joint realignment, and the digit immobilized ith a foam-padded splint.

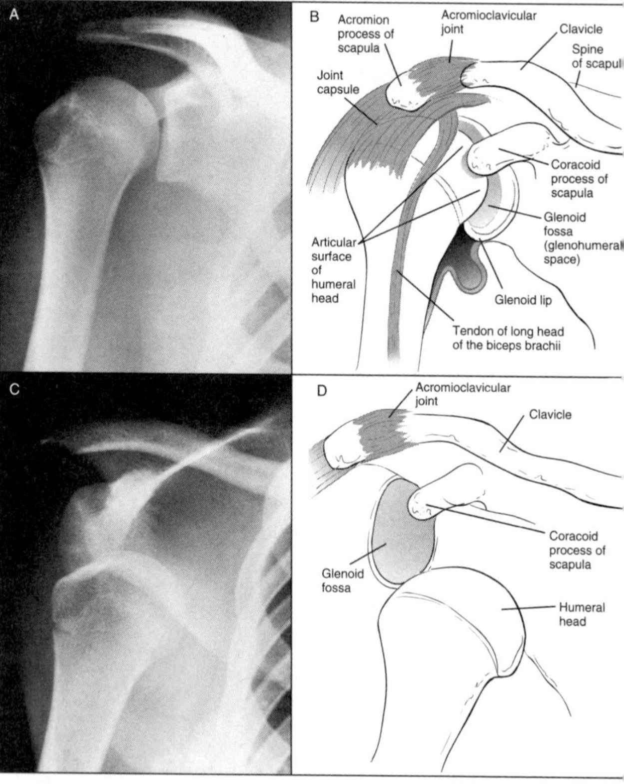

FIGURE 60.4 Radiographic and anatomic views of normal shoulder (**A**,**B**) and anteri dislocation of the shoulder (**C**,**D**) in the anteroposterior view.

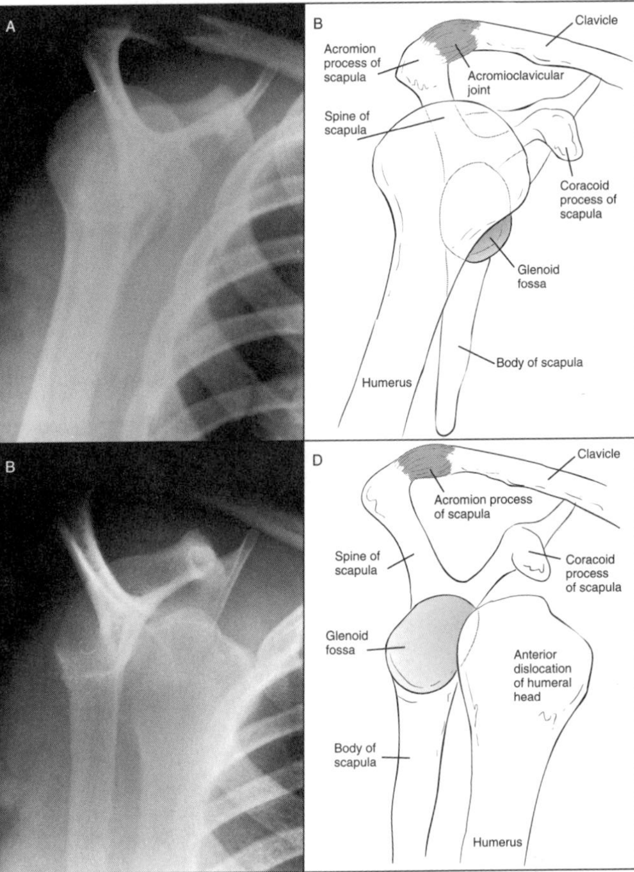

FIGURE 60.5 Radiographic and anatomic views of normal shoulder (**A**,**B**) and anterior dislocation of the shoulder (**C**,**D**) in the scapular Y view.

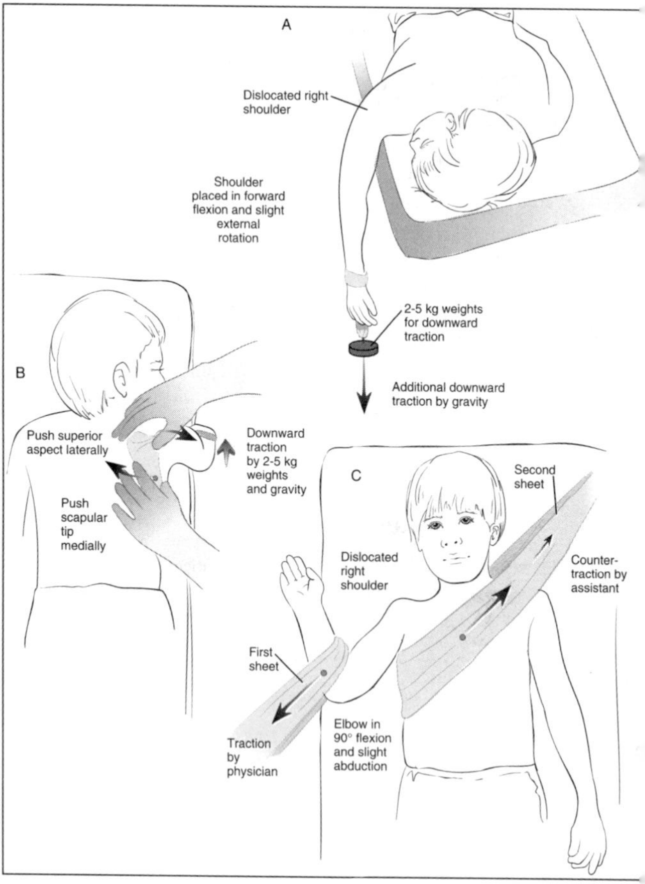

A
Dislocated right shoulder
Shoulder placed in forward flexion and slight external rotation
2-5 kg weights for downward traction
Additional downward traction by gravity
B
Push superior aspect laterally
Downward traction by 2-5 kg weights and gravity
Push scapular tip medially
C
Second sheet
Dislocated right shoulder
Counter-traction by assistant
First sheet
Traction by physician
Elbow in 90° flexion and slight abduction

Apply slight pressure to patella in medial direction
Extend leg at knee slowly
Supine position with hips in slight flexion

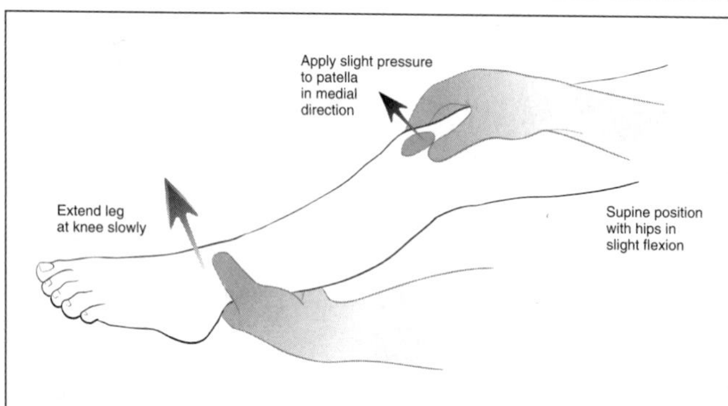

FIGURE 60.6 Reduction of anterior shoulder dislocation. Before attempting shoulder reduction, radiographs are obtained to examine for associated fractures or intraarticular bony fragments. The following reduction maneuvers are appropriate for children and adolescents. Reduction may be achieved with the forward flexion–gravity technique; if unsuccessful, this may be followed by attempts using the scapular manipulation or traction–countertraction techniques. **A:** Reduction by forward flexion–gravity. This reduction technique requires minimal exertion or strength, and no other assistance usually is needed. Although patience and a stable patient are required, the maneuver is atraumatic, simple, and safe. The patient is placed prone with the affected arm hanging vertically over the edge of the stretcher. The shoulder is in forward flexion and slight external rotation. In this position, gravity offers downward traction. Additional traction is applied with 2- to 5-kg weights strapped to the wrist. With sufficient time (20 to 30 minutes), muscle relaxation, and analgesia, the shoulder muscles fatigue and the humeral head gradually relocates into the glenoid fossa. When reduction occurs, the affected arm swings freely and painlessly in the forward position. **B:** Reduction by scapular manipulation. The patient is placed in a prone position with the affected arm hanging vertically over the edge of the stretcher. Downward traction using 2- to 5-kg weights for 5 minutes produces muscle fatigue and relaxation of the shoulder muscles. To achieve reduction, the scapula is rotated gently by simultaneously pushing its tip medially and its superior aspect laterally. A palpable or audible "clunk" is detected with a successful reduction. This technique may also be performed with the patient seated. When this approach is used, the patient sits facing the back of a chair. The patient rests his or her chest against the chair back, and an assistant applies traction to the affected arm. Manipulation of the scapula is performed as previously described. Scapular manipulation reduction may require less sedation and analgesia than other techniques. **C:** Reduction by traction–countertraction. The patient is placed in the supine position. The elbow of the affected side is held in slight abduction and 90 degrees of flexion. With the physician next to the patient's hip on the side of the affected shoulder, one sheet is looped around the flexed forearm just distal to the elbow and around the physician. A second sheet is wrapped around the patient's chest under the axilla of the affected side and around the assistant; using this sheet, the assistant provides countertraction. Continuous and gradually increasing longitudinal traction on the abducted arm with countertraction across the chest gradually achieves reduction. Both the physician and the assistant may gain mechanical advantage by leaning back on the sheets. As the shoulder muscles fatigue, reduction may be assisted by gentle internal and external rotation of the shoulder. Reduction is often clearly observed and may be accompanied by a palpable or audible "clunk." This technique requires more physical strength, and a minimum of two people.

FIGURE 60.7 Reduction of patellar dislocation. Reduction of a clinically apparent typical lateral patellar dislocation without suspicion for fracture or other serious pathologic process may precede radiographic evaluation. The patient is placed supine with the hips in flexion to relax the quadriceps muscles. The knee is slowly brought to full extension; slight pressure on the laterally displaced patella applied in a medial direction facilitates reduction. After reduction, radiographs are obtained and the knee immobilized in extension.

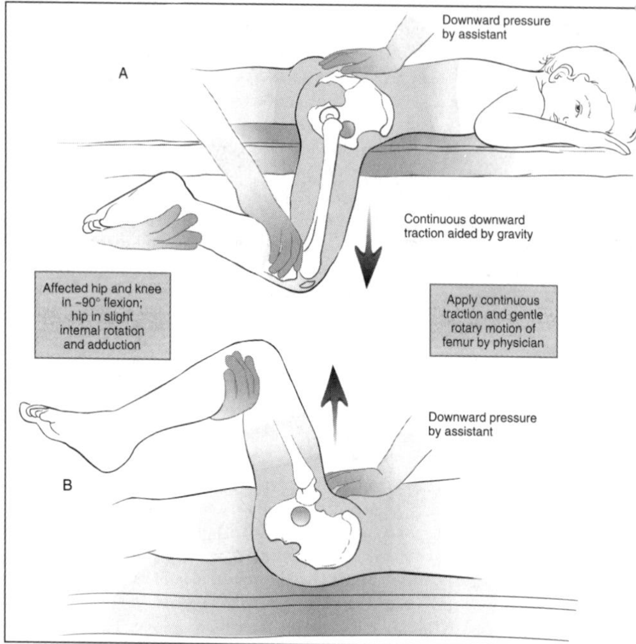

FIGURE 60.8 Techniques for reduction of posterior hip dislocation. Reduction of hi[p] dislocation follows initial trauma resuscitation in a patient with multiple trauma, and af[ter] adequate radiographic evaluation in all cases. To be successful, adequate analgesia an[d] muscle relaxation are necessary, but the use of parenteral medications for this purpos[e] may compromise an unstable patient, and thus general anesthesia and operating room re[duction] may be required in some cases. To achieve reduction, the femoral head must b[e] maneuvered laterally and anteriorly from its position posterior and medial to the acetab[ular] rim. With the prone technique, the patient is placed prone with the affected le[g] hanging off the edge of the stretcher (**A**). The knee and hip are flexed 90 degrees, wit[h] the hip also in slight adduction and internal rotation. An assistant stabilizes the pelvi[s] with downward pressure. Continuous downward traction, aided by gravity, to the dista[l] femur in line with the deformity fatigues and overcomes muscle spasm. The femora[l] head, aided by gentle rotatory motion of the femur, is gradually brought over the poste[rior] acetabular rim and into the acetabulum. Alternatively, the patient may be place[d] supine (**B**), and comparable upward traction applied with the physician mounting th[e] stretcher to gain mechanical advantage while an assistant applies downward pelvic pres[sure] for countertraction. Postreduction, radiographs are obtained to confirm successfu[l] reduction and the hip is immobilized in anatomic position with slight abduction and ex[ternal] rotation.

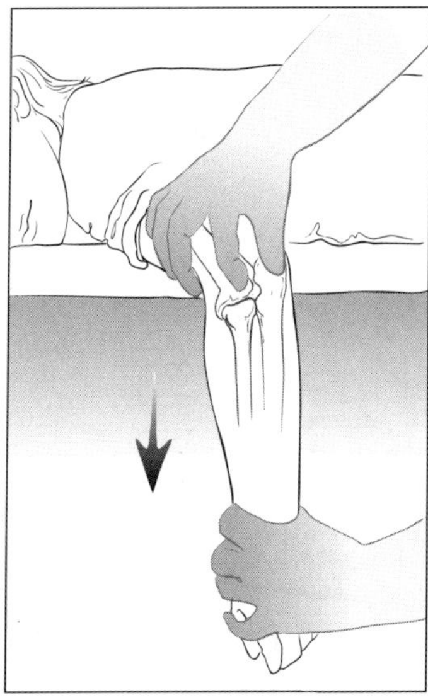

FIGURE 60.9 Reduction of posterior elbow dislocation. Isolated elbow dislocation is rare in children but has high risk of neurovascular compromise. This dislocation is typically referred for immediate orthopedic management, but emergent reduction may be attempted by the emergency physician or pediatrician if the injured limb demonstrates compromised neurovascular status and an orthopedist is not immediately available. Reduction should optimally occur within 2 hours of dislocation to minimize the incidence of complications. Radiography to examine for associated fractures is indicated, but may be deferred until after reduction in the context of acute neurovascular compromise.

The patient is positioned prone, and either the entire arm or only the forearm is allowed to hang over the side of the stretcher. Traction is applied to the proximal forearm with the elbow in 70 to 80 degrees of flexion, either by the physician or with weights for 15 to 20 minutes. Gentle countertraction on the humerus may be applied by an assistant. Forward and downward force applied to the olecranon with the physician's thumbs with simultaneous gentle elbow flexion usually effects reduction. Postreduction, radiographs are obtained and the elbow is immobilized in 90 degrees of flexion. Arteriography may also be indicated.

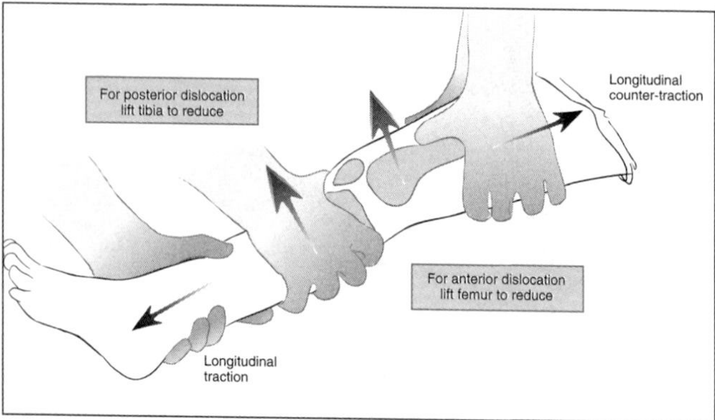

FIGURE 60.10 Reduction of knee dislocation. Isolated knee dislocation is rare in children but has high risk of neurovascular compromise. This dislocation is typically referred for immediate orthopedic management, but emergent reduction may be attempted by the emergency physician or pediatrician if the injured limb demonstrates compromised neurovascular status and an orthopedist is not immediately available. Reduction should optimally occur within 6 hours of dislocation to minimize the incidence of complications. Radiography and arteriography to examine for associated fractures and subclinical vascular damage is indicated, but may be deferred until after reduction in the context of acute neurovascular compromise.

To reduce a knee dislocation, gentle longitudinal traction is applied to the lower leg. For anterior dislocation, reduction is effected by lifting the femur anteriorly while the proximal tibia is pushed posteriorly into anatomic position. For a posterior dislocation extension at the knee and lifting the proximal tibia into the reduced position follows longitudinal traction. Postreduction, radiography and arteriography are done and the knee is immobilized in 15 degrees of flexion.

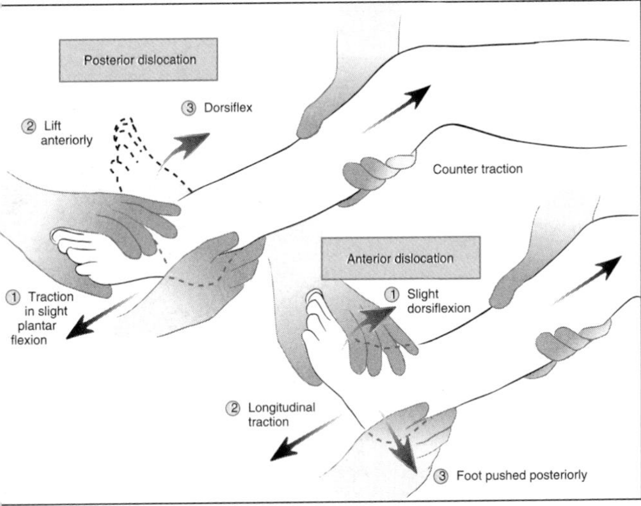

FIGURE 60.11 Reduction of ankle dislocation. Isolated ankle dislocation is rare in children but has high risk of neurovascular compromise. This dislocation is typically referred for immediate orthopedic management, but emergent reduction may be attempted by the emergency physician or pediatrician if the injured limb demonstrates compromised neurovascular status and an orthopedist is not immediately available. Radiography to examine for associated fractures is indicated, but may be deferred until after reduction in the context of acute neurovascular compromise.

The patient is placed supine with the knee in slight flexion (30 to 45 degrees). Traction is applied to the foot by the physician while countertraction in the long axis of the limb is applied to the calf and proximal lower leg by an assistant. The physician's dominant hand holds the heel and the other hand grasps the forefoot. Traction and countertraction are applied with the foot in slight plantar flexion for a posterior dislocation, or in slight dorsiflexion for an anterior dislocation. To reduce a posterior dislocation, the foot is then lifted anteriorly and dorsiflexed gently. For an anterior dislocation, the foot is brought into further dorsiflexion, then pushed posteriorly and plantar flexed gently. A second assistant may apply additional force on the distal tibia: posteriorly directed in a posterior dislocation, or anteriorly directed in an anterior dislocation. Successful reduction is evident by the position of the talus in the mortise with a joint line that is parallel to the ground. Postreduction radiographs are obtained and the patient is immobilized in neutral position. Arteriography may also be indicated.

CHAPTER 61

Measurement of Compartment Pressure and Reduction of Fractures with Neurovascular Compromise

OVERVIEW

1. Stabilize patient; ensure airway-breathing-circulation (ABCs) under advanced trauma life support (ATLS) protocol.
2. Remove all clothing (including footwear) and jewelry covering and distal to injured extremity.
3. Stop active bleeding with direct-pressure dressing.
4. Observe child and inspect injury: note position extremity maintained, note gross deformities, findings consistent with an open fracture, color. Always examine contralateral limb in same manner.
5. Unless obvious neurovascular compromise is present, gently apply temporary, simple, padded splint to injured part, initially leaving it in its deformed position. Include joints above and below suspected fracture to provide adequate stability. Elevate and ice injured limb (if neurovascular compromise is present, see 12 and 14, later).
6. Observe movements distal to injury. Have child move fingers and toes. Specifically, assess radial nerve function through finger and wrist extension and test median nerve with thumb-to-fingers apposition; ulnar nerve can be assessed by spreading and adducting fingers. For lower extremity injuries, have child dorsiflex and plantarflex toes.
7. Palpate extremity distal to injury by assessing temperature, capillary perfusion, and quality of distal pulses.
8. Carefully palpate injured part, noting deformity pattern, hematoma, and crepitus. Listen for bruits. In upper extremity, pay careful attention to cubital fossa, and in lower extremity injuries, closely examine popliteal fossa Evaluate for tenderness and swelling over associated compartments.
9. Assess sensation distal to injury. In upper extremity, test on dorsum of hand (radial nerve), thumb or index finger (median nerve), and fifth finger

(ulnar nerve). In the leg, always assess sensation in web space between first and second toes (deep peroneal nerve).

10. Passively stretch injured part to evaluate further for compartment syndrome.
11. Administer anesthesia if not already done and if child is in pain.
12. Adequately splint injured part—if neurovascular impairment exists before splinting, an attempt should be made to reduce the fracture. Reassess neurovascular status after traction splint or appliance is in place to ensure that no new deficits are present.
13. Obtain appropriate radiographs with comparison views as needed.
14. Consult orthopedic surgery.

CLINICAL TIPS

1. Do not focus on the injured extremity at the expense of the ABCs.
2. Do not be afraid to remove dressings and splints applied elsewhere to ensure a good examination.
3. Do not be afraid to attempt reduction of a fracture that is causing vascular compromise, particularly when an orthopedic surgeon cannot be available in a timely fashion.
4. When reducing such a fracture, remember that the goal is restoration of blood flow, not definitive reduction.
5. When unsure how to reduce such a fracture, gentle longitudinal traction is usually the most effective technique.
6. Do not fail to consider a compartment syndrome simply because pulses are present.

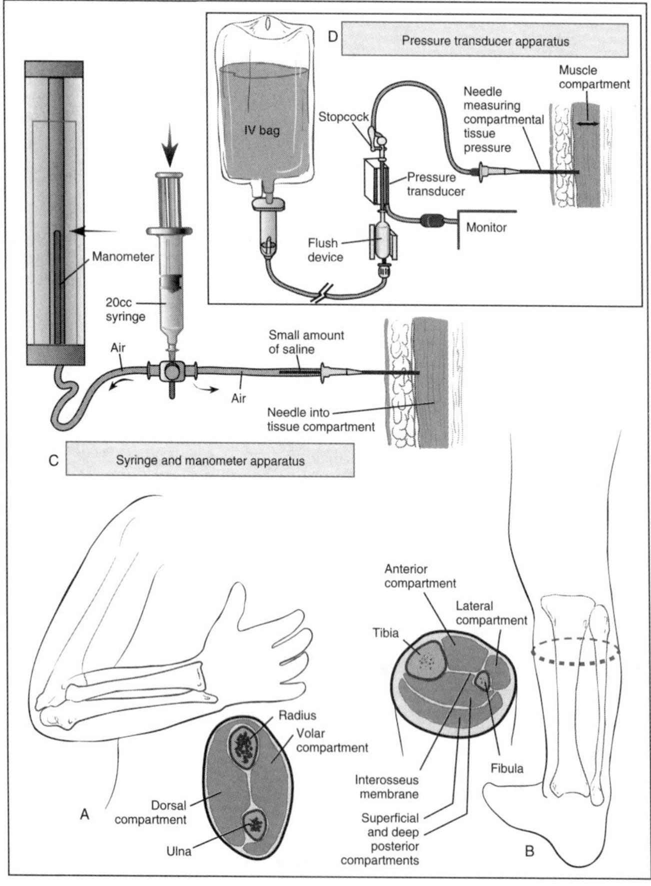
D
Pressure transducer apparatus
IV bag
Stopcock
Needle
measuring
compartmental
tissue
pressure
Muscle
compartment
Pressure
transducer
Monitor
Flush
device
Manometer
20cc
syringe
Air
Small amount
of saline
Air
Needle into
tissue compartment
C
Syringe and manometer apparatus
Anterior
compartment
Lateral
compartment
Tibia
Radius
Volar
compartment
Fibula
Interosseus
membrane
A
Dorsal
compartment
Ulna
Superficial
and deep
posterior
compartments
B

FIGURE 61.1 Compartment pressure measurement. Compartment syndrome represents any condition that leads to elevated tissue pressure within muscle groups enveloped by a fascial sheath. This can lead to restricted blood flow and subsequent ischemic insult, which can be limb threatening. Early recognition of possible compartment syndrome and timely diagnosis by tissue compartment pressure measurement allow for timely intervention with emergent fasciotomy. Normal intramuscular pressure at rest approximates zero. Abnormally high pressures requiring surgical decompression are typically greater than 30 mm Hg (some authorities recommend decompression when the intracompartmental pressure approaches 10 to 30 mm Hg of the diastolic blood pressure). **A:** Anatomy of the forearm compartments. **B:** Anatomy of the lower leg compartments. **C:** A system for measuring intracompartmental pressure using simple equipment available in any emergency department.[a] The skin over the involved compartment is prepared with antiseptic. The skin site of needle insertion is anesthetized with local anesthetic, while care is taken to avoid intracompartmental injection. The manometer device is assembled as illustrated. First, intravenous extension tubing is connected to the front and rear ports of a three-way stopcock, and a 20-mL syringe with the plunger at the 15-mL mark is connected to the upper port. A sterile 18-gauge needle is used to release the vacuum of a bottle of bacteriostatic normal saline. Once the vacuum has been released, this needle is connected to the front port of the stopcock. The front port of the stopcock is opened and the plunger of the syringe slowly withdrawn until saline fills approximately half the length of the tubing attached to the front port. The saline should be withdrawn slowly and smoothly to minimize bubble formation within the extension tubing and ensure that saline fills only half the extension tubing; the syringe should contain only air. The stopcock is then used to close the front port, and the needle is removed from the saline bottle. This needle is carefully removed and replaced with a new, sterile needle. Keeping the front port stopcock closed during needle transfer prevents loss of saline from the extension tubing. Next, the extension tubing attached to the rear port is connected to the manometer. The needle is inserted into the desired muscle compartment space and the stopcock is opened to both extension tubes and the syringe. This produces a closed system whereby air is free to flow into both extension tubes as the pressure increases. The plunger is then depressed slowly, forcing pressure to rise within the system. As this is done, the mercury column in the manometer slowly rises until the pressure within the system is equivalent to that in the tissue compartment. Then, as the pressure within the system surpasses tissue pressure, the saline contained in the extension tubing is forced toward the needle, which causes visible movement of the saline in the extension tubing. The reading on the mercury manometer at the time the saline begins to move represents the compartmental pressure. **D:** Alternatively, compartmental pressure can be measured using standard electronic arterial blood pressure transducers and monitoring systems. The system is assembled as for typical arterial pressure monitoring, with two exceptions. First, the fluid to be infused need not be heparinized, and second, it is not necessary for the bag of intravenous fluid to be placed into a pressure infuser. As described, a needle is placed on the distal end of the infusion setup, instead of an intraarterial catheter. The system is then zeroed just as it would be before measuring intraarterial pressure. When the needle is inserted into the compartment, the pressure reading obtained from the monitor is the intracompartmental pressure.

---

[a] Whitesides TE Jr, Haney TC, Harada H, Holmes HE, Morimoto K. A simple method for tissue pressure determination. *Arch Surg* 1975;110:1311–1313.

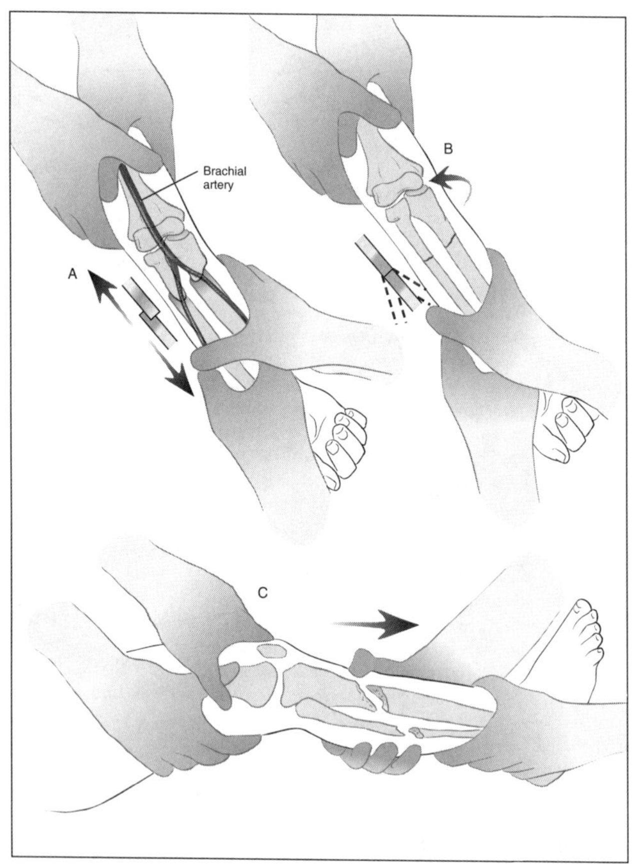

FIGURE 61.2 Emergency reduction of fractures with neurovascular compromise. Severe fractures of the long bones, especially complete fractures with significant displacement or angulation, may compromise neurovascular structures. Such fractures warrant immediate orthopedic consultation for emergency reduction. If an orthopedist is not available, the emergency physician or pediatrician should attempt reduction to restore blood flow and function. This may need to be done even before obtaining radiographs. Most patients require parenteral analgesia and muscle relaxation. Gentle longitudinal traction is the mainstay of such reduction. This figure illustrates emergency reduction of such fractures occurring in the radius and ulna of the forearm (**A**,**B**) and the tibia and fibula of the lower leg (**C**). An assistant grasps the upper arm above the elbow to stabilize it (**A**). The physician then exerts gentle longitudinal traction on the arm distal to the fracture, overcoming muscle spasm- induced shortening and allowing release of brachial artery tenting (**B**). The procedure is successful if circulation to the hand is restored. Definitive reduction need not be accomplished until later. Similarly, gentle longitudinal traction is applied to the lower leg (**C**). The leg may need to be turned from the plane of deformity while applying traction. When aligning a tibial fracture, the second toe should align with the tibial tubercle.

CHAPTER 62 •

Laceration Repair

OVERVIEW

Wound Preparation

1. Provide conscious sedation as needed.
2. Anesthetize wound.
3. Provide hemostasis.
4. Explore wound for foreign bodies or injuries to underlying structures.
5. Remove contaminated or devitalized tissue through debridement and excision.
6. Thoroughly cleanse wound.
7. Undermine wound edges when necessary to reduce tension.

Using Needle Holder

1. Grasp needle away from swage and closer to tip for tougher tissue.
2. Hold needle perpendicular to needle holder.
3. Enter skin perpendicular to surface.
4. Stabilize or manipulate skin edges with skin hook or nontraumatic forceps.
5. Retrieve needle after each pass with needle holder or forceps.

Instrument Tie

1. Pull suture through wound, leaving a few centimeters at insertion site.
2. Grasp longer (needle) length of suture in dominant hand.
3. Loop suture twice *over* tip of needle holder.
4. Grasp free end of suture with needle holder.
5. Pull shorter (free) end through loops and away from side of wound initially entered.
6. Tighten knot so that skin edges just come together.
7. Loop needle end of suture once *under* tip of needle holder.
8. Grasp free end of suture with needle holder.
9. Pull free end through loop and back to initial needle entry side of wound.

10. Repeat single loop tie, first in over and then in under manner, for a total of four throws.
11. Cut both ends of suture, allowing adequate length to retrieve suture at time of removal.

Simple Interrupted Skin Sutures

1. Enter skin with needle directed downward or angled slightly away from wound edge.
2. Drive needle to a depth greater than its width.
3. Trace a symmetric path through both sides of wound.
4. Secure suture with an instrument tie.

Inverted Subcutaneous Sutures

1. Insert needle from within wound at dermal-fat junction.
2. Rotate needle up through tissue and exit in dermis.
3. Insert needle in opposing dermis at an equal vertical and horizontal level.
4. Rotate needle down through tissue and exit at dermal-fat junction.
5. Bring both ends of suture to same side of loop.
6. Secure suture with a knot consisting of three throws.

Interrupted Mattress Sutures

1. Vertical mattress
   - A. Place a wide, deep stitch across wound—use two steps (retrieving needle from within wound) when necessary.
   - B. Reverse directions from previous stitch, entering same side as recent exit but at a point closer to wound edge and in line with previous pass.
   - C. Complete a smaller and shallower pass on same side as initial entry site and equidistant from wound edge as second entry site.
   - D. Tie knot on side of wound that was initially entered.
2. Horizontal mattress
   - A. Place an initial stitch of same dimensions as a simple interrupted suture pass.
   - B. Reenter skin lateral to exit point and equidistant from wound edge.
   - C. Perform a second pass, reversing directions from previous stitch and exiting at a point lateral to initial entry site and equidistant from wound edge, so that free and needle ends of suture remain on same side of wound.

   D. Tie knot on side of wound that was initially entered.

3. Half-buried mattress or corner stitch
   A. Enter skin below and just lateral to point of V.
   B. Exit within wound.
   C. Evert tip of flap with skin hooks or forceps.
   D. Pass needle through dermis of flap tip, parallel to skin surface.
   E. Enter wound on opposite side of point of V.
   F. Exit through skin at a point below and lateral to point of V, symmetrically across from initial insertion site.
   G. Secure suture with an instrument tie.

Continuous Skin Sutures

1. Simple running stitch
   A. Place a simple interrupted suture at one end of laceration without cutting needle end of suture.
   B. Travel length of laceration, performing sequential passes perpendicular to laceration and equidistant from each other.
   C. Maintain tension on needle end of suture after each pass.
   D. Reverse direction of needle pass when end of laceration is reached.
   E. Enter skin close to previous exit site, and leave a narrow loop on that side by only partially pulling suture through.
   F. Secure end of suture with an instrument tie using narrow loop as free end of suture.

2. Running subcuticular stitch
   A. Pass suture through skin at one end of wound and exit in dermis.
   B. Travel length of wound making small passes (<1 cm in width) within dermis and parallel to skin surface.
   C. Alternate sides of wound with each entry site slightly behind previous exit point and at same vertical level of dermis.
   D. Complete suture by bringing needle out through skin surface at end of wound.
   E. Cut needle from suture.
   F. Tape free ends of suture to skin surface using skin adhesive.

CLINICAL TIPS

1. Adequate immobilization, sedation, and anesthesia are crucial to successful laceration repair in children.
2. Natural landmarks should be used. Shaving eyebrows and using epinephrine in anesthetizing the vermilion border obscures two important landmarks.

3. Shaving the hair usually is unnecessary in the repair of scalp wounds.
4. The intrinsic and extrinsic tension forces across a laceration must be considered when planning the repair.
5. Wound edges must be everted at the time of closure. *Eversion* means that the wound edges are rolled slightly outward with two edges of the wound lined up exactly. To achieve wound edge eversion, the path of the needle must be directed down or angled slightly away from the wound edge. In addition, the depth of the suture path must be greater than the width. The needle must trace an equal path through both sides of the wound to ensure accurate apposition of the wound.
6. Only skin hooks, nontraumatic forceps, or fingers should be used in handling wound edges.
7. The fewest number of sutures that provide an adequate closure should be used.
8. Three layers support sutures best: the fascial-fat junction, the dermal-fat junction, and the level just below the dermal-epithelial junction. Fat and muscle do not hold a stitch.
9. Wounds under greater tension should have more skin sutures placed and these should be closer to the wound edge.

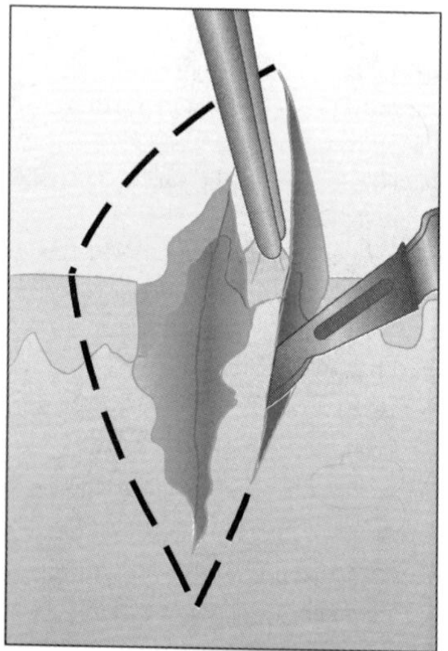

FIGURE 62.1 Debridement can be an important step in wound management before laceration repair. It should be used to remove heavily contaminated tissue and also to remove devitalized tissue that fosters bacterial growth. However, debridement can also cause problems with wound healing. Removal of tissue may result in excessive tension at the wound margins and subsequently increased scar formation. If complete debridement of the wound is contraindicated because of the presence of vital structures or the probability of a poor cosmetic result, high-pressure irrigation should be used. This should be followed by meticulous debridement of all clearly nonviable tissue.

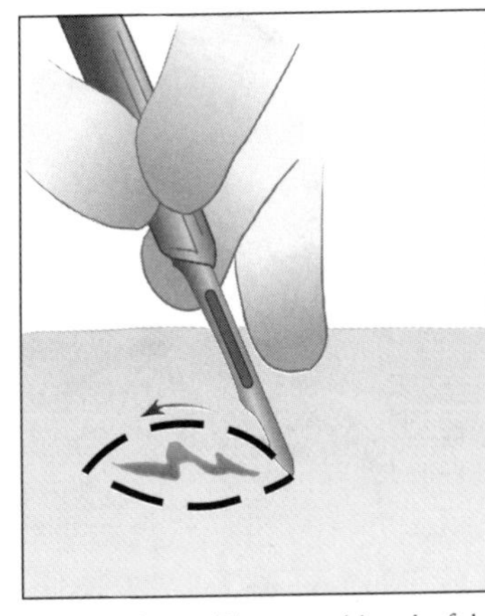

IGURE 62.2 When appropriate, ebridement may be accomplished by xcising the entire wound, which is ometimes referred to as wound elipsing. This method should be used nly in the following circumstances: a) when cosmetic outcome is not a igh priority compared with possible nfection; (b) when there are no vital nderlying structures; (c) when there s sufficient excess tissue to allow closng the wound without undue tenion; and (d) when excision can be lone in a manner that will closely parllel the natural skin tension lines. The wound is excised by making a mooth, elliptical cut around the vound as shown. It is important to btain a perpendicular cut completely through the dermis. The eventual length of the xcision exceeds the width by a factor of three.

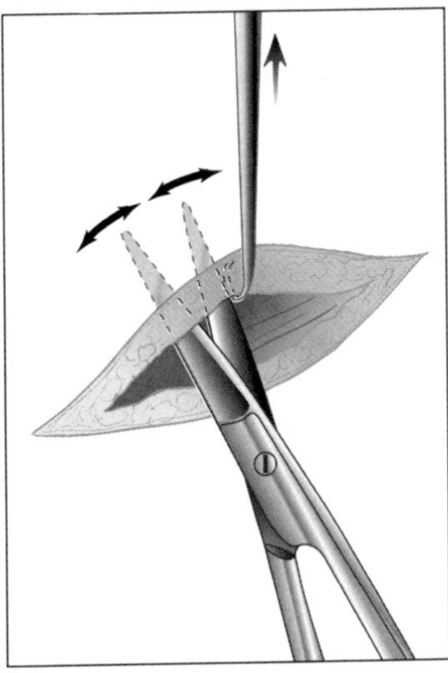

FIGURE 62.3 Undermining a wound reduces the degree of tension present after the repair. This is done using a pair of scissors or a scalpel to loosen the subdermal fatty tissue. Undermining is performed in the plane of the subcutaneous fat to a distance of several millimeters or up to twice the width of the wound. With contaminated wounds, disruption in blood supply that results from undermining may lead to an increased risk of infection and offset any cosmetic improvement.

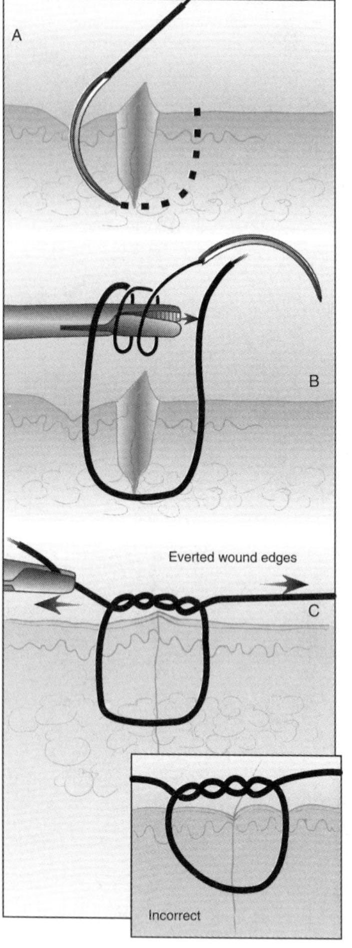

FIGURE 62.4 The easiest method of knot tying is the instrument tie. This is best accomplished by pulling most of the suture though the wound so that only a few centimeters of thread is exposed at the first insertion site. At this stage, the remaining longer length of thread attached to the needle is grasped in the nondominant hand. The needle holder, grasped in the dominant hand, is placed across the longer (needle) length of the thread, and the thread is then looped twice over the tip. The needle holder then grasps the short (free) end of the suture and pulls this away from the side of the wound initially entered, which lays the double knot flat. The knot is tightened so that the skin edges just come together. The process is now reversed, with the needle holder again placed across the longer length of suture, which is then looped once under the tip. The needle holder then grasps the free end of the suture and returns it to the initial needle entry side of the wound, while the needle length of suture is carried back to the initial needle exit side of the wound. For monofilament sutures, this process is repeated (using one loop around the needle holder each time after the first throw) for a total of four throws to secure the knot.

10. Wound edges should be approximated to accommodate the edema that occurs after closure. Strangulation of tissue must be avoided.
11. Wound edges should always be everted, not inverted.
12. A pass that is wider at the base than the surface ensures eversion of the edges.
13. The use of colored sutures in hair improves visibility for eventual removal.

14. Suture ends should be cut long enough to allow easy handling for removal.
15. Parents should be told that the healing process and scar appearance will not be complete until 6 months after the repair.
16. Leaving sutures in place for prolonged periods of time or under excessive tension results in stitch marks.
17. Skin tapes can provide useful reinforcement to sutures, or continued support after suture removal.
18. The general schedule for suture removal is 3 to 5 days for the face, 7 days for the scalp and anterior trunk lacerations, and 10 to 14 days for the extremities and back.

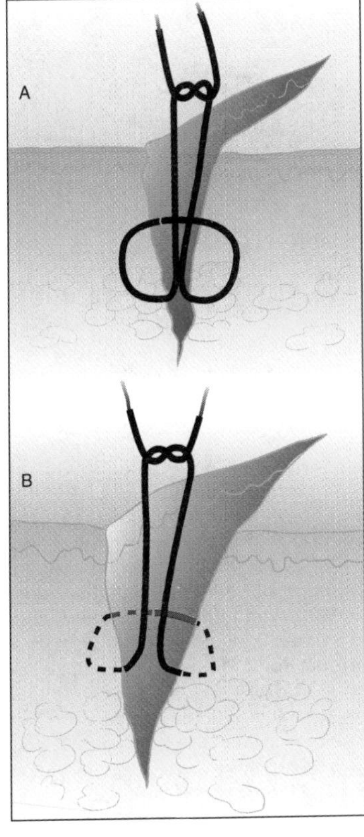

FIGURE 62.5 Subcutaneous sutures should be inverted (i.e., with the knot buried) where the skin is thin or cosmetic appearance is important. The initial insertion point of these subcutaneous sutures is in the depths of the wound, typically at the fat-dermal junction. Exposure of the correct entry point can be facilitated by using tissue forceps or a skin hook. **A:** For a traditional subcutaneous suture, the needle is rotated up through the tissue to exit the dermis. At this point, it is essential to pause and make sure that the second insertion point in the opposing dermis is at an equal vertical and horizontal level with the exit point of the first pass. Once this is ascertained, the downward pass of the suture becomes a mirror image of the first pass, exiting at the same level as the original insertion. The needle end and free end of the suture must be on the same side of the loop to correctly bury the knot. The knot is then tied, usually with only three throws to minimize suture material in the wound. **B:** A simple but useful variation is the horizontal dermal stitch. With this technique, the dermis is aligned by placing a simple stitch in the horizontal plane. The loop and knot are at the same level in the subcutaneous tissue. This suture provides a nice approximation of the wound edge before skin closure, but carries the disadvantage of an inability to bury the knot.

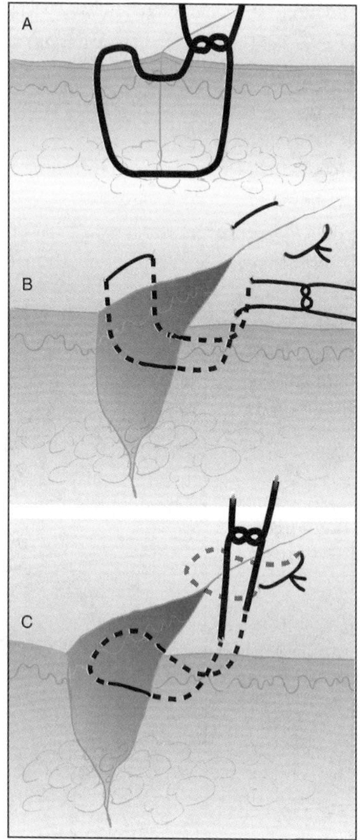

FIGURE 62.6 Mattress sutures are useful for providing eversion of the wound edges, particularly with larger wounds. However, it is important to avoid the tendency to apply excess tension when using this type of stitch. **A:** The traditional vertical mattress suture involves taking a large, deep course with the first pass of the needle and then making a smaller stitch close to the wound edge. The knot is tied on the side of the wound entered initially. The vertical mattress suture is especially prone to result in ischemia of the wound edge when excessive tension is used. **B:** The horizontal mattress suture closes a greater length of wound than the vertical mattress suture but usually results in a less accurate approximation of the wound edges. **C:** The half-buried horizontal mattress stitch offers some advantages in that the number of skin punctures is halved and less tension is on the free edge of the wound opposite the knot, but the tensile strength of this suture is less than that of the other mattress sutures.

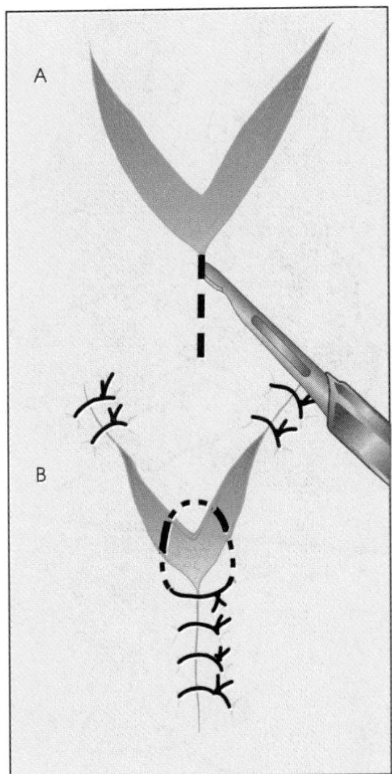

FIGURE 62.7 The skin at the tip of a V-shaped laceration has a tenuous vascular supply. Consequently, a cutaneous stitch at this point is prone to result in tissue ischemia and a poor outcome. The corner stitch and V-Y advancement flap techniques are designed to overcome this problem. **A:** A corner stitch is simply a variation on the half-buried mattress suture, in which the subcutaneous path passes through a relatively large segment of the V-shaped skin flap. **B:** It is sometimes necessary to extend the apex of the V-shaped laceration to form a Y, which releases some of the tension on the corner. The extension into a Y shape can be complemented with undermining to decrease tension further. Simple interrupted stitches are used to close the remainder of the wound.

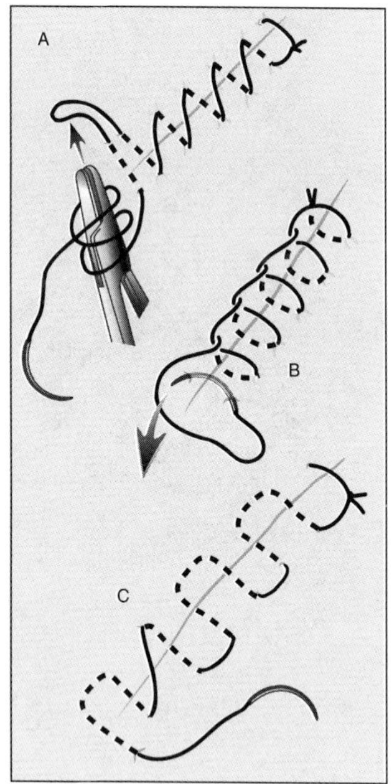

FIGURE 62.8 Continuous skin sutures. **A:** The most useful continuous stitch is the simple running stitch, which is started by making a simple interrupted stitch and cutting only the end of thread not attached to the needle. The clinician then performs sequential passes perpendicularly across the wound the same distance apart as normally placed interrupted sutures. Once the desired length is closed, the running stitch is most simply ended by reversing the direction of the needle pass using an entry site close to the previous exit site. This allows a loop to be formed on one side that can be tied with the final pass on the opposite side. **B:** The continuous interlocking stitch is conducted in virtually the same manner as the simple running stitch except that the needle is passed through a loop created by pulling the length of thread down in the direction the clinician is suturing. **C:** A variation of the running stitch that exploits the eversion characteristics of a mattress stitch is the running lateral mattress stitch or continuous half-buried horizontal mattress stitch. It is recommended in this technique that a loop be intermittently run over the top of the wound to facilitate removal of this suture.

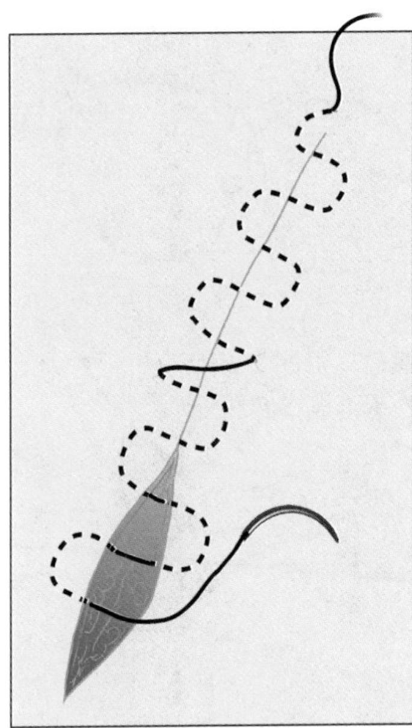

IGURE 62.9 The continuous subcuticular stitch is usually begun by passing the suture hrough the skin at one end of the wound to exit in the dermis. The wound is then closed y making small passes, usually less than 1 cm in width, in alternating sides of the wound n the dermal layer parallel to the skin surface. Placement of each pass must be at the same evel of dermis throughout the wound to ensure a good result. If the clinician must sew long distance, it is advisable to bring the suture up to the surface on occasion to allow or easier removal. The clinician can end the suture by bringing it out through the skin urface; the two ends of exposed suture can then be taped in place using skin tapes.

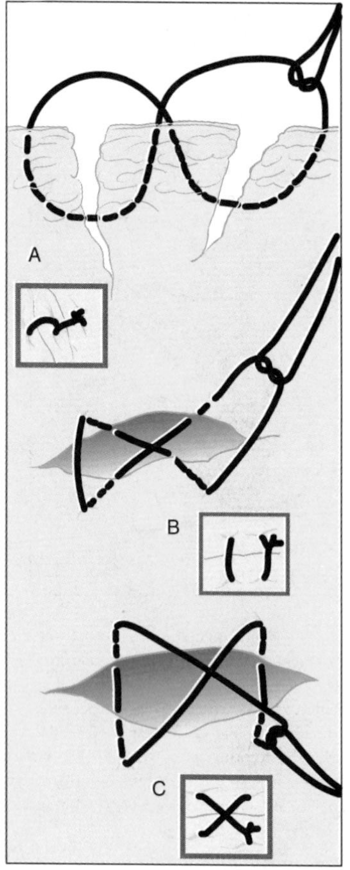

FIGURE 62.10 Large lacerations with significant bleeding from a vessel can be close with a figure-of-eight stitch. This stitch compresses the tissue surrounding the bleedin vessel and tamponades the hemorrhage. **A:** A vertical figure-of-eight stitch. **B,C:** Tw types of horizontal figure-of-eight stitches.

Management of Plantar Puncture Wounds

OVERVIEW

1. Obtain radiographs to identify potential foreign body or fracture, or to evaluate for osteomyelitis if late presentation.
2. Place patient in prone position.
3. Prepare wound in an antiseptic fashion.
4. Administer local or peroneal block.
5. Coring: remove 2-mm rim of full-thickness skin from around puncture site.
6. Remove any debris or foreign bodies.
7. Irrigate wound with saline under high pressure.
8. Pack wound with iodoform gauze.
9. Apply bulky dressing.
10. Administer tetanus toxoid and tetanus immune globulin when indicated.
11. Encourage non-weight bearing for 5 days and elevation of extremity.
12. Administer antistaphylococcal antibiotics if evidence of cellulitis.
13. Refer for surgical management if retained foreign body or osteomyelitis is present.
14. Follow-up in 24 to 48 hours.

CLINICAL TIPS

1. Clean or superficial wounds need not undergo coring.
2. Wounds of the forefoot and those with late presentations are more likely to become infected.
3. A high index of suspicion must be maintained for a retained foreign body and for osteomyelitis in late presentations.

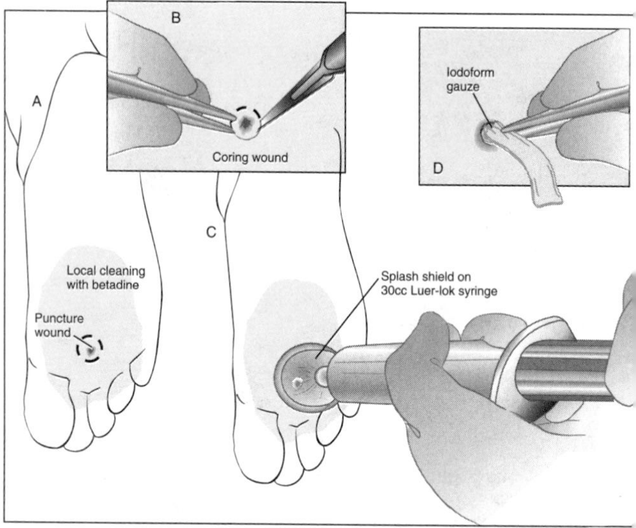

FIGURE 63.1 Before coring a plantar puncture wound, the external surface is tho oughly cleaned with povidone-iodine. Wounds that require coring should receive loc or regional anesthesia. Probing is not recommended because this may result in a foreig body being pushed deeper into the foot and also may cause damage to underlying nerv and vessels. With a no. 11 scalpel blade (or 4-mm punch biopsy corer or cuticle scissors a 2-mm circular rim of full-thickness skin is removed from around the puncture woun Irrigation into the wound tract with normal saline may be performed using a 30-mL sy ringe and an 18-gauge angiocathether or splash shield. Any debris or foreign objec should be removed with care. The clinician may also opt to pack the tract with iodofor gauze before applying a bulky dressing.

CHAPTER 64 •

Subcutaneous Foreign Body Removal

OVERVIEW

1. Use appropriate radiographic technique and surface markers to identify possible foreign body.
2. Examine extremity proximal and distal to wound to ensure that tendon function, neurologic function, and vascular status are intact.
3. Examine tendons through their entire range of motion to ensure that potential overlapping tissue planes present during injury are reproduced.
4. Provide adequate local analgesia, consider conscious sedation, and immobilize patient and extremity.
5. Control for hemostasis by applying proximal tourniquet or blood pressure cuff expanded to 20 mm Hg above systolic blood pressure for no more than 30 minutes at a time.
6. Set time limit of 30 minutes for exploration of wound.
7. Explore wound so that entire foreign body location is known, including any anatomic relationships with important structures.
8. Remove entire foreign body including devitalized or infected tissue.
   A. Removal of objects parallel to skin surface.
      1) Incise skin perpendicular to midpoint of object's long axis.
      2) Spread tissues with hemostat to locate object.
      3) Grasp object with hemostat and remove through original entrance site or new incision.
   B. Removal of objects perpendicular to skin surface.
      1) Make elliptical incision with entrance site of foreign body in center.
      2) Undermine surrounding skin 0.25 to 0.50 inch in all directions.
      3) Compress adjacent skin surface to displace foreign body into center of wound.
      4) Grasp and remove foreign body with hemostat.
   C. *En bloc* removal.
      1) Make sure no tendons, nerves, or vessels are within surgical field.
      2) Make an elliptical incision around wound.
      3) Undermine surrounding skin 0.25 to 0.50 inch in all directions.
      4) Extend initial incision to a depth greater than foreign body.
      5) Remove block of tissue with hemostat or forceps by applying gentle traction.

9. Reexplore wound to ensure no damage to important structures or any re maining fragments of foreign body.

10. Irrigate and consider closing wound if not old or dirty.

CLINICAL TIPS

1. The presence of a foreign body should be considered in every laceration an puncture wound.

2. Every persistent infection, draining sinus, and culture-negative absce should be considered to be caused by a foreign body until definitivel proven otherwise.

3. A normal plain radiograph does not rule out the presence of a nonra diopaque foreign body.

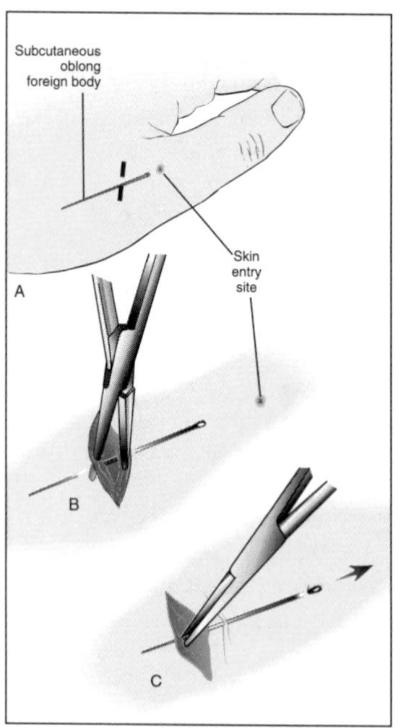

FIGURE 64.1 Difficult-to-find, rela tively clean embedded objects that a parallel to the skin, such as a lon thin needle or a piece of glass, are be approached by incising the skin pe pendicular to the midpoint of the ob ject's long axis. Gentle spreading tissues with a hemostat aids in loca ing the object. The object then can b grasped with the hemostat and re moved through its original entran site or through the newly created inc sion. The incision is then closed.

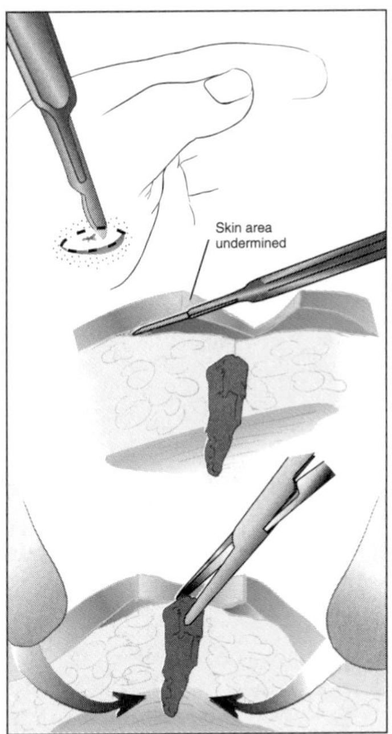

FIGURE 64.2 If a foreign body enters perpendicular to the skin and is difficult to find, attempted localization through a linear incision is not recommended. This displaces the foreign body to one side of the wound. Instead, a small, elliptical incision (large enough to ensure that the foreign body can be removed) should be made with the entrance site of the foreign body at its center. The skin is then undermined circumferentially 0.25 to 0.50 inch. The foreign body can be displaced into the middle of the wound by compressing the skin surface. It then can be grasped and removed with a hemostat. If no contamination is evident, thorough irrigation should by followed by closure of the wound.

4. Examination of tendon, neurologic, and vascular function should be performed before and after the administration of any anesthetic or sedating agent and before and after wound exploration.
5. If the skin must be incised to retrieve a foreign body, the clinician should attempt to incise along natural skin folds and not perpendicular to skin creases. The wound can be carefully explored by spreading the soft tissue with a hemostat.
6. Blind probing with any instrument should be avoided, especially in areas where vital structures are located, such as the hand, foot, or face.
7. Provision of adequate analgesia and immobilization allows the wound to be thoroughly evaluated without patient movement or discomfort.
8. The field being evaluated should be bloodless with appropriate hemostasis.
9. Consultants should be involved if the exploration involves complex structures or will take a prolonged amount of time.

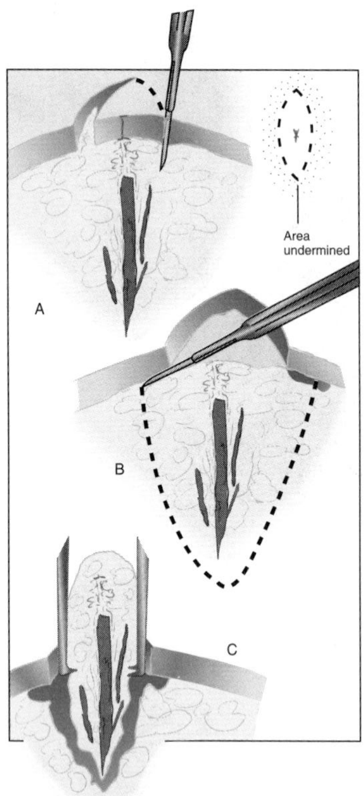

FIGURE 64.3 *En bloc* removal can be performed with a foreign body that is likely to fragment, leaving multiple pieces in the wound (e.g., vegetable matter or wooden splinters). Before performing *en bloc* removal of a foreign body and surrounding tissue, the clinician must first ensure that no tendons, nerves, or vessels are present in the surgical field. An elliptical incision is then made around the wound, including the entire area to be removed to a depth below the foreign body. The surrounding skin is undermined circumferentially 0.25 to 0.50 inch. The entire block of tissue then can be removed by grasping the piece of tissue and applying upward traction. If performed properly, no fragments are left behind and contaminated tissue is excised.

CHAPTER 65

Hair Tourniquet Removal

OVERVIEW

1. Grasp loose fibers and gently unwind.
2. Insert blunt probe or curette beneath hair or thread.
3. Isolate fiber from underlying soft tissue.
4. Remove fiber.
   A. Cut fiber with fine-tipped scissors,
   OR
   B. Cut through fiber and onto probe or curette with no. 11 scalpel blade.
5. Explore for presence of additional strands.
6. Evaluate neurovascular status or tendon function.

Incisional Approach

1. Digit
   A. Perform digital nerve block on involved digit.
   B. Prepare and drape digit and surrounding area in sterile fashion.
   C. Incise along digit perpendicular to tourniquet to the depth of bone.
      1) Incise laterally at 3-o'clock or 9-o'clock position,
      OR
      2) Incise dorsally at 12-o'clock position.
2. Penis
   A. Apply local or regional anesthesia.
   B. Prepare and drape penis and surrounding area in sterile fashion.
   C. Incise lateral inferior surface at either 4-o'clock or 8-o'clock position.

CLINICAL TIPS

1. Hair tourniquets frequently involve multiple strands and multiple digits.
2. When in doubt, an incision should be performed to ensure complete disruption of the tourniquet.
3. The possibility of a hair tourniquet should be considered in the evaluation of the irritable infant.

4. Scarring or reepithelialization may hide the strand below the skin surface.
5. Urologic assistance should generally be obtained before embarking on incisional removal of a penile hair tourniquet, unless the penis is deemed to be at immediate risk.
6. Evidence of reperfusion usually occurs within several minutes after release of the constricting band; however, depending on the tissue insult caused by the constriction, it may be days before normal perfusion has returned completely.
7. When any question remains as to whether the circumferential constriction has been completely removed, surgical consultation should be obtained.
8. Reevaluation in 24 hours helps ensure that all constricting bands have been removed and that the soft tissue is adequately perfused and free from infection.

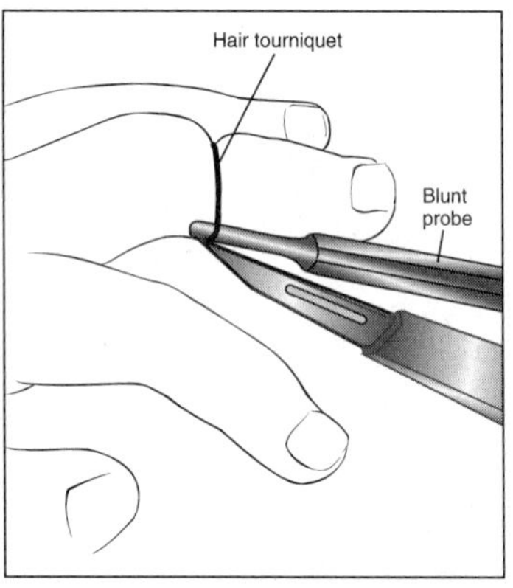

FIGURE 65.1 If a hair tourniquet has not embedded too deeply into the tissue, a blunt metal probe or metal ear wax curette can sometimes be gently inserted beneath the constriction. Once the strand is isolated with a metal object, it can be cut with fine-tipped scissors. Alternatively, a scalpel blade may be used to cut through the hair onto the probe or curette, which serves to protect the underlying skin.

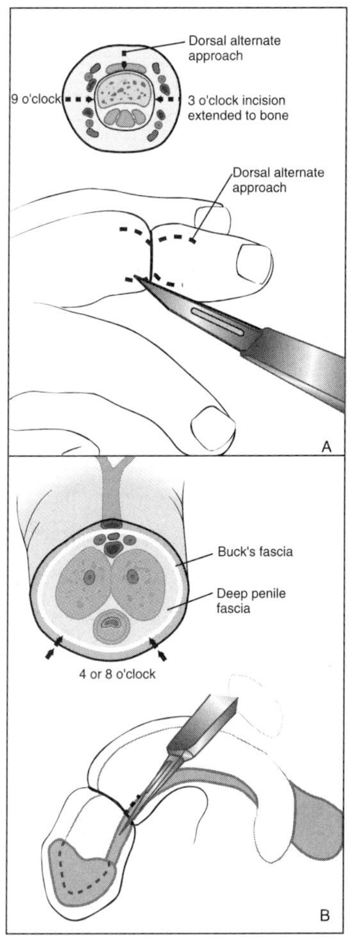

FIGURE 65.2 Incisional removal of a hair tourniquet. **A:** Because the neurovascular bundles lie at the dorsal and palmar aspects of the radial and ulnar portions of the digits, one recommended approach is to make the incision between the bundles using a no. 11 scalpel blade at either the 3-o'clock or 9-o'clock position. The incision is made in a proximal-to-distal direction, and should be extended to the bone to ensure incision of the fiber. An incision on the dorsal surface provides an acceptable alternative approach. Although this may result in a small incision into the extensor tendon, a longitudinal incision parallel to the direction of the tendon fibers should heal well with splinting and general wound care. This incision has the advantage of avoiding the neurovascular bundles completely. **B:** In the penis, the main neurovascular bundles are adjacent to the dorsal surface and the urethra is adjacent to the ventral surface. For this reason, the recommended site for an incision is on the lateral inferior surface at the 4-o'clock or 8-o'clock position. Attempts should be made to stay in the deep penile fascia at the junction of the corpus cavernosum and spongiosum. Given that the fascia is a relatively tough layer, the clinician may elect to make light incisions of the skin cutting slightly deeper with successive strokes through the same initial incision, with the goal of cutting the constricting band without penetrating the fascial layer into the lumen of the corpora.

CHAPTER 66

Burn Management

OVERVIEW

Major Burns

1. Initiate necessary resuscitation measures.
2. Provide adequate analgesia.
3. Remove clothing.
4. Perform emergent escharotomy if indicated.
   A. Incise full length of burn down to subcutaneous fat.
   B. Incise along lateral or medial aspect of limb, or bilaterally in anterior axillary line for chest.
5. Irrigate burns with saline.
6. Cover burns with sterile dry sheets or saline-soaked gauze.
7. Maintain body temperature with overhead warmers as needed.
8. Administer tetanus immunoprophylaxis when indicated.
9. Contact burn center as necessary.

Minor Burns

1. Provide adequate analgesia.
2. Prepare wound.
   A. Irrigate burns with saline.
   B. Debride necrotic or clearly nonviable tissue using forceps and scissors.
   C. Gently clean burns with mild soap or quarter-strength povidone-iodine.
   D. Pat dry with sterile sponges.
3. Apply wound dressing.
   A. Open.
      1) Apply antibiotic ointment (e.g., bacitracin/polymyxin B) to face, neck, or small (<1 cm) extremity burns.
   B. Closed.
      1) Apply inner dressing.
         a) Conventional.
            - Coat burn with a layer of silver sulfadiazine.
            - Cover area with sterile gauze.

b) Synthetic.
- Cut material to fit burn with a slight overlap of adjoining healthy skin.
- Apply material without wrinkles or trapped air.
- Secure material with tape.

2) Apply outer dressing.
a) Wrap inner dressing in several layers of roller gauze.
b) Cover dressing with a stockinette or elastic bandage.

4. Splint extremities with partial- or full-thickness burns that extend across joints.
5. Administer tetanus immunoprophylaxis when indicated.

CLINICAL TIPS

1. Appropriate burn management depends on the depth and extent of the burns.
2. Burns in children may be a manifestation of abuse.
3. Most major burns in children require the expertise of a burn center.
4. Initial resuscitation measures should be addressed before definitive burn care.
5. Analgesia should be provided as early as possible.
6. Aspiration of blisters should be avoided.
7. A final covering of stockinette or burn netting limits the ability of the young child to remove the dressing.
8. The young burn victim is at significant risk of heat loss because of the relatively high ratio of body surface area to volume.
9. Children who are transported to a burn center usually should have only a sterile sheet applied over the burned areas. In most cases, silver sulfadiazine or antibacterial ointment applied at the initial treatment facility will have to be removed at the burn center so that the depth and types of burns can be appropriately assessed.

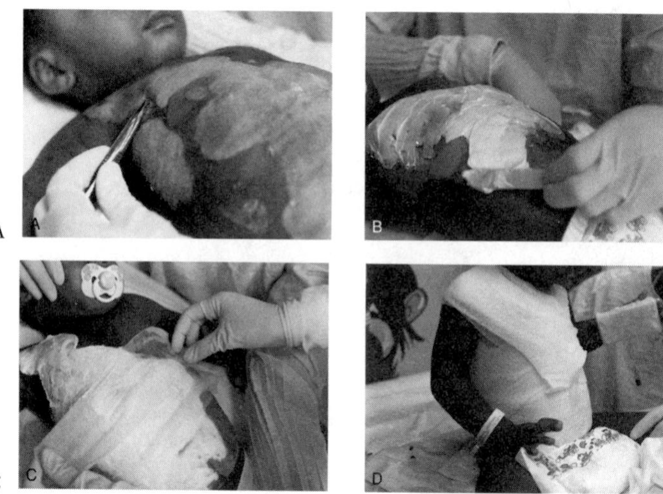

FIGURE 66.1 Application of a conventional burn dressing. **A:** Careful debridement of devitalized tissue significantly decreases the likelihood of infection. **B:** Antibacterial cream such as silver sulfadiazine is applied to the cleansed and debrided wound to a thickness of approximately 2 to 3 mm using a sterile tongue blade, covering the entire surface. **C:** A nonadherent type of dressing (petrolatum gauze) is then placed over the area of injury to facilitate later removal of the dressing. **D:** Finally, the area is wrapped with several layers of roller gauze to create a bulky, absorbent outer dressing.

TABLE 66.1 Classification of Burns in Children

Classification	*Burn*		*Associated Factors*	*Disposition*
Major	2°: >20% BSA		Potential loss of function	Burn center
	3°: >10% BSA	or	Increased risk of infection	
	Circumferential		Severe deformity	
	Crosses flexion crease		e.g., burns of hands, face, ears, nose, feet, perineum, genitalia	
			e.g., immunosuppressed child	
			High-voltage injury	PICU
		or	Smoke inhalation	
Moderate	2°: 10%–20%	+	None of above	Hospitalization or close follow-up by specialist
	3°: 2%–10%	or	Parental inability to care for burn	
		or	Child abuse suspected	
Minor	2°: <10% BSA	+	None of above	Outpatient treatment
	3°: <2% BSA			

BSA, body surface area; PICU, pediatric intensive care unit.

CHAPTER 67

Incision and Drainage of a Cutaneous Abscess

OVERVIEW

1. Optimize approach to and visualization of abscess site.
2. Anesthetize around abscess site and along proposed incision course by intradermal infiltration with 1% lidocaine without epinephrine.
3. Perform percutaneous needle aspiration for Gram stain and culture when indicated.
4. Incise entire length of abscess cavity.
5. Spread open abscess cavity bluntly with hemostat clamp or fingers. Clear all loculations of purulent material. Irrigate copiously and evacuate cavity completely.
6. Pack remaining cavity loosely with gauze packing strip and cover with dry gauze dressing.
7. Consider need for antibiotics (cephalexin, amoxicillin-clavulanate, or erythromycin).
8. Provide tetanus toxoid immunization when indicated.
9. Change gauze packing strip and check wound within 24 to 48 hours or earlier.
10. Encourage warm soaks 15 to 20 minutes several times daily after gauze packing strip is removed.
11. Reevaluate frequently.

CLINICAL TIPS

1. Evaluation of the inflammatory mass is necessary to ensure that it is an acute, superficial, and localized cutaneous abscess without extension to deeper structures. Incision and drainage of an inflamed mass that is not an abscess should be avoided.
2. General anesthesia and an intraoperative procedure should be considered for the child who is uncooperative or has other conditions that may preclude outpatient management.

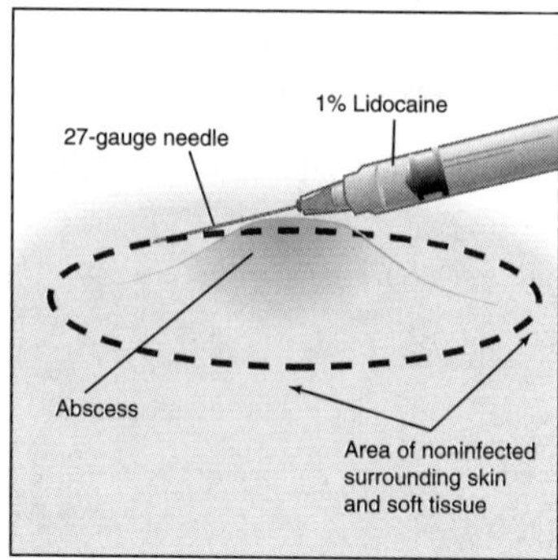

FIGURE 67.1 In preparation for incision and drainage of an abscess, the surrounding noninfected skin and subcutaneous tissue is first anesthetized using 1% lidocaine without epinephrine by local infiltration or regional block.

3. A sufficiently wide incision with adequate blunt spreading and copious irrigation are necessary to ensure complete drainage of the abscess cavity. The risk of progression or recurrence of an abscess increases with suboptimal incision and drainage.
4. Oral or parenteral antibiotics may be indicated for the complicated patient.
5. Close follow-up should be emphasized.

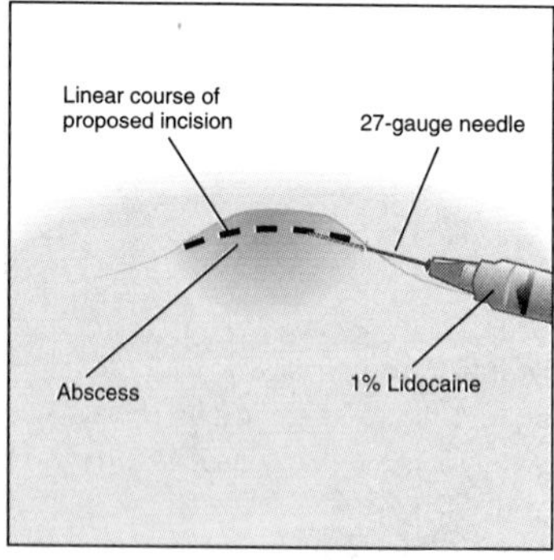

FIGURE 67.2 After the surrounding skin is anesthetized, the roof of the abscess is then infiltrated with anesthetic along the linear course of the proposed incision.

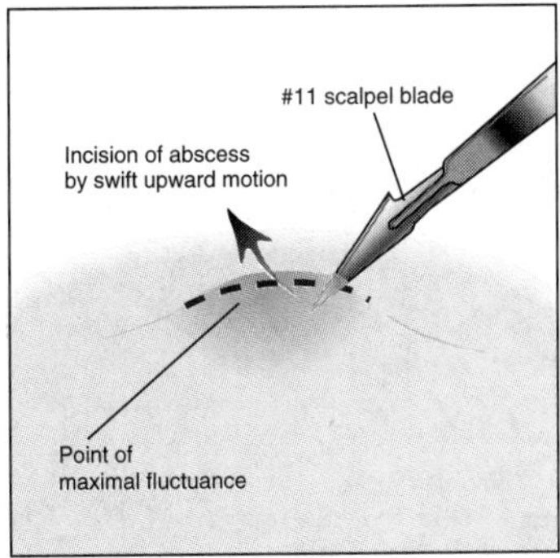

FIGURE 67.3 For a smaller (<1 cm) abscess, a no. 11 scalpel blade is used to make a stab opening directed toward the point of maximal fluctuance, followed by one swift upward motion across the entire abscess to complete the incision.

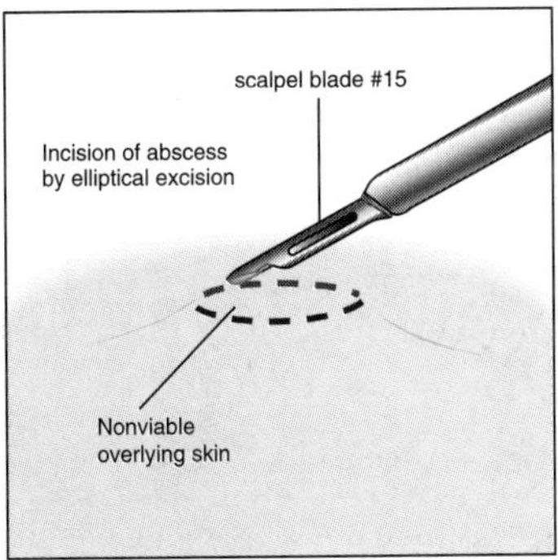

FIGURE 67.4 For a larger (>1 cm) abscess, a no. 15 scalpel blade is preferred for making an elliptical excision of the thin, nonviable, or necrotic overlying skin and to facilitate drainage. An opening sufficiently wide to allow complete drainage of pus is crucial to the successful evacuation of the abscess cavity.

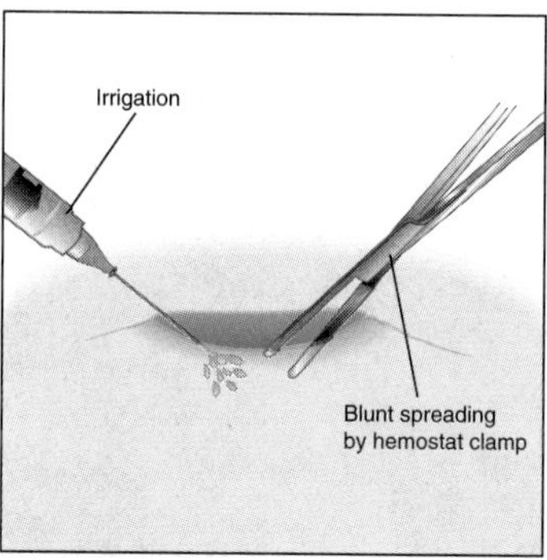

FIGURE 67.5 After the abscess is incised, the cavity is probed; any loculations of pus and necrotic debris are cleared by blind spreading with a hemostat clamp, or with the clinician's finger if the size of the cavity permits. Copious irrigation of the abscess follows with normal saline, sterile water, or peroxide solution to remove all pus and necrotic tissue.

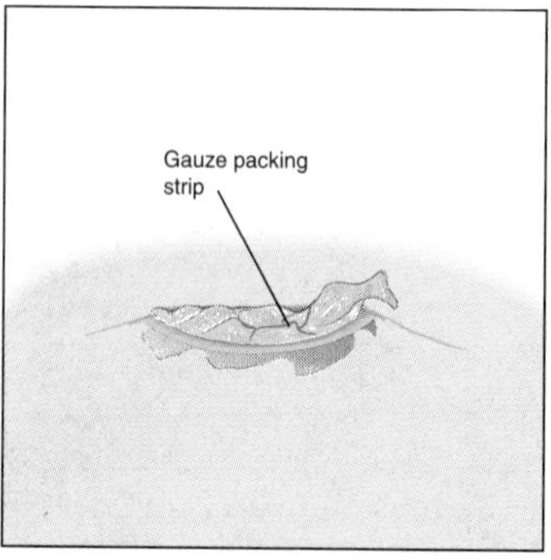

FIGURE 67.6 Many superficial abscesses empty completely after incision and irrigation, and have no remaining cavity. These require warm soaks to keep the incision open until healing occurs. If a cavity remains, it is filled loosely with a gauze packing strip to ensure continued drainage of blood and coagulum. Tightly packing the cavity with a large amount of gauze does not enhance healing. A 1-cm end is left external to the wound edges to act as a wick and to aid subsequent removal of the packing strip.

CHAPTER 68

Paronychia and Felon Repair

OVERVIEW

Paronychia Repair

1. Restrain child when necessary.
2. Prepare antiseptic field.
3. Apply ethyl chloride/digital block anesthesia.
4. For proximal, superficial involvement, lift eponychium and use packing as needed. Minimal anesthesia may be necessary in this setting.
5. For subungual purulence, lift eponychium and remove part of nail plate.
6. Cover site with outer, bulky gauze dressing.
7. Consider local or oral antibiotics.
8. Encourage warm soaks (when packing removed).
9. Follow up in 24 to 48 hours for more complex procedures to evaluate site and remove packing, or 5 to 7 days for simple repairs.
10. Refer to subspecialist for persistence beyond 10 days or continued recurrence.

Felon Repair

1. Immobilize involved digit.
2. Administer conscious sedation as needed.
3. Perform digital or metacarpal nerve block of affected digit.
4. Sterilely prepare and drape digit.
5. Apply tourniquet to provide hemostasis.
6. Incise area of maximal tenderness with no. 11 scalpel blade.
   A. Use longitudinal incision of anterior surface if fluctuance is located at center of terminal pulp.
   B. Use lateral incision in a plane parallel to fingernail when fluctuance is along radial or ulnar aspect of distal pulp.
7. Disrupt loculations at base of abscess gently with small hemostat.
8. Irrigate wound with sterile saline through 18-gauge intravenous catheter.

9. Place loose gauze wick in wound.
10. Remove tourniquet.
11. Apply nonstick dressing, splint, and sling.

CLINICAL TIPS

Paronychia Repair

1. Early drainage of pus is the basic intervention—err on side of early procedure.
2. For most small, localized paronychia, simple lifting of the edge of the cuticle can be accomplished without anesthesia.
3. Follow-up is critical because complications may occur even when treatment is optimal.

Felon Repair

1. A tense fingertip or pointing abscess requires incision and drainage.
2. Excessive disruption of septa as caused by a fishmouth incision may result in an unstable touch pad.
3. Lateral incisions should be made on one side only and just below the fingernail and phalanx to avoid injury to the digital nerves.
4. Incision type and location are determined by the point of maximum fluctuance.

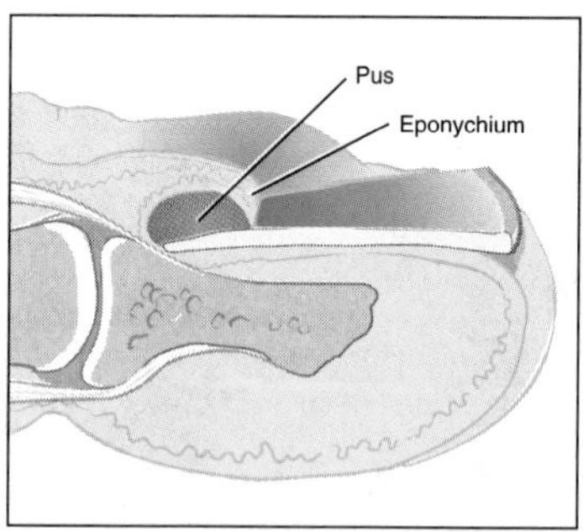

FIGURE 68.1 A paronychia is an infection of the soft tissue structure in the space surrounding the nail. As infection evolves, pus may accumulate under the eponychium (cuticle) and under the nail fold along the sides of the nail plate.

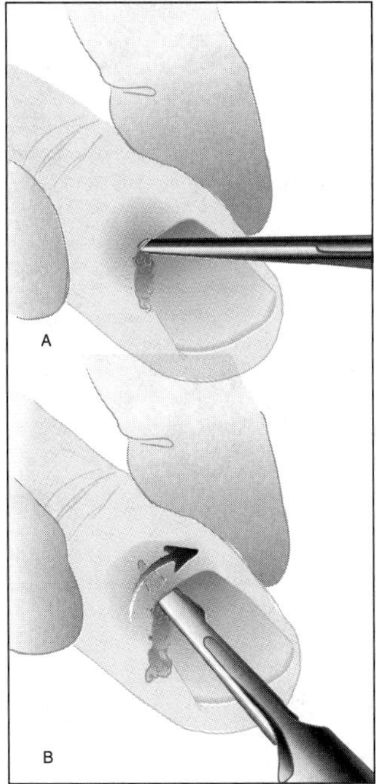

FIGURE 68.2 Drainage of a paronychia. **A:** A no. 11 blade or the tip of a small hemostat is introduced under the eponychial fold, parallel to the surface of the nail plate, and extended into the depth of the enclosed pocket of pus. Because the overlying skin is usually thin and devitalized, this can often be done with one quick pass of the scalpel blade or hemostat, causing a minimal amount of pain. **B:** For larger paronychias involving most of the nail base, the blade or hemostat tip may by fanned through the range of the pus pocket.

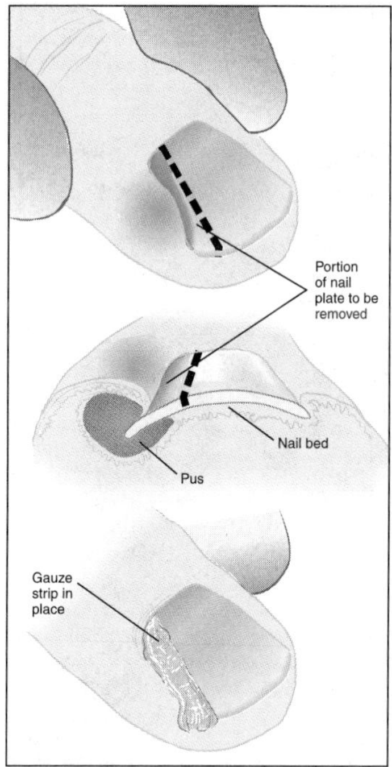

FIGURE 68.3 If the evolution of a paronychia has resulted in pus below the lateral edge of the nail, the nail skin fold should be gently lifted, and a thin longitudinal strip of nail is incised and removed. When the nail is so incised, or if a deep pocket remains after simple lifting of a large proximal paronychia, a small strip of gauze packing should be left in place to ensure continued drainage.

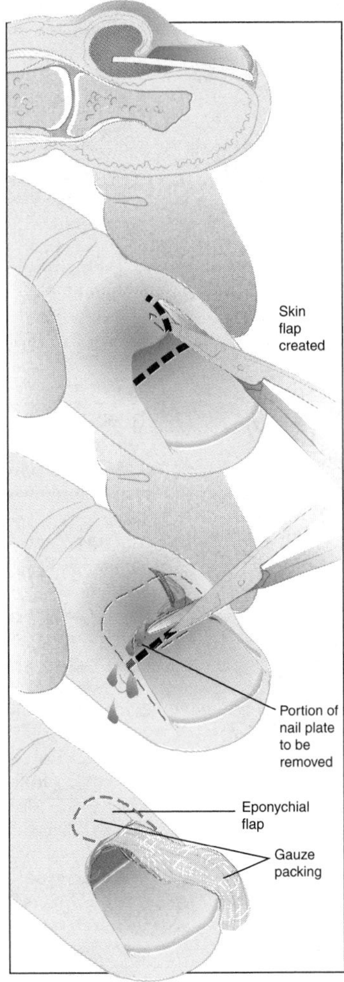

FIGURE 68.4 If the pus of a paronychia has dissected below the proximal base of the nail, the proximal one third of the nail is removed in a strip perpendicular to the long axis of the nail. A small, superficial incision in the eponychium in the longitudinal plane at the corner of the nail may facilitate lifting the nail plate. Gauze packing is then placed below the eponychium.

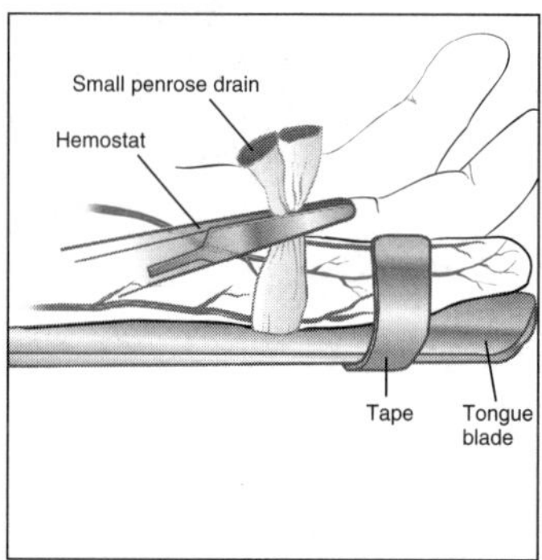

FIGURE 68.5 Before repair of a felon, immobilization and hemostasis of the finger may be accomplished using a sterile tongue depressor secured at the level of the middle phalanx and again more proximally on the hand to minimize movement of the fingertip. A bloodless field is achieved with a digital tourniquet such as a Penrose drain clamped at the base of the finger, or simple manual pressure along the radial and ulnar digital arteries. The tourniquet should be released briefly every 20 to 30 minutes to avoid prolonged ischemia of the finger.

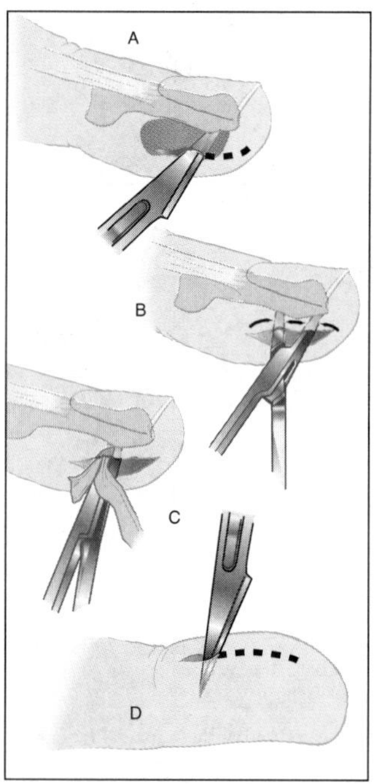

FIGURE 68.6 Drainage of a felon. **A:** A felon with maximal fluctuance located on the radial or ulnar aspect of the distal pulp is incised along the lateral surface using a no. 11 scalpel blade with the bevel facing distally. The incision is made midway between the fingertip and the distal flexor crease and just below the nail. The scalpel blade is advanced into the pulp space, where pus is most likely to be found. The incision may be carried in a J-shaped fashion along the involved side of the digit. In general, the length is approximately 0.5 to 1.0 cm. **B:** Using a small hemostat, the loculations are gently disrupted to drain all the pus adequately. The wound is then irrigated with sterile saline though an 18-gauge intravenous catheter or comparable splash shield. **C:** A sterile gauze wick (plain or antibiotic-impregnated umbilical tape or 0.25-inch iodophor gauze) is loosely packed in the depth of the wound. **D:** A felon with maximal tenderness at the center of the terminal pulp should be incised longitudinally. This incision must not cross the distal interphalangeal joint because this may extend the infectious process proximally to the tendon sheath of the flexor digitorum profundus.

CHAPTER 69

Ingrown Toenail Repair

OVERVIEW

Conservative

1. Administer digital nerve block anesthesia.
2. Clean nail groove with alcohol pad.
3. File central nail peak as needed.
4. Elevate nail edge from groove.
5. Remove debris from nail groove with curettage and debridement.
6. Apply silver nitrate to granulation tissue as needed.
7. Pack cotton or gauze beneath nail edge.
8. Apply bulky dressing.
9. Emphasize follow-up home care.
10. Change packing as needed until nail extends beyond distal aspect of nail fold.
11. Initiate warm-water soaks after 24 hours.
12. Trim nail transversely.
13. Wear loose-fitting shoes.
14. Follow up with physician for wound evaluations at 24 to 48 hours and again after 1 to 2 weeks.

Angular Nail Resection

1. Administer digital nerve block anesthesia.
2. Clean nail groove with alcohol pad.
3. Cut triangular wedge from distal nail.
4. Remove nail wedge and spicule.
5. File remaining nail edge.
6. Remove debris from nail groove with curettage and debridement.
7. Apply antibacterial ointment.
8. Apply bulky dressing.
9. Emphasize follow-up home care as for conservative method.
10. Follow up with physician for wound evaluations at 24 to 48 hours and again after 1 to 2 weeks.

Partial Nail Resection

1. Administer digital nerve block anesthesia.
2. Clean nail groove with alcohol pad.
3. Place digital tourniquet for hemostasis.
4. Cut the nail longitudinally through eponychium.
5. Remove resected nail edge with a hemostat, ensuring total nail root removal.
6. Remove debris from nail groove with curettage and débridement.
7. Apply antibacterial ointment.
8. Apply bulky dressing.
9. Consider oral antibiotics.
10. Emphasize follow-up home care as previously discussed.
11. Follow up with physician for wound evaluations at 24 to 48 hours and again after 1 to 2 weeks.

CLINICAL TIPS

1. Surgical approaches in young infants should be avoided.
2. Digital block anesthesia should be considered even with the most conservative treatment.
3. Nail edge elevation with gauze packing is effective for most patients.
4. Wedge or lateral nail plate resections should be reserved for the more severe cases.

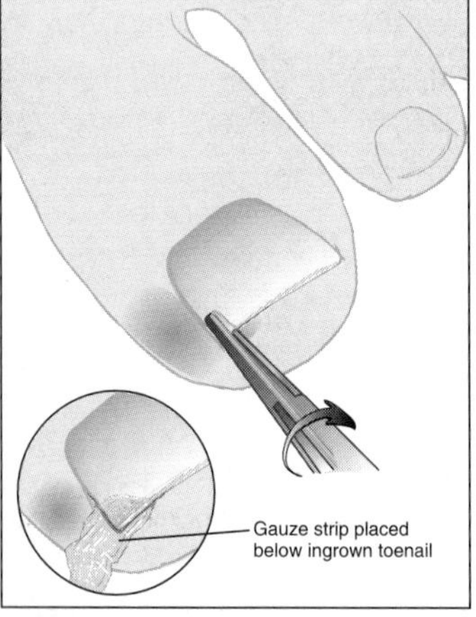

FIGURE 69.1 Conservative management of an ingrown toenail consists of lifting the nail edge out of the nail groove with a hemostat, rotating away from the nail fold. A small piece of cotton soaked in alcohol or petrolatum gauze is then firmly packed under the nail edge. If the nail is curved to form a central peak, the central portion of the nail surface may be filed down until the nailbed matrix is visible through the thinned nail, allowing for release of the curvature pressure.

FIGURE 69.2 For more advanced cases, angular resection of the nail may be performed. The nail is cleansed and a triangular wedge of nail is excised to a point one-third to two-thirds the distance from the eponychium. The nail wedge and the nail spicule must be completely removed. The remaining nail edge should be filed down so that it will grow smoothly along the nail groove. Trauma to the nail groove must be avoided because this can lead to scarring and obliteration.

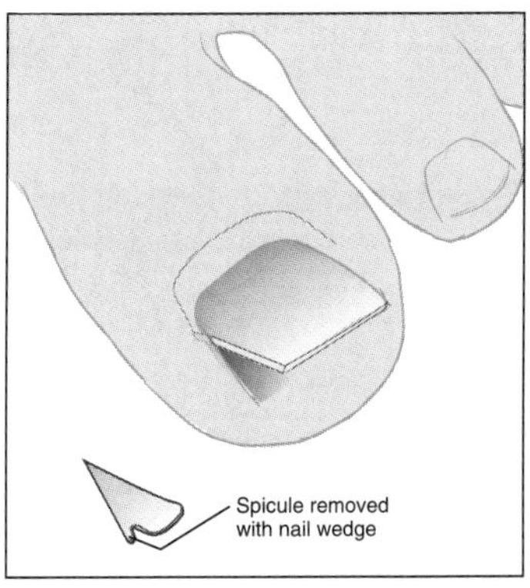

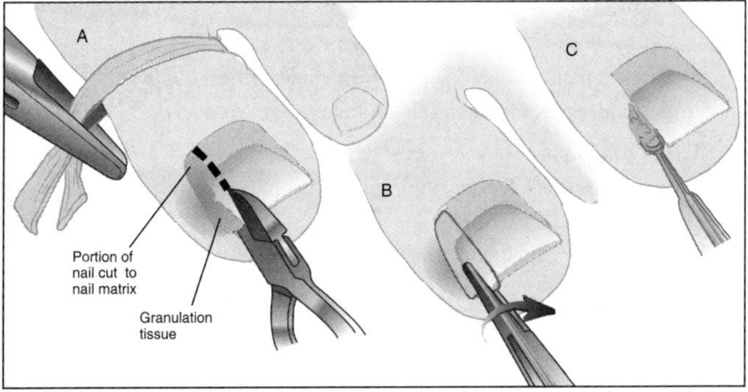

FIGURE 69.3 For the patient with a recurrence after wedge resection, or for more severe cases with hyperkeratosis and granulation, partial nail resection may be required. **A:** The nail is cut longitudinally, approximately one-third the distance from the lateral edge using a nail cutter or a scalpel. The incision must advance toward and continue through the eponychium so that the entire nail portion inclusive of the nail root may be resected. **B:** The resected nail is then carefully removed using a hemostat, with a slow, steady, rotating motion toward the intact nail edge to minimize damage to the nailbed. **C:** The exposed nailbed is gently debrided and cleansed to remove all the keratotic and granulation tissue. Additional pressure may be applied during this stage of the procedure to ensure hemostasis.

CHAPTER 70

Fishhook Remova

OVERVIEW

1. Remove attached lures and additional hooks from embedded hook.
2. Prepare field in antiseptic fashion.
3. Inject local anesthesia or perform a digital block.
4. Push-through method.
   A. Push tip of hook through anesthetized skin.
   B. Clip barb.
   C. Back shank and belly of fishhook out of wound.
5. String technique.
   A. Secure body part involved.
   B. Loop string around belly of fishhook.
   C. Wrap ends of string around index finger.
   D. Depress shank of hook with opposite index finger and thumb.
   E. Forcefully jerk string to remove hook.
6. Needle technique.
   A. Insert 18-gauge needle along inside of fishhook belly.
   B. Engage barb with needle opening.
   C. Back needle and hook out of skin together.
7. Administer tetanus booster if indicated.

CLINICAL TIPS

1. The push-through method works best when the point of the hook is nea the skin surface, minimizing additional tissue damage as the barb is advanced through the skin.
2. The needle technique works best when the hook is superficially embedded
3. The string technique is simple enough to be done in the field and, whe performed correctly, requires no anesthesia.

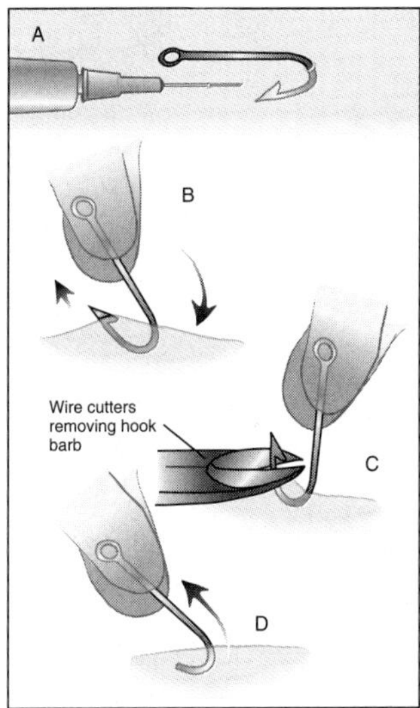

FIGURE 70.1 Push-through method. **A:** This method of fishhook removal requires a digital block or local infiltration of the skin overlying the point of the hook with lidocaine. **B:** The point of the hook is advanced and pushed through the skin. **C:** The barb is clipped off with a wire cutter. **D:** The remainder of the shank and belly are then backed out of the wound. The exit site is usually small and therefore suturing is not indicated.

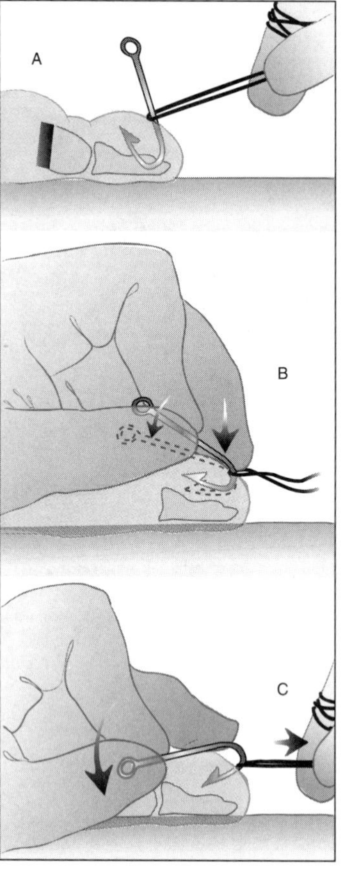

FIGURE 70.2 String technique. **A:** The body part containing the fishhook is firmly secured against a table or flat surface to prevent movement during the procedure. A piece of string (e.g., suture silk) approximately 3 feet long should be looped around the belly of the fishhook. The ends of the string should be wrapped securely around the clinician's right index finger (or left index finger if the clinician is left handed). **B:** The eye and shank of the fishhook should be firmly grasped between the clinician's left index finger and thumb and then depressed, disengaging the barb from the surrounding tissue. The left middle finger applies slight pressure downward on the shank toward the patient's skin. The loop is then pulled slowly away from the hook, horizontally in the plane of the shank's long axis until just taut. **C:** Using the right index finger, the loop is allowed to relax slightly and then, reversing direction, jerked suddenly away from the fishhook, flicking the hook from the skin. Because the hook often flies out of the wound, protective goggles should be worn by both patient and clinician, and bystanders should be cleared from the expected flight path.

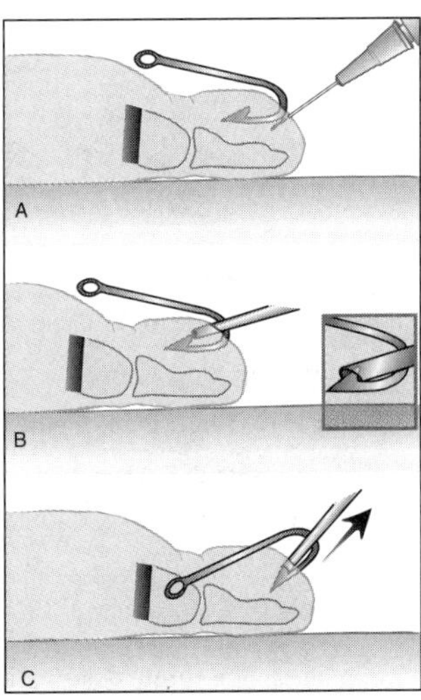

FIGURE 70.3 Needle technique. **A:** The area where the hook is embedded is first infiltrated with lidocaine using a 27-gauge needle. **B:** An 18- or 20-gauge needle is then inserted through the wound along the shaft of the hook. With the bevel of the needle facing the inside of the hook's belly, the needle is advanced along the hook's belly until the needle opening slides over (engages) the barb of the hook. **C:** Once the barb has been covered, the needle and hook are held firmly together while backing the hook and needle out of the wound as a unit.

CHAPTER 71

Ring Removal

OVERVIEW

General

1. Explain procedure to child and parents.
2. Elevate hand.
3. Apply ice to finger for 5 minutes to see if swelling will diminish.
4. Cleanse area with sterile water and keep hand elevated as much as possible during procedure.

String Pull

1. Slip one end of suture or string beneath ring and pull through until both ends are of equal length. A hemostat may be used to grasp suture under ring.
2. Lubricate ring and distal finger.
3. Grasp suture with fingers or a hemostat.
4. Pull in a circular motion. Slip suture around to different sections of ring, and pull as ring gradually moves off of finger.
5. Clean digit and reassess perfusion (color, capillary refill).

String Wrap

1. Administer a digital block.
2. Pass end of suture of string under ring so 5 inches remains on proximal side of finger. A hemostat may be used to slide suture under ring.
3. Tightly wrap remaining suture around swollen finger beginning just distal to ring.
4. Continue wrap beyond proximal interphalangeal (PIP) joint.
5. Pull proximal end of string toward fingertip with fingers or a hemostat. As it gradually unwinds, it should ease ring over PIP joint and off of finger.
6. Remove suture from finger.
7. Repeat procedure as needed.
8. Clean digit and assess perfusion (color, capillary refill).

Ring Cutter

1. Administer a digital block.
2. Examine ring cutter to ensure that swath wheel is sharp, approximates cutter guard, and turns easily.
3. Clean ring cutter with alcohol and then dry with gauze.
4. Turn ring, if possible, until thinnest section is on palmar surface of finger.
5. Place cutter guard under ring.
6. Place wheel on ring, grasp handle of ring cutter and apply pressure while turning wheel. If ring begins to heat up, stop until metal cools.
7. When ring is cut, manually pull apart ring, or spread ends using a hemostat or clamp, and remove ring.
8. When necessary, make a second cut 0.5 to 1.0 cm from first cut. Protect finger from sharp edges of first cut with a think piece of gauze or a Band-Aid slipped underneath ring. Once second cut is complete, remove free piece and pull ends of ring apart using hemostats.
9. Examine finger for cuts, clean finger, and check perfusion.

CLINICAL TIPS

1. The ring cutter should be tested before beginning the procedure, including a visual inspection or a test on a piece of plastic.

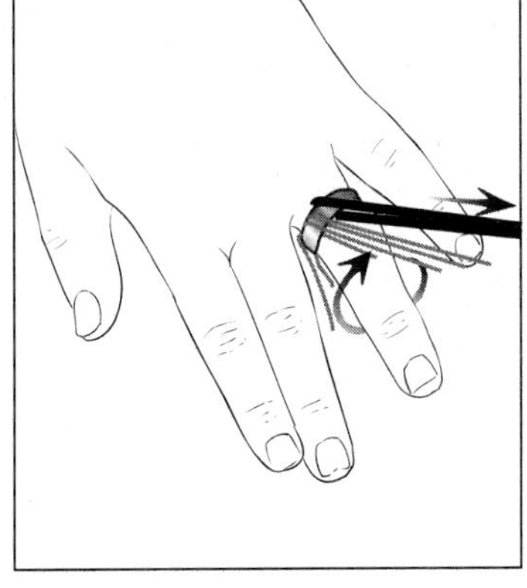

FIGURE 71.1 With the string-pull method, one end of a suture (string) is slipped beneath the ring and pulled through until both ends are of equal length. A hemostat may be used to grasp the suture under the ring to pull one end through. The ring and distal finger are then lubricated. Both ends of the suture are grasped with the clinician's fingers or a hemostat and pulled in a circular motion. The suture should be rotated around to different sections of the ring and pulled along the axis of the finger gradually to advance the ring off.

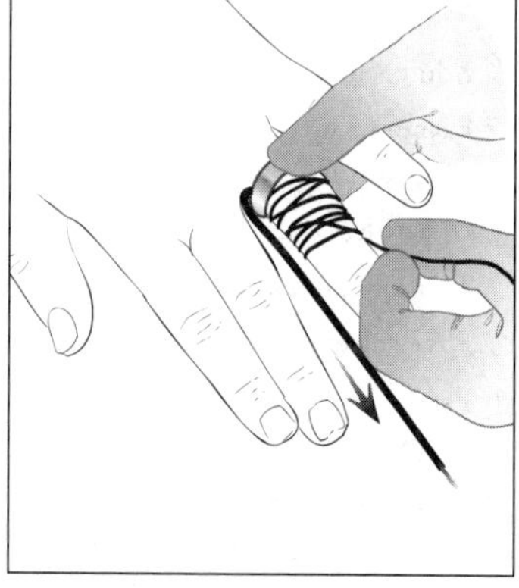

FIGURE 71.2 With the string-wrap method, one end of thick silk suture (or umbilical tape) is passed under the ring so that 5 inches remains on the proximal side of the finger. A hemostat may be used to slide the suture under the ring. The remaining suture is wrapped tightly around the swollen finger beginning just distal to the ring. Each loop of the suture should touch so that no tissue bulges between loops. The wrap should be continued beyond the proximal interphalangeal (PIP) joint. When the wrap is complete, the proximal piece of string (under the ring) is pulled toward the fingertip with the clinician's fingers or a hemostat. As the string gradually unwinds, it should ease the ring over the PIP joint and off the finger.

2. The patient or parents should be informed before the procedure that one of the options includes cutting the ring. Some prefer that this be tried first.
3. The decision to use a digital block should be based on the patient's degree of discomfort, level of cooperation, and the likelihood of the ring removal by the first method chosen. In some cases with young children, the use of string and ring cutters far outweighs the threat of a needle.

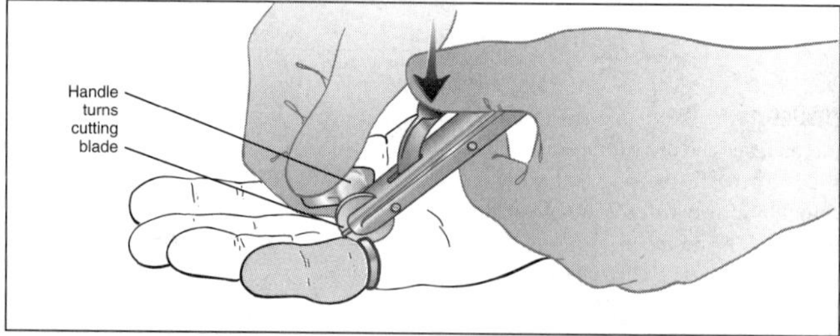

FIGURE 71.3 When a ring cutter is used, the cutter guard is first placed under the ring. Because of swelling of the tissue, this frequently causes pain. The easiest place to cut is the thinnest portion of the ring, but the best position to perform this procedure is usually on the palmar surface. If possible, the ring should be turned until the thinnest section is on the palmar surface. The wheel is placed on the ring, the handle of the ring cutter is grasped, and pressure is applied while the wheel is turned. If the ring begins to heat up, the procedure should be stopped until the metal cools.

CHAPTER 72

Envenomation and Tick Removal

OVERVIEW

Nematocyst Deactivation and Removal After Jellyfish Stings

1. Wear double gloves before handling wound to avoid accidental envenomation.
2. Do not wipe or rub wound.
3. Soak lesions from all species except Chesapeake Bay sea nettle in 5% acetic acid solution (vinegar) for 30 minutes to deactivate nematocysts.
4. Treat Chesapeake Bay sea nettle wounds with paste of bicarbonate of soda.
5. Remove tentacle fragments with forceps.
6. Apply shaving cream and shave wound to remove residual nematocysts.

CLINICAL TIPS

Jellyfish Stings

1. Fresh water or isopropyl alcohol increases nematocyst discharge and should not be used.
2. Meat tenderizer is commonly used but also may promote nematocyst discharge.
3. Life-threatening anaphylactic reactions rarely occur from jellyfish stings in the United States.
4. Delayed pruritus and hives localized to the sting site are common.

OVERVIEW

Tick Removal

1. Grasp tick as close to skin as possible using blunt, curved forceps held in gloved hand.
2. Steadily pull firmly and directly away from skin.
3. Examine skin to ensure all tick parts have been removed.
4. Remove residual material with forceps or excise it with large-gauge needle.
5. Thoroughly clean skin with soap and water.

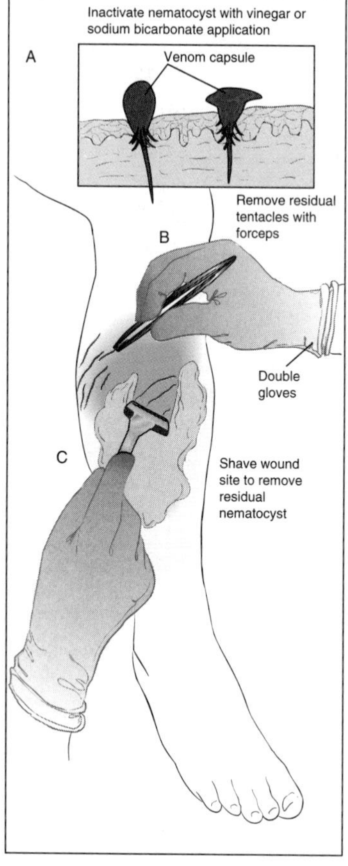
Inactivate nematocyst with vinegar or sodium bicarbonate application
A
Venom capsule
Remove residual tentacles with forceps
B
Double gloves
C
Shave wound site to remove residual nematocyst

FIGURE 72.1 Management of jellyfish stings. For severe jellyfish stings, attention to cardiorespiratory support and significant allergic reactions must precede wound management. In addition to supportive care and analgesia, attention is focused on deactivation of nematocysts (**A**), removal of retained tentacle fragments, and skin care. The clinician should double glove to avoid accidental nematocyst envenomation (**B**). The sting site should not be washed, scrubbed, or wiped. When providing first aid at the scene, rinsing with sea water may help remove some nematocysts. Lesions from North American species, except those due to the Chesapeake Bay sea nettle (found only in bays on the Atlantic coast), should be soaked for 30 minutes in 5% acetic acid (vinegar) to deactivate nematocysts. The Chesapeake Bay sea nettle is better treated with a paste of baking soda. Wounds should not be washed with fresh water, which may cause more nematocysts to discharge. Alternative first aid measures such as isopropyl alcohol or meat tenderizer are no longer recommended. Tentacle fragments should be removed with forceps (**B**), followed by application of shaving cream and delicate shaving of the affected area (**C**). Local wound care includes daily application of Burow's solution, and possibly therapy with topical corticosteroids.

CLINICAL TIPS

Tick Removal

1. Crushing the tick increases the potential exposure to the patient and clinician.
2. All material must be carefully removed from the skin.
3. Universal precautions should be observed to avoid contamination by human or tick secretions.

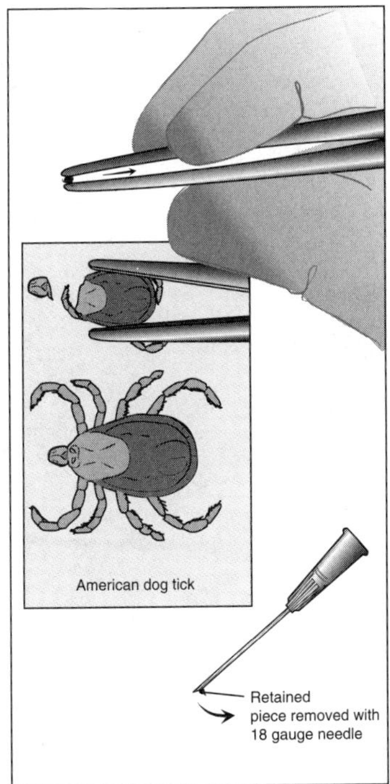

FIGURE 72.2 Tick removal. All ticks should be removed when discovered because length of time of attachment correlates with likelihood of transmission of tick-borne infections such as Lyme disease. Despite considerable folklore, mechanical tick removal is the only recommended technique. The tick should be grasped as close to the skin as possible using blunt, curved forceps held in a gloved hand (upper and middle frames). The tick is then pulled out of the skin using a firm, steady motion directed perpendicular to the body. The skin should then be closely examined to ensure that all tick parts have been removed. Any remaining material should be removed with forceps or an 18-gauge needle (lower frame). Finally, the site is thoroughly cleansed with soap and water.

Index

Page references for figures are followed by an f, page references for tables are followed by a t.